A Colour Guide to the

Nursing

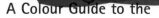

W9-APH-473

Management

of

Chronic

Wounds

Second Edition

edited by

Moya Morison PhD MSc BSc BA RGN PGCE
Lecturer, School of Social and Health Sciences
University of Abertay, Dundee

Christine Moffatt MA RGN DN
Director, Centre for Research and Implementation of Clinical Practice
Thames Valley University, London

Jane Bridel-Nixon BSc RGN DN
Head of Nursing Research and Development
St James's and Seacroft University Hospitals NHS Trust, Leeds

Sue Bale BA RGN NDN RHVDipN
Nursing Director, Wound Healing Research Unit
University of Wales College of Medicine, Cardiff

M Mosby

London Chicago Philadelphia St Louis Sydney Tokyo

Project Manager:	Sarah Gray
Development Editor:	Georgina Massy
Publisher:	Nicola Horton
Design:	Lara Last
Cover Design:	Lara Last
Illustrations:	Sandie Hill, John Cheung

Published in 1997 by Mosby, a division of Times Mirror International Publishers Limited.

Printed by Grafos SA, Arte sobre papel, Barcelona, Spain.

ISBN 0 7234 25574

For full details of all Times Mirror International Publishers Limited titles, please write to Times Mirror International Publishers Limited, Lynton House, 7–12 Tavistock Square, London WC1H 9LB, UK.

A CIP catalogue record for this book is available from the British Library.

Library of Congress Cataloging-in-Publication Data applied for.

Contents

Contributors

Sue Bale
Wound Healing Research Unit
University of Wales College of Medicine
Cardiff

Jane Bridel-Nixon
Nursing Research and Development
St James's and Seacroft University
   Hospitals NHS Trust
Leeds

Janice Cameron
Department of Dermatology
Oxford Radcliffe Hospital
Oxford

Madeleine Flannagan
University of Hertfordshire
Hatfield

Peter Franks
Centre for Research and Implementation
   of Clinical Practice
Thames Valley University
Wolfson School of Health Sciences
London

Brian Gilchrist
Department of Nursing Studies
School of Life, Basic Medical
   and Health Sciences
King's College
London

Sheenan Kindlen
Department of Health and Nursing
Queen Margaret College
Edinburgh

Susan McLaren
Department of Nursing
Joint Faculty of Healthcare Sciences
Kingston University and St George's
   Hospital Medical School
Kingston upon Thames

Christine Moffatt
Centre for Research and Implementation
   of Clinical Practice
Thames Valley University
Wolfson School of Health Sciences
London

Moya Morison
School of Social and Health Sciences
University of Abertay
Dundee

Sue Spence
St Leonard's Hospice
York

Preface

Knowledge of how to facilitate the natural healing processes is growing rapidly. The challenge for us, as healthcare professionals, is to keep up-to-date with this burgeoning knowledge-base in order to optimize outcomes, both for patients and for the purchasers of our services.

In whatever context, the findings from an ongoing process of assessment should form the basis for rational decision-making. Wound care has, for the most part, been researched at the individual, cellular and molecular system levels, and it is all too easy for the assessment process to focus on the wound itself to the detriment of wider issues. Throughout this book the emphasis is shifted from the wound towards assessment of the patient with a wound, and the environmental and social factors that may influence the healing process are acknowledged.

The book begins with an extensively revised chapter on the physiology of wound healing, including the role of growth factors and an explanation of the ways in which local and systemic responses to injury are integrated. The chapters on wound infection, wound cleansing and dressing selection have been completely reorganized and up-dated and there are valuable new chapters on nutrition and the dermatological aspects of wound and skin care. These chapters support the extensively updated chapters on pressure sores, leg ulcers, and other chronic wounds such as sinuses, fistulae and fungating wounds.

Healthcare professionals are becoming increasingly aware of the pervasive effects that chronic wounds can have on the individual's quality of life. This is acknowledged in the final chapter.

We have attempted to adopt sound educational principles and every chapter includes further activities, including self-assessment questions and case studies. These case studies emphasize the importance of healthcare professionals gaining some understanding of the unique context within which each individual's wound is to be managed. The book concludes with ten advanced case studies which should challenge even the more experienced practitioner.

No enterprise such as this is undertaken without a personal cost to those involved both directly and indirectly. It is a tribute to the contributors that each has seen this complex undertaking through to its conclusion. I would like to extend my warmest thanks to them for their outstanding contributions, encouragement and forbearance; thanks should also go to their families and friends for their forbearance while this work was completed.

Dr Moya J Morison
School of Social and Health Sciences
University of Abertay
Dundee

Foreword

The pace of change in nursing practice has accelerated over the past decade. A variety of influences have combined to stimulate review, innovation and experimentation in nursing practice: the development of strategies to provide individualized care; the emphasis on building a sound knowledge base for nursing care; advances in knowledge, research and technology; the emerging role of the nurse with regard to other health workers, together with changing demands and expectations of society. Valuable initiatives have been taken, not least by the contributors to this book. Traditional ideas on treating wounds are challenged and all the contributors have actively furthered developments in wound care; their contributions demonstrate the considerable progress that has been made in this area. This book is undoubtedly a valuable text for nurses working in a wide range of healthcare contexts.

Professor Sally Glen
School of Nursing and Midwifery
University of Dundee

Foreword

The large number of books and publications on wound management is a reflection of the increasing attention being paid to this area of clinical practice. Wounds are one of the most expensive problems in healthcare delivery, with non-healing a matter for serious concern. This text has an important contribution to make. Moya Morison has brought together ten experts in the field, including Susan McLaren at Kingston, Jane Bridel–Nixon at Leeds, Christine Moffatt at London and Sue Bale at Cardiff. The authors share with us their fascination and enthusiasm for, and expertise in, wound management.

The subject of wound management is a potentially confusing one. There have been rapid advances and changes in recommended practice based on a new understanding of the subject, and numerous choices for action are now available. Many healthcare professionals have a responsibility for the management of patients with wounds, and almost all specialties can be involved. This book provides a clear account of this difficult subject for them. Chapters look at patient assessment, wound cleaning, wound dressing and patient education. Particular problems discussed are pressure sores, leg ulcers and other chronic wounds.

The concept of the 'reflective' practitioner is well-documented. The book provides the necessary background information and advice that allows readers to function as 'reflective' wound-patient carers, and to base their clinical decisions on the best information available, which is important in the context of the recognized need to practice evidence-based medicine. Some of the many topics addressed are the factors which may delay wound healing, the nutritional factors that may be relevant and the causes of a wound becoming infected.

Quality assurance is as important in managing patients with wounds as it is in other areas of practice. A discussion of this topic is included in the book and readers are asked to consider the factors affecting the translation of theory into practice. Evidence-based medical practice is now receiving much attention. As part of this trend there is the need to assess the impact of disease on patients' lives. Chapter 13, on quality of life as an outcome indicator, summarizes the current research on health-related quality of life in chronic wound healing.

Those who purchase books now have high expectations, not only with regard to the content covered, but also in relation to the educational strategies adopted and layout and design. In this second edition, the reader is presented with an attractive design with careful page layout, judicious use of headings and clear illustrations and colour photographs. The book encourages the reader to engage actively with the text, and every chapter includes self-assessment questions and activities. The final chapter gives more in-depth case studies and readers may choose to work their way through these diagnostically before reading the text, or after reading the text as a test of their mastery of it.

A key question with any book on this subject is, 'Will the reader be better able to manage patients with wounds?'. With this book the answer must be a definite 'Yes'.

Professor RM Harden
Postgraduate Dean and Director
Centre for Medical Education
University of Dundee

The Physiology of Wound Healing

The physiological response to wounding has evolved into an elegant and immensely complex series of processes which are only now beginning to be fully understood. In the past decade great progress has been made in understanding the ways in which each stage of the healing process is regulated, how the progress from one stage to the next is controlled and how the responses at the wound site relate to those elsewhere in the human body. These issues are addressed in this chapter.

The relationships between local and systemic activities are extremely complex. Local effects at the site of a wound are visible and familiar to both patient and carer, but, particularly when the wound is relatively minor, there may be no visible sign of systemic activity, although there will be biochemical evidence of such activity. A simplified representation of the integration of the sequence of local and systemic events in response to wounding is shown in Figure 1.1.

This chapter begins with a description of local tissue responses to injury and is followed by an overview of systemic response to injury and a consideration of how local and systemic responses are integrated. The chapter concludes with a discussion of the wide range of biological, psychological and social factors that can affect the healing process.

LOCAL TISSUE RESPONSES TO INJURY

The same basic cellular and biochemical processes are involved in the healing of all soft-tissue injuries, whether they are traumatic wounds, such as lacerations, abrasions and burns, surgically made wounds or chronic ulcerative wounds such as pressure sores or leg ulcers.

The physiological processes involved in wound healing were traditionally divided into four main phases, which follow on from the haemostatic processes involved in the initial arrest of any bleeding:

1. Acute inflammatory phase: the release of histamine and other mediators from damaged cells and the migration of white blood cells (polymorphonuclear leucocytes and macrophages) to the damaged site.
2. Destructive phase: the clearance of dead and devitalized tissue by polymorphs and macrophages.
3. Proliferative phase: the infiltration of the wound by new blood vessels, supported by connective tissue.
4. Maturation phase: re-epithelialization, wound contraction and connective tissue re-organization.

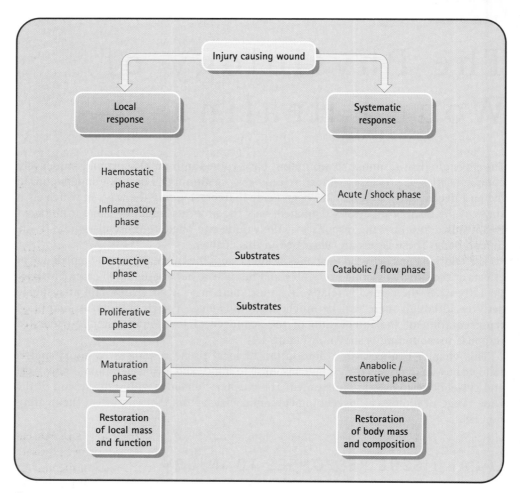

Figure 1.1 The relationship between the local and systemic responses to injury in outline (see also Figure 1.6).

In practice, these phases of healing overlap; the duration of each phase and the total duration of wound healing will depend on many factors, such as the site, size and degree of contamination of the wound and the physiological, immunological and nutritional status of the patient. A chronic wound may fluctuate in its response to the initial injury by moving forward and backward across the phases many times during the healing process. The interventions aimed at promoting healing may or may not facilitate the healing process. These factors are considered in more detail at the end of this chapter.

A variety of mediators that control and orchestrate the processes involved in tissue healing are referred to in this chapter. They can be classified into several groups, such as neurotransmitters, hormones and cytokines. Of these, the cytokines are perhaps the least well understood and have generated a great deal of interest in recent years.

The group name 'cytokines' is now commonly accepted but various names have been used for the group in the past, such as monokines, lymphokines, interleukins and interferons. These names are now, correctly, applied to subgroups or to individual cytokines. The individual name usually describes a function of the substance or, more usually, the first function discovered, for example, 'transforming growth factor' (TGF). The name can sometimes indicate both the origin and a function of the cytokine, for example, 'platelet-derived growth factor' (PDGF).

Cytokines control the processes of inflammation, communication between cells and subsequent repair and regrowth of the tissue. They may act singly or in concert and their actions can vary depending on the other cytokines present and the individual concentrations of each. To make the situation even more difficult to disentangle, the functions of a number of cytokines overlap.

Cytokines are released by the cells that synthesize them in response to an appropriate stimulus which may be tissue damage or the presence of a chemical mediator such as a hormone. They may act on the tissue close to the area in which they are secreted (a paracrine action) or at a distance from the site at which they are secreted (an endocrine action). They interact with specific receptor sites on target cells and, once bound, they alter the target cell behaviour. All cytokines are extremely potent and are present in the human body in extremely low concentrations. Many cytokines have been commercially synthesized and are being successfully used in clinical practice (Cox, 1993).

The biochemical and cellular events involved in the local tissue response to injury are now described in more detail and the implications for practice are clearly indicated.

Haemostasis

When blood vessels are damaged, collagen is exposed and platelet adhesion is increased by agents such as tumour necrosis factor (TNF) and nitric oxide (NO) which are released by the damaged cells. The platelets stick to one another and to the surface of the vessel, forming a plug. This platelet plug may be enough to stop blood loss in a minor injury.

Cut blood vessels that have smooth muscle constrict in response to signals from the autonomic nervous system and constrictors such as serotonin, which are released by platelets. The narrowing of the vessel temporarily reduces blood loss and increases the likelihood of the platelet plug remaining in place.

Contact of the platelets with exposed collagen triggers the release of a number of platelet factors, including adenosine diphosphate (ADP), serotonin and platelet-factor 3, which stimulate:

- Further platelet aggregation.
- Continued but temporary local vasoconstriction.
- A cascade of enzymatic reactions which results in the formation of a clot whose strong fibrin matrix reinforces the platelet plug.

The coagulation cascade, illustrated in Figure 1.2, is initiated in two ways: by the intrinsic pathway, just described, triggered by abnormalities in the blood vessel lining and by an extrinsic pathway triggered by factors released as a result of tissue damage. The two pathways converge to activate factor X and the final common pathway results in the conversion of the inactive precursor prothrombin to the active enzyme thrombin.

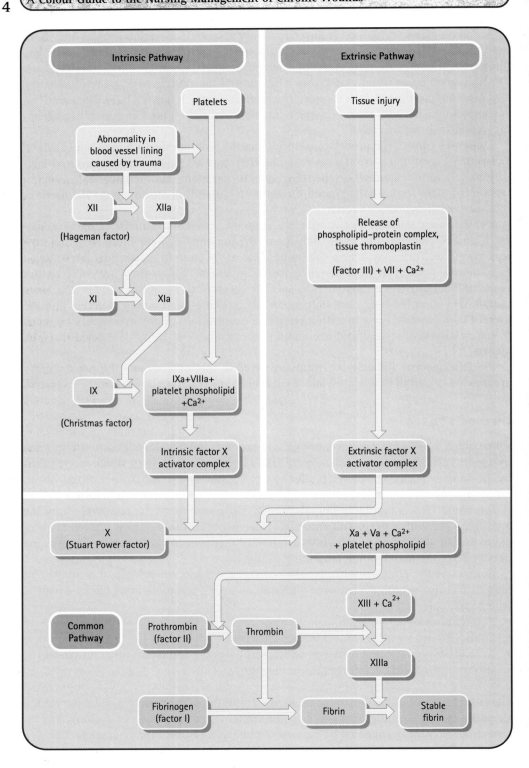

Thrombin then converts soluble fibrinogen into fibrin. Initially, soluble fibrin is formed; this is then polymerized and cross-linked to form insoluble stable fibrin, which is a physically stronger structure.

Implications for practice

The formation of fibrin requires the presence of calcium ions and the full complement of coagulation factors. Any factor missing or deficient will cause a failure in the mechanism. Vitamin K is necessary for the synthesis of several factors (II, VII, IX, X) by the liver. Deficiency of vitamin K can lead to slow haemostasis and vitamin K supplements may be given to patients judged to be deficient, for instance, before major surgery. Conversely, competitive inhibitors of vitamin K, which reduce the synthesis of vitamin K-dependent factors, are used as anti-thrombotic drugs. This is a relatively slow process because the pre-existing factors must first be metabolized and removed from the system before any significant effect is seen. An example of this group, the coumarins, is warfarin. It can be taken orally and is used in ongoing treatment when there is increased risk of thrombus formation.

Heparin inhibits the coagulation process more rapidly. Its effect is to interfere with the conversion reactions that produce active factors such as thrombin and fibrin. Its effects are short-lived and because it is destroyed in the gut, it must be given by regular injection or continuous infusion. It is used in the prevention of unwanted thrombi, especially in the deep veins of the legs.

A coagulation factor may be deficient because of one of a number of inherited genetic defects resulting in a number of clotting-defect disorders, collectively known as haemophilia. The most common forms are the result of deficiencies of factors VIII or IX. The genes are sex-linked recessive genes on the 'X' chromosome, which is why almost all haemophiliacs are male. The effects of a defective coagulation mechanism include the risk of major haemorrhage after minor trauma such as dentistry and a tendency to internal bleeding from minor injuries, especially into the joints where blood vessels are continually being subjected to mechanical distortion.

After normal haemostasis it is important not to disturb the blood clot formed. There is an adage: 'It takes two clots to make a haemorrhage, the clot on the vessel and the clot who knocks it off!' In the case of a major traumatic wound, prematurely dislodging the blood clot before fibroblasts have moved into the area and formed a permanent connective-tissue seal can be fatal.

Fibrinolysis

After the danger of haemorrhage has passed, the fibrin matrix of the blood clot must be dissolved; if the clot is allowed to remain it represents a hazard because it will act as a nucleus for further platelet aggregation and clot formation or it may narrow the vessel further and impede perfusion. If the clot becomes detached from the vessel surface and moves into the circulation it may lead to embolism. In any case, fibrin is continuously being formed in small quantities in response to tiny and unsuspected injuries, therefore, a mechanism for its removal is essential.

← **Figure 1.2** The coagulation cascade; coagulation factors are given in roman numerals. 'a' indicates that the factor has been converted into the active form. The stable insoluble fibrin fibres reinforce the platelet plug at the site of blood vessel injury.

Fibrin removal is achieved by the process of fibrinolysis (Figure 1.3). Evidence of fibrinolytic activity can be found by measuring the level of fibrinogen and fibrin degradation products (FDP) in the blood. Fibrinogen and fibrin degradation products can be found in any sample of blood but the level is substantially increased after injury.

Plasminogen has been found, in close association with macrophages and fibroblasts, throughout the entire period of wound healing and it has been suggested that, in addition to its role in the dissolution of fibrin associated with the clot, it has a role in the later removal of the fibrin-containing provisional matrix which supports granulation tissue (Schafer, 1994).

Implications for practice

Therapeutically, plasminogen activators, such as tissue plasminogen activator (TPA) or the enzymes streptokinase and urokinase, can be given to patients with unwanted thromboses to facilitate rapid dissolution of clots. Inhibitors of fibrinolysis, such as tranexamic acid can be given when it is necessary to maintain the presence of the clot.

Surgery or injury to the kidneys and urinary tract may need extra nursing vigilance because this is an area with higher levels of urokinase and, consequently, increased tendency to bleed.

Inflammatory phase (Phase 1, 0–3 days)

Release of histamine and other mediators from damaged cells and the migration of white blood cells (polymorphonuclear leucocytes and macrophages) to the damaged site

'Calor, rubor, turgor, dolor' is the classical description of inflammation, that is, the affected area is hot, red, swollen and painful.

On injury, damaged cells immediately release mediators such as histamine, TNF, which is a cytokine, and substance P which, as its name suggests, causes pain. The cells of the vascular endothelium release NO. Nitric oxide, histamine and TNF are potent vasodilators and have the effect of increasing blood-vessel permeability. This vasodilation, plus the local axon reflex dilator effects, reduces the pressure inside the vessel and further limits blood loss. The local dilation makes the area warm and red, with the beginnings of swelling.

Increased blood vessel permeability allows the easy passage of both fluid and phagocytes into the surrounding tissue space (Figure 1.4). The extravasated fluid may raise extravascular pressure enough to stop further blood loss into the tissue space. The local area is now clearly swollen and there may be blistering or dysfunction if the oedema occurs in the area of a joint. These are sometimes referred to as the vascular effects of inflammation and they are closely related to the cellular effects described below.

In addition to forming a plug and donating coagulation factors, platelets produce PDGF. This cytokine is a potent growth promoter that stimulates the growth of blood vessels and new structural tissue. The wound-healing process has started even at this very early stage, while the clot is still forming.

Neutrophils (polymorphonuclear leucocytes) are attracted to the site of the wound in large numbers by several factors released by damaged cells and by factors produced by platelets. Neutrophils serve an important role as very active phagocytes which can move easily between blood and tissue; they can be regarded as the first line of defence

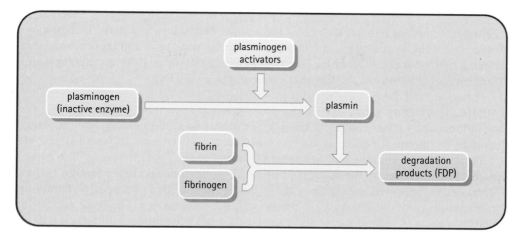

Figure 1.3 Fibrinolysis.

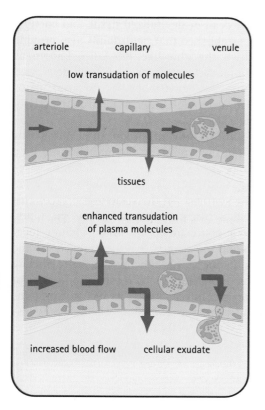

Fig. 1.4 Inflammation. The diagram shows normal tissue (upper), and three major alterations that occur when inflammation develops (lower): increased blood supply, increased capillary permeability to plasma components and migration of leucocytes (initially neutrophils and macrophages and then lymphocytes) into the surrounding tissues. (Reproduced from Roitt *et al.* 1995.)

against infection entering at the site of the wound. Monocytes and tissue macrophages at the site of the wound are stimulated by a number of platelet and leucocyte factors, to release their mediators which are chemotaxic and stimulatory to macrophages. Macrophages are required for the next stage of wound healing.

Implications for practice

The inflammatory phase is an essential part of the healing process and no attempt should be made to subdue it, unless it occurs in a closed compartment in which important structures may be compressed, for example, burns to the neck. However, if it is prolonged, for example, by the continued presence of devitalized tissue, foreign bodies, excess slough, recurrent trauma or by the injudicious use of topical wound preparations, healing is delayed and the wound's tensile strength remains low. The large number of cells attracted to the site of the wound compete for available nutrients. Too much inflammation can lead to excessive granulation in Phase 3 and to hypertrophic scarring. Discomfort caused by oedema and throbbing at the site of the wound is also prolonged and can affect the patient's quality of life. PDGF has been used as a therapeutic intervention when the inflammatory process has become chronic (Robson *et al.* 1993).

Destructive phase (Phase 2, 1–6 days)

Clearance of dead and devitalized tissue by polymorphs and macrophages

This phase is characterized by the clearance of dead or devitalized tissue and bacteria by neutrophils and macrophages. It has been established that neutrophils also provide at least one of the enzymes that break down the glue-like substance known as fibronectin (Grinnell & Zhu, 1994); fibronectin binds together damaged and denatured tissue and without this breakdown the solid mass of debris at the wound site remains longer and hinders the growth of new tissue. However, high levels of neutrophil activity are short-lived and healing can proceed in their absence.

In contrast, healing ceases if macrophages are significantly reduced in number or activity. Macrophages are attracted to the site of the wound by factors produced by a number of cell types, including platelets. Macrophages are not only able to destroy bacteria and remove devitalized tissue and excess fibrin but also produce growth factors that stimulate the formation of fibroblasts, the synthesis of the structural protein collagen and the process of angiogenesis. They also, in common with many other cell types, produce interleukin-1 (IL-1). This cytokine has many functions which include local effects, such as an increase in tissue adhesion and the attraction of lymphocytes to the site of infection, and systemic effects such as the induction of acute-phase proteins by the liver. Interleukin-1 also plays a role in stimulating the increased production of adrenocorticotrophic hormone (ACTH) and cortisol. Interleukin-1, its receptor proteins and the naturally produced receptor–antagonist proteins constitute one of many systems involved in the integration of local and systemic activities in injury (Dinarello & Thomson, 1990), as discussed later in this chapter.

Implications for practice

A fall in temperature at the wound site, as can occur when a wet wound is left exposed or when a wound is swabbed with fluid below body temperature, affects cellular processes and the cells' activity may fall to zero. Cell activity can also be inhibited by chemical agents, hypoxia and by the build up of metabolic waste because of poor tissue perfusion.

Proliferative phase (Phase 3, 3–24 days)

Infiltration of the wound site by new blood vessels, supported by connective tissue

It is a generally accepted biological principle that cells in an early stage of a process recruit cells that will be involved in later stages of that process. The process of wound healing is a good example of this principle.

Platelet activity (Phase 1) and macrophage activity (Phase 2) have been found to result in the recruitment of increased numbers of fibroblasts and other cells at the site of wounds and to stimulate their activity. Fibroblasts lay down ground substances and collagen fibres at the site of the wound which result in a rapid increase in the tensile strength of the wound. New blood vessels start to infiltrate the wound and capillaries are formed by endothelial budding. This process, called angiogenesis, is stimulated by several factors including PDGF (Robson *et al.*, op. cit.). The fibrin clot produced in Phase 1 is removed as the new capillaries provide a supply of the necessary enzymes. The signs of inflammation begin to subside.

The bright red tissue formed from the new capillary loops, supporting collagen and ground substance, is called granulation tissue because of its granular appearance. Growth factors are required for the increase in cell numbers and cell synthetic activity. Substrates, such as glucose, amino acids and the vitamins and minerals that contribute to tissue formation (*see* Chapter 2), are ineffective in the absence of growth promoters which regulate their incorporation and retention. There are several families of growth factor, a number of which are important in wound healing. Many cell types produce both growth factors and growth inhibitors and the balance between the two influences normal cell replication.

The factors called 'insulin-like growth factors' (IGF), which include IGF-1 and IGF-2, have been extensively studied. These are produced by a wide range of cells including macrophages and fibroblasts and promote many anabolic processes (Bennett & Schultz, 1993a,b). Insulin-like growth factor-1 attracts endothelial cells and is therefore involved in angiogenesis. It is also mitogenic to fibroblasts and is therefore required for tissue construction.

Epidermal growth factor (EGF) is probably one of the most thoroughly investigated cytokines. It too is found in many tissues and has been found to be secreted by platelets in large enough quantities to stimulate mitosis and migration of cells, indicating that its local effects are important to the early stages of wound healing (Brown, 1993). Epidermal growth factor is also found in saliva, being produced by the submandibular cells, perhaps endorsing the practice of licking one's wounds!

Proliferation must not develop into hypertrophy. To prevent hypertrophy the growth factors are controlled by a series of inhibitors that prevent overgrowth. These are cytokines such as 'transforming-growth factor beta' (TGFβ) and enzymes such as the collagenases.

The balance between promoters and inhibitors is finely adjusted and in the proliferative phase, the balance is in favour of the growth factors. However, when the balance is disturbed, the result may be an ugly hypertrophy or poor healing and the development of a chronic wound.

The cells being laid down at the site as granulation or other tissue are supported by an extracellular matrix (ECM). The major components of the ECM of skin are the collagen family of proteins, elastin, the proteoglycans, fibronectin and the integrins (Hopkinson, 1992).

Recent work on the ECM suggested that the major role of this material is not simply in supporting cells but also in providing a means of regulating cell-to-cell communication. Work on the composition of ECM showed that in addition to water and dissolved components, it contains small soluble proteins provided by both fibroblasts and keratinocytes which become attached to the ECM and apparently act as a signalling system between different structural components (MacNeil, 1994). Particular interest is being shown in the group of substances called the integrins. These are cell-adhesion molecules located on the cell surface which provide mechanical connection between the components of the matrix and act as transducers for the signals between cells (Gailit & Clark, 1994).

The signalling system and the integrins may be parts of a system that match the size, shape and direction of orientation of the parts which make up the area being repaired. Epithelialization, for example, takes place from the margins of the wound towards the centre of the wound and blood vessels and muscles become correctly aligned. Research in this area is clearly important to the understanding of wound contracture and scarring and also to the factors that affect graft 'take'.

Implications for practice

The new blood capillary loops formed in the proliferative phase are numerous. They are very fragile and are easily damaged by rough handling, as can occur on pulling off an adherent dressing. Vitamin C is essential for collagen synthesis (Dickerson, 1993). Without it, collagen synthesis ceases, the unsupported new blood capillaries break down and bleed and wound healing ceases. Other systemic factors that delay healing at this stage include iron deficiency, hypoproteinaemia and hypoxia. The proliferative phase proceeds more slowly with increasing age (Gerstein et al., 1993).

Maturation phase (Phase 4, 3 weeks–many months)

Re-epithelialization, wound contraction and connective tissue re-organization

This phase involves completion of epithelialization, contraction of supporting tissue, and connective tissue re-organization.

In any injury involving skin loss, epithelial cells at the wound margins and from remnants of hair follicles, sebaceous glands and sweat glands divide and begin to migrate over the newly granulating tissue. As this process is dependent on regulation by factors within the ECM, the cells can only move over living tissue. They pass under any eschar. When such cells meet other migrating epithelial cells mitosis ceases because of the effect of inhibitory factors such as TGFβ which become dominant as their concentrations rise when advancing cells come together. Wound contraction is the result of contractile myofibroblasts which help to bring the wound edges together. There is a progressive decrease in the vascularity of the scar tissue as angiogenesis is inhibited. This changes the appearance of the tissue from dusky red to white. The collagen fibres are reorganized and the wound's tensile strength increases. Figure 1.5 illustrates the location of collagen fibres in the dermis, as they appear in normal intact skin. After injury and repair, the scar tissue differs somewhat from that of the original healthy tissue and is not as strong or as flexible.

Implications for practice

The wound is still very vulnerable to mechanical damage, often only 50% of the normal skin tensile strength being regained within the first 3 months after injury.

Epithelialization occurs up to three times faster in a moist environment (under an occlusive or semipermeable dressing) than in a dry environment (Field & Kerstein, 1994).

Wound contraction is normally a helpful phenomenon (Butterworth, 1993), reducing the surface area of the wound and leaving a relatively small scar, but it proceeds poorly in certain areas, such as over the tibia, and can cause distortion of the features in facial injuries. Occasionally, fibrous tissue in the dermis becomes grossly hypertrophic, red and raised, leading in the extreme to unsightly keloid scarring (Thomas *et al.* 1994; Munro, 1995).

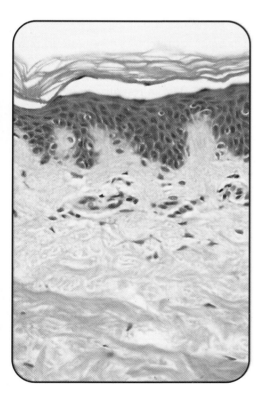

Figure 1.5 Micrograph showing the different natures of the loose pale-staining papillary dermis and the more densely collagenous reticular dermis. (Reproduced from Stevens & Lowe, 1997.)

SYSTEMIC RESPONSES TO INJURY

When an injury occurs the whole body is affected and a wise carer should be able to recognize or even anticipate systemic responses as well as the more obvious local effects.

At injury, the hypothalamic stress response is activated by stimuli such as pain and fear from higher brain centres and by other conscious stimuli associated with injury. The hypothalamus also responds to autonomic stimuli, such as a change in blood pressure, and to chemical mediators, such as the cytokines, produced in response to damage to tissue cells. Although moderated, the stress response occurs even in the deeply unconscious state.

The stress hormones released, that is, catecholamines (adrenaline and noradrenaline), glucagon and cortisol, provide increased glucose availability which protects brain metabolism. This glucose is initially made available by the action of glucagon on glycogen and the suppression of insulin by the catecholamines and later by the breakdown of skeletal muscle, mainly by cortisol. This breakdown is obligatory and is an automatic reaction to injury. Body fat is broken down and used as an alternative energy source and also makes a small contribution to new glucose production (gluconeogenesis). The normally large mass of body fat makes it an important contributor to survival.
Protein has several uses:

- Some of the protein provides the continued glucose supply necessary for brain and nerve metabolism. The provision of glucose from protein in this way is expensive because the nitrogen part of the amino acids used is detached and lost by excretion.
- Some of the protein is used as a source of nitrogen for amino acid synthesis and for repair at the wound site and replacement of proteins lost at injury such as the clotting factors and plasma albumin.
- Yet more nitrogen is used to produce the 'acute-phase proteins'. These proteins play a part in the inflammatory and immune response as inflammatory mediators, complement components and scavenger proteins such as haptoglobins. They are produced by the liver and the cells of the immune system in response to cytokine stimuli.

The presence of the hormone cortisol is essential to survival in circumstances of stress. One of its important effects is to moderate the inflammatory response which may otherwise overwhelm the individual who has a severe wound; at the same time cortisol also suppresses the immune response. The wounded individual is therefore more likely to survive but will be more vulnerable to infection in the short term.

Pain is a powerful stimulus to mechanisms for systemic catabolism, therefore, inadequate or ineffective analgesia will inhibit wound repair, leaving the patient nutritionally diminished and likely to be prone to infection. As described in more detail in Chapter 2, the weight loss induced by these catabolic activities cannot be reversed by simply increasing energy and protein intake. The hormonal balance must favour energy and nitrogen retention. As long as the effect of catabolic hormones, such as the catecholamines and cortisol, outweigh the anabolic effects of insulin and growth hormone, little headway can be made in the accretion of new body mass, although losses can at least be minimized by adequate nutrition.

Poor nutritional status diminishes both the effectiveness of the systemic response and the healing of the wound. Evidence of catabolism is clear, especially in a large wound, where there is very marked weight loss. Small wounds show little evidence of the systemic response to injury, but even a moderately sized wound that persists becomes a drain on the nutritional economy (*see* Chapter 2). At the wound site there is an analogous situation. Substrates provided by the systemic response may be present but the balance between local growth-promoting cytokines and inhibitors of various kinds must be favourable before normal healing can take place.

THE INTEGRATION OF LOCAL AND SYSTEMIC RESPONSES TO INJURY

As already described, the processes involved at a wound site do not occur in isolation. Just as it has long been good clinical practice to adopt a holistic approach to the management of the patient with a wound, so an understanding of the physiological processes occurring during wound healing is facilitated by taking a broader view which encompasses the systemic processes that impinge on it.

As illustrated in outline in Figure 1.1, the local effects produced at the wound site are integrated with and dependent on the systemic response that maintains homoeostasis in the body as a whole during and after injury and provides the substrates for wound repair. Figure 1.6 expands on this model by including some of the agents that regulate the sequence of the steps involved. It cannot be emphasized enough that the local effects cannot take place without the supply of materials provided from the systemic response to injury.

WOUND HEALING BY PRIMARY AND SECONDARY INTENTION

Although the same basic cellular and biochemical processes are involved, it can be helpful for practical purposes to make a distinction between wounds healing by primary and secondary intention.

Primary intention

When there is little tissue loss, as in a clean surgically made wound or a minor laceration, the edges of which are held together by skin tapes, healing is said to occur by *primary intention*, that is, by the union of two closely opposing wound edges (Figure 1.7). Very little granulation tissue is produced. Within 10–14 days, re-epithelialization is normally complete and usually only a thin scar remains, which rapidly fades from pink to white. However, it may take many months for the tissues to regain anything like their former tensile strength.

Secondary intention

In open wounds where there is significant tissue loss, healing is said to occur by *secondary intention*. Granulation tissue, composed of new blood capillaries supported by connective tissue develops in the base of the wound (Figure 1.8) and epithelial cells

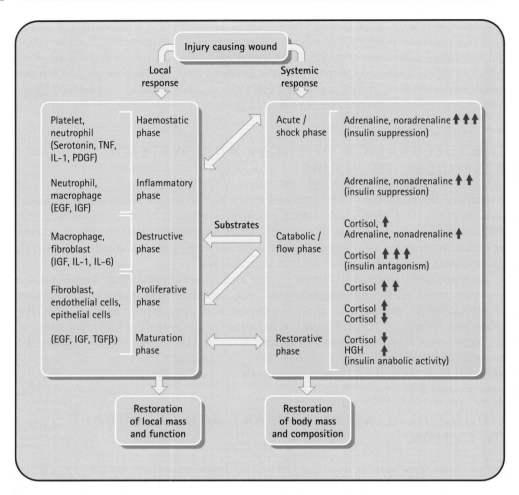

Figure 1.6   A model illustrating some of the relationships between local and systemic effects after injury.
HGH, human growth hormone; HGF, epidermal growth factor; IL-1, interleukine 1;
IL-6, interleukine 6; IGF, insulin-like growth factor; PDGF, platelet derived growth factor;
TGFβ, transforming growth factor β; TNF, tumour necrosis factor.
Arrows indicate increase or decrease.

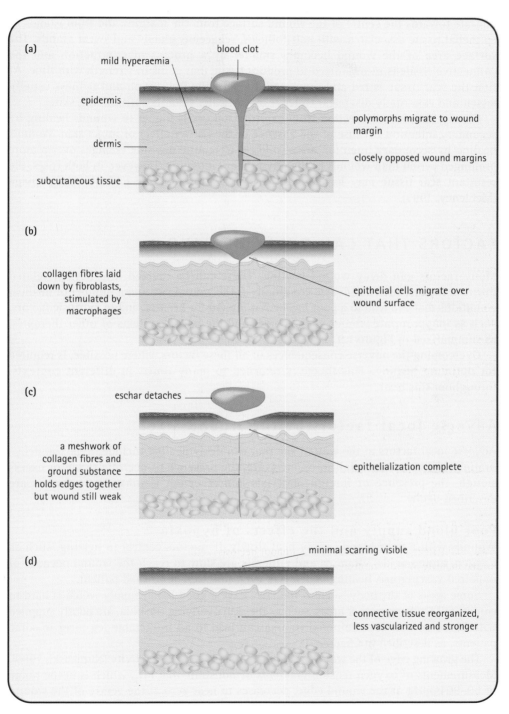

(a)
- mild hyperaemia
- blood clot
- epidermis
- polymorphs migrate to wound margin
- dermis
- closely opposed wound margins
- subcutaneous tissue

(b)
- collagen fibres laid down by fibroblasts, stimulated by macrophages
- epithelial cells migrate over wound surface

(c)
- eschar detaches
- a meshwork of collagen fibres and ground substance holds edges together but wound still weak
- epithelialization complete

(d)
- minimal scarring visible
- connective tissue reorganized, less vascularized and stronger

Figure 1.7   Wound healing by primary intention, such as a surgically closed wound or minor laceration closed with skin tapes (a) immediately following injury, (b) 2–3 days later, (c) 10–14 days later, (d) 1 year later. (Reproduced from Morison, 1992.)

migrate towards the centre of the wound surface from the margins and from islands of epithelial tissue associated with hair follicles, sebaceous glands and sweat glands. The surface area of the wound becomes smaller by a process of contraction and the connective tissue is re-organized to produce tissue that gains in strength with time. At first the scar tissue is red and indurated. In time, the induration and redness usually lessen and eventually disappear to leave a scar, paler than its surrounding skin.

Clearly, the risk of infection from external sources is higher in wounds healing by secondary intention because of the absence of the barrier effect of intact skin. Wounds healing by secondary intention are also likely to require dressing changes over a more prolonged period than wounds healing by primary intention. However, in both cases, the resultant scar tissue may have important implications for the patient's body image (McEleney, 1993).

FACTORS THAT CAN DELAY HEALING

Many factors can delay wound healing. These can be divided into patient-related intrinsic factors, such as adverse conditions at the wound site and a number of medical conditions that can lead to a poor local environment for healing, and to extrinsic factors, such as inappropriate wound management and the adverse effects of other therapies, as summarized in Figure 1.9.

Overcoming the adverse consequences of all these factors, where possible, is required for optimum healing. This theme is returned to many times, in different contexts, throughout this book.

Adverse local factors at the wound site

Adverse local factors at the wound site that can delay healing include: hypoxia, dehydration, excess exudate, fall in temperature, the presence of necrotic tissue or excess slough, the presence of foreign materials and recurrent trauma. These factors are described below.

Poor blood supply and the effects of hypoxia

Wounds with a poor blood supply heal slowly. If factors central to healing, such as oxygen, amino acids, vitamins and minerals are slow to reach the wound because of impaired vasculature, healing is delayed, even in a well-nourished patient.

Some areas of the body, such as the face, have a good blood supply which is hard to compromise, whereas other areas, such as the skin overlying the tibia, are poorly supplied with blood so that even minimal trauma can lead to an intractable leg ulcer in some patients, as described in Chapter 10.

The growing edge of the wound is an area of high metabolic activity (Niinikoski, 1980). Measurements of oxygen tension gradients demonstrate that PO_2, which is in the range of 60–90 mmHg at the wound edge, decreases to near zero at the centre of the wound (Silver, 1980). Almost no cell division can be found where the oxygen tension is consistently below 20 mmHg (Niinikoski *et al.*, 1991). According to Silver (op. cit.), maximum synthetic and collagen cross-linking activity takes place in a zone where the PO_2 is 20–60 mmHg. Hypoxia inhibits collagen synthesis and the ability of macrophages to

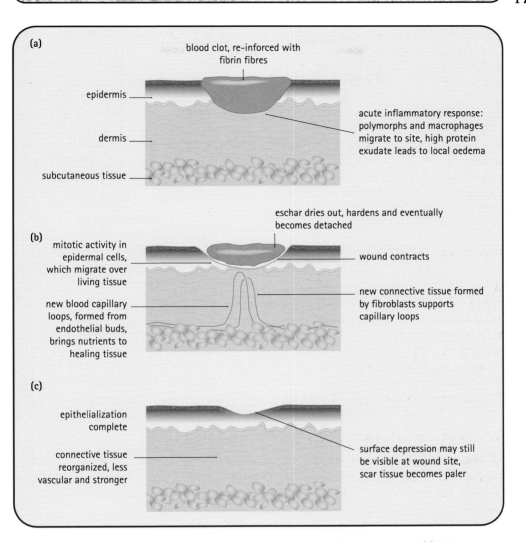

Figure 1.8 Wound healing by secondary intention, where there is initial tissue loss. (a) 0–3 days, (b) 1 week later, (c) 6 months later. (Reproduced from Morison, 1992.)

destroy ingested material. However, when the partial pressure of oxygen at the wound site is low, macrophages produce a factor that stimulates angiogenesis. By stimulating the growth of new blood capillaries the local problem of hypoxia may be overcome (Cherry & Ryan, 1985).

Thus, there appears, at first, to be a paradox. Overall, increased oxygen tension promotes healing whereas local hypoxia acts as a stimulus to repair. Niinikoski *et al.* (op. cit.) suggest that this paradox disappears when the role of lactate is considered. Lactate levels in blood rarely rise above 1 mmol/l in normal circumstances, but in

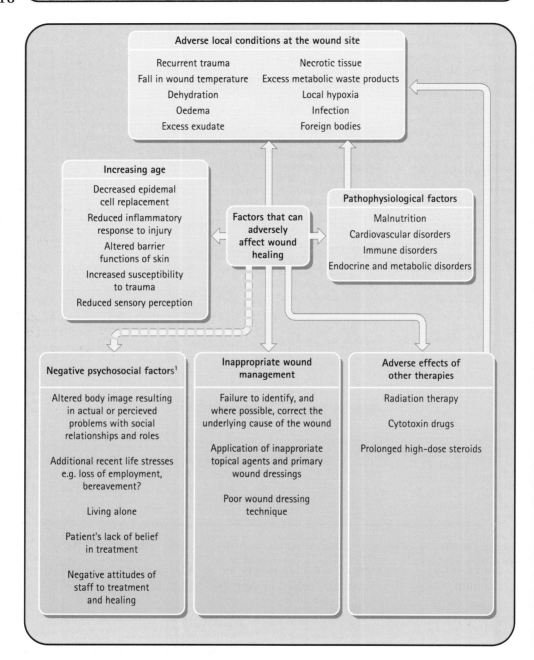

Figure 1.9 Factors that can adversely affect wound healing. (Note: [1] the direct link between delayed healing and negative psychosocial factors has yet to be unequivocally demonstrated.) (Reproduced from Morison & Moffatt, 1994.)

wounded tissue they can rise to 5–15 mmol/l. At these high levels, lactate causes macrophages to produce and release an angiogenic factor (Jensen *et al.*, 1986). When more oxygen is supplied, lactate levels at the wound site fall only slightly and angiogenesis continues to be enhanced.

In summary, hypoxia in the wound centre helps to *drive* tissue repair but oxygen is required to *respond* to the hypoxic stimulus, that is for capillary proliferation, collagen synthesis and for the functioning of the white blood cells involved in the functioning of the immune system (Doughty, 1992).

Dehydration

If an open wound is exposed to the air the surface layers dry out. Epithelial cells at the wound margins move downwards, beneath these layers, until they reach moist conditions that favour mitosis and migration of the cells across the damaged surface. The long-term results of letting the wound dry out are more pronounced tissue loss and scarring and delayed healing. If a wound is kept moist, under a semipermeable or occlusive dressing, healing is likely to occur much more rapidly (Field & Kerstein, op. cit.).

Excess exudate

There is a delicate balance between the need for a moist wound environment and the need to remove excess exudate that can result in sloughing of tissue. Exotoxins and cell debris present in the exudate can retard healing by perpetuating the inflammatory response.

Fall in temperature

Phagocytic and mitotic activity are particularly susceptible to a fall in temperature at the wound site. Below about 28°C leucocyte activity can fall to zero. Long exposure of wet wounds during dressing changes, or while the patient is waiting for the doctor's round, can reduce the surface temperature to as low as 12°C. Recovery of the tissue to body temperature and full mitotic activity may take several hours.

Necrotic tissue, excess slough and foreign bodies

The presence of necrotic tissue and excess slough at a wound site delay healing and increase the risk of a clinical infection developing. So, too, does the presence of any foreign body including suture materials and wound drains. It is therefore important to remove organic and inorganic contaminants as quickly as possible but with the minimum of trauma to the intact tissues, as described in Chapter 5.

Haematoma

Where a wound has been surgically closed, whether by primary suture, skin grafting or a transposed flap of tissue, the development of a haematoma is a significant cause of delayed healing.

A haematoma can cause complications in several ways:

- It provides an excellent culture medium for micro-organisms, which might otherwise merely be commensal, increasing the risk of clinical infection and wound breakdown.
- It increases the tension on the wound.
- It acts as a foreign body, which can lead to excessive fibrosis and scar tissue in the long term.
- By preventing the rapid vascular link-up between the raw surfaces, it can cause skin graft or flap failure.

Recurrent trauma

In an open wound, mechanical trauma can easily damage highly vascular granulation tissue and delicate newly formed epithelium and can cause the wound to revert to the acute inflammatory-response phase of healing.

Recurrent trauma can be caused in many ways. For example, if a patient with a pressure sore is placed on the sore while in bed or in a chair, then the forces of pressure, shearing and friction, which led to the breakdown of the overlying skin initially, will inevitably damage the even more delicate healing tissues and the condition of the wound will deteriorate (*see* Chapter 9).

Trauma can also be caused by the careless removal of an adherent dressing. Even when the greatest care is taken a degree of trauma to the wound is possible if a low adherent dressing is left in place for too long, especially if strike-through of exudate occurs and the wound dries out (*see* Chapter 6). Bleeding of a wound on removal of a dressing is an obvious sign of trauma.

General pathophysiological factors

A number of medical conditions are associated with poor wound healing. The mechanisms by which these conditions affect repair are often complex but many delay healing by reducing the availability of substances, such as oxygen, amino acids, vitamins and minerals, that are required for the healing processes to occur.

Reduced oxygen supply

Oxygen plays a critical role in the formation of collagen, new capillaries and epithelial repair, as well as in the control of infection (La Van & Hunt, 1990; Niinikoski *et al.* op. cit.) as previously described. The amount of oxygen delivered to a wound depends on the partial pressure of oxygen in the blood, the degree of tissue perfusion and the total blood volume.

The oxygen demands at a wound site are high. Reduced oxygen supply to the wound can be caused by:

- *Respiratory disorders:* reduced efficiency of gaseous exchange in the lungs, for whatever reason, can lead to a reduced partial pressure of oxygen in the blood and therefore reduce the availability of oxygen to the tissues.
- *Cardiovascular disorders*: these can reduce the degree of tissue perfusion. This is especially significant where the peripheral circulation is compromised, as in diabetes mellitus, if there is microangiopathy or in rheumatoid arthritis, if there is arteritis or where there are damaged valves in the deep and perforating veins leading to chronic venous hypertension and local oedema (*see* Chapter 10).

- *Anaemia:* whatever the cause of the anaemia, there is a reduction in the blood's oxygen carrying capacity. This can significantly affect wound healing when associated with hypovolaemia, for example, after haemorrhage.
- *Haemorrhage:* to maintain adequate blood pressure and blood supply to the heart, brain and other vital organs, peripheral vasoconstriction usually accompanies major haemorrhage. The degree of peripheral shutdown depends on the severity of the blood loss. Reduced peripheral blood supply leads to delayed healing until the blood volume is restored. This is normally a temporary phenomenon but tissue necrosis can occur during this time. In established shock, perfusion of the wound margins ceases almost entirely and the PO_2 falls to zero (Niinikoski *et al*, op. cit.).

Malnutrition

Whether a wound is traumatic, surgically made or a chronic open wound, such as a pressure sore, one of the most common causes of delayed healing is malnutrition. The importance of nutrition in relation to wound healing has been briefly commented on in this chapter and is discussed further in Chapter 2.

Decreased resistance to infection

Immunosuppression by cortisol is an integral part of nature's response to injury. The effects are more pronounced in patients with immune disorders, diabetes or chronic infection, in whom healing is delayed because of the reduced and now suppressed efficiency of the immune system. Chronic infection also results in catabolism and depletion of the protein pool and is an ever-present source of endogenous wound infection.

Wound healing across the life span

There are significant differences in the structure and characteristics of skin across the life span which, coupled with normal age-associated physiological changes in other body systems, can affect predisposition to injury and the efficiency of the wound-healing mechanisms. Some of these differences and their clinical implications are discussed chronologically, beginning with the preterm neonate.

The preterm neonate

Problems resulting from a defective skin barrier in the mature neonate are rare but the preterm baby has a much less effective skin barrier system (Young, 1995) and the skin is very susceptible to trauma, because of a thin, poorly developed stratum corneum and to epidermal–dermal instability. This has important implications for many aspects of the nursing care of preterm babies (Gavin, 1990):

- The selection and use of soap and bath frequency.
- The use of topical agents, such as antiseptics, steroid creams and emollients, which may be excessively absorbed percutaneously.
- The prevention of pressure necrosis, especially on the occiput.
- The choice of methods for securing equipment and appliances. It is particularly important not to attach equipment to preterm babies with tapes that contain strong adhesives, as considerable epidermal damage can result on their removal.

As a result of the relative incompetence of their immune system, preterm babies are particularly vulnerable to infection, including infection of the umbilical stump by Gram-negative organisms, *Staphylococcus aureus* and *Candida* infections.

The full-term infant

The skin of the full-term neonate is much more robust and less prone to infection than that of the preterm infant. This is because the stratum corneum and dermis are much thicker than in the preterm neonate; the immune system is also more fully developed in the full-term infant. Although the skin is virtually sterile at birth, colonization occurs rapidly and within 6 weeks the infant's skin has microbial flora at levels comparable with that of an adult.

The dermis increases in thickness during the years 1–3 and doubles in thickness during the years 4–7.

From adulthood to old age: the physiological effects of the normal ageing process

Intact skin in the healthy young adult forms a good barrier against mechanical trauma and infection and the efficiency of the immune, cardiovascular and respiratory systems in young people means that wound healing is likely to be rapid.

Different body systems age at different rates but over the age of 30 years a significant decline in some functions becomes evident, such as reduced cardiac efficiency, vital capacity and immune system efficiency, which in part can contribute to longer healing times with increasing age. There are also significant, normal, age-associated changes in the skin itself that predispose to injuries such as pressure sores and to poor wound healing. Changes that worsen with increasing age include decreases in epidermal cell replacement rate, inflammatory response to injury, sensory perception, mechanical protection and barrier functions of the skin. Coupled to these, the increased frequency of age-associated pathological disorders can delay wound healing through many mechanisms.

Arterial disease and the development of chronic venous hypertension in the lower limb predisposes to leg ulceration (*see* Chapter 10). Chronic sun damage increases the risk of skin cancer and nutritional deficiencies, as is common in elderly people, and delays wound healing (Lewis & Harding, 1993). Recognition of the increased vulnerability of elderly people to tissue damage is reflected in many risk-assessment scoring systems for pressure sores (*see* Chapter 9) but whether sufficient recognition of the age-related phenomena just described is reflected in the planning and implementation of nursing care in general is a vexed question.

Psychosocial factors

The closeness of the relationship between mind and body is becoming increasingly recognized. It has been demonstrated, for instance, that when patients are anxious, the efficiency of their immune system is reduced and they are physiologically less able to deal with any pathological disturbances. Conversely, in a placebo study of a pressure sore treatment, Fernie and Dornan (1976) demonstrated that positive attitudes of staff to the patients' treatment had a highly significant part to play in healing.

Where wound healing is likely to be prolonged, for instance in the case of a large, long-standing leg ulcer in an elderly patient (*see* Chapter 10), a number of social factors can influence the process. These include the availability of social support and practical help, where necessary, for example, to facilitate the application of compression hosiery. As described in Chapters 2, 8 and 10, social factors can also have a very important bearing on the patient's nutritional status and their ability positively to engage in health-promoting activities.

Adverse effects of other therapies

Cytotoxic drugs, radiotherapy and in some circumstances steroid therapy can delay wound healing. Cytotoxic drugs can have marked effects on wound healing by interfering with cell proliferation (Stevenson & Mathes, 1988). Furthermore, many patients receiving chemotherapy are neutropenic and more prone to wound infection, which further impairs healing (Carrico *et al.*, 1984).

Prolonged steroid therapy can also delay healing during certain phases of the healing process, by suppressing the multiplication of fibroblasts, collagen synthesis and capillary budding (Mast, 1992). In contrast, non-steroidal anti-inflammatory drugs (NSAIDs) appear to have very little effect on wound healing in normal therapeutic doses (Westaby, 1985).

Radiation therapy used, for example, in the treatment of malignant disease can produce local damage, retard healing and cause long-term weakness in tissues, especially in the skin. It may cause loss of vascularity and in extreme cases skin ulceration can occur.

Inappropriate wound management

Failure to identify the underlying cause of a wound or to identify local problems at the wound site, the injudicious use of antiseptics, topical antibiotics and other wound-care preparations and careless wound-dressing technique are examples of avoidable causes of delayed wound healing that can be classified as inappropriate wound management. The principles of patient assessment are discussed in Chapter 4. Guidance on the selection of the most appropriate wound-cleansing agents and primary dressings is given in Chapters 5 and 6, where the emphasis is placed on both the efficacy of the treatments used and the avoidance of unnecessary complications. Chapters 9–11 are concerned with the assessment and treatment of patients with particular types of chronic wound. Professional issues impinging on the decision-making process regarding the treatment of wounds are discussed in Chapters 12 and 13.

SELF-ASSESSMENT QUESTIONS AND ACTIVITIES

1. *With the help of Figure 1.9, which summarizes a number of factors that can delay wound healing, list the factors that may be delaying wound healing for three patients currently within your care. Which of the factors identified are within your sphere of responsibility? Have you identified any factors that may require medical intervention or intervention from another health-care professional? What are you going to do next?*

2. *Using examples from your own clinical experience, where possible, list eight reasons why wound healing may be delayed in:*
    *   *An elderly, hospitalized patient.*
    *   *An elderly person, living alone in the community.*

    Indicate which of the reasons listed are avoidable. Make a note of how the effects of any unavoidable factors could be minimized.

REFERENCES

Bennett NT, Schultz GS(a). Growth factors and wound healing: part I. Biochemical properties of growth factors and their receptors. *Am J Surg* 1993, 165:728–737.

Bennett NT, Schultz GS(b). Growth factors and wound healing: part 2. Role in normal and chronic wound healing. *Am J Surg* 1993, 166:74–81.

Brown GL. Enhancement of wound healing by topical treatment of chronic wounds with epidermal growth factor. *N Engl J Med* 1993, 321:76–79.

Butterworth RJ. Wound contraction: a review. *J Wound Care* 1993, 2(3).172–175.

Carrico TJ, Mehrhof AI, Cohen IK: Biology of wound healing. *Surg Clin North Am* 1984, 64:721–733.

Cherry GW, Ryan TJ. Enhanced wound angiogenesis with a new hydrocolloid dressing. In Ryan TJ, ed. *An environment for healing: the role of occlusion*. London: Royal Society of Medicine International Congress and Symposium Series (No.88); 1985:61–68.

Cox DA. Growth factors in wound healing. *J Wound Care* 1993, 2(6):339–342.

Dickerson JWT. Ascorbic acid, zinc and wound healing. *J Wound Care* 1993, 2(6):350–353.

Dinarello CA, Thomson RC. Blocking IL-1: interleukin 1 receptor antagonist in vivo and in vitro. *Immunol Today* 1990, 12(11):404–410.

Doughty DB. Principles of wound healing and wound management. In: Bryant RA, ed. *Acute and chronic wounds: nursing management*. St. Louis: Mosby; 1992:31–68.

Fernie GR, Dornan J. The problems of clinical trials with new systems for preventing or healing decubiti. In: Kenedi RM *et al.* eds. *Bedsore biomechanics*. London: Macmillan; 1976:315–320.

Field FK, Kerstein MD. An overview of wound healing in a moist environment. *Am J Surg* 1994, 167 (1A) (supplement):2–6.

Gailit J, Clark RA. Wound care in the context of extracellular matrix. *Curr Opin Cell Biol* 1994, 6(5):717–725.

Gavin G. Skin care considerations in the neonate. *J Enterostom Ther* 1990, 17:225–230.

Gerstein AD, Phillips TJ, Rogers GS, Gilchrist BA: Wound healing and ageing. *Dermatol Clin* 1993, 11(4):749–757.

Grinnell F, Zhu M: Identification of neutrophil elastase as the proteinase in burn wound fluid responsible for the degradation of fibronectin. *J Invest Dermatol* 1994, 103(2):155–161.

Hopkinson I. Molecular components of the extracellular matrix. *J Wound Care* 1992, 1(1):52–54.

Jensen JA, Hunt TK, Schevenstuhl H, Banda MJ. Effect of lactate, pyruvate and pH on secretion of angiogenesis and mitogenesis factors by macrophages. *Lab Invest* 1986, 54:574–578.

La Van F, Hunt TK. Oxygen and wound healing. *Clin Plast Surg* 1990, 3:463–472.

Lewis BK, Harding KG. Nutritional intake and wound healing in elderly people. *J Wound Care* 1993, 2(4):227–229.

MacNeil S. What role does the extracellular matrix play in skin grafting and wound healing? *Burns* 1994, 20 (supplement 1):67–70.

Mast BA. The skin. In: Cohen IK, Diegelmann RF, Lindblad WJ, eds. *Wound healing: biochemical and clinical aspects.* Philadelphia: WB Saunders; 1992:344–355.

McEleney M: The psychological effects of head and neck surgery. *J Wound Care* 1993, 2(4):205–208.

Morison, MJ: *A colour guide to the nursing management of wounds.* London: Mosby; 1992.

Morison MJ, Moffatt CJ: *A colour guide to the assessment and management of leg ulcers,* 2nd ed. London: Mosby; 1994.

Munro KJG. Hypertrophic and keloid scars. *J Wound Care* 1995, 4(3):143–148.

Niinikoski J. The effect of blood and oxygen supply on the biochemistry of repair. In: Hunt TK *et al.,* eds. *Fundamentals of wound management.* New York: Appleton-Century Crofts; 1980: 56–70.

Niinikoski J, Gottrup F, Hunt TK. The role of oxygen in wound repair. In: Janssen H, Rooman R, Robertson JIS, eds. *Wound healing.* Petersfield: Wrightson Biomedical Publishing; 1991:165–174.

Robson MC, Phillips LG, Thomson A, Robson LE, Pierce GF. Platelet derived growth factor BB for the treatment of chronic pressure ulcers. *Lancet* 1993, 339:23–25.

Roitt I, Brostoff J, Male D. *Immunology,* 4th Ed. St Louis: Mosby; 1995.

Schafer BM, Maier K, Eickhoff U, Todd RF, Kramer MD. Plasminogen activation in healing human wounds. *Am J Pathol* 1994, 144(6):1269–1280.

Silver JA. The physiology of wound healing. In: Hunt TK *et al.,* eds. *Wound healing and wound infection: theory and surgical practice.* New York: Appleton-Century Crofts; 1980:11–31.

Stevens A, Lowe J. *Human Histology,* 3nd ed. London: Mosby; 1997.

Stevenson TR, Mathes SJ. Wound healing. In: Miller TA, Rowlands BJ, eds. *Physiologic basis of modern surgical care.* St Louis: CV Mosby; 1988:1010–1013.

Thomas DW, Hopkinson I, Harding KG, Shepherd JP. The pathogenesis of hypertrophic/keloid scarring. *Int J Oral Maxillofac Surg* 1994, 23(4):232–236.

Westaby S, (ed). Wound Care, London: Heinemann Medical Books; 1985.

Young T. Wound healing in neonates. *J Wound Care* 1995, 4(6):285–288.

FURTHER READING

Books, book chapters and proceedings

Berne RM, Levy MN. *Physiology.* Chapter 50, 3rd Ed. St Louis: Mosby-Yearbook; 1993.

Cohen IK, Diegelmann RF, Lindblad WJ. *Wound healing: biochemical and clinical aspects.* Philadelphia: WB Saunders; 1992.

Daly TJ. The repair phase of wound healing — re-epithelialization and contraction. In: Kloth LC, McCulloch JM, Feedar JA, eds. *Wound healing: alternatives in management.* Philadelphia: FA Davis; 1990:14–30.

Ganong WF. *Review of medical physiology.* Chapter 27, 17th Ed. Lange Med: Prentice Hall; 1995.

Janssen H, Rooman R, Robertson JIS, eds. *Wound healing.* Petersfield: Wrightson Biomedical Publishing; 1991.

Kloth LC, Miller KH. The inflammatory response to wounding. In: Kloth LC, McCulloch JM, Feedar JA, eds. *Wound healing: alternatives in management.* Philadelphia: FA Davis; 1990:3–13.

Journal articles

Herndon DN, Habermann B, Cheresh DA. Growth factors: local and systemic. *Arch Surg* 1993, 128(11):1227–1233.

Kirsner RS, Eaglstein WH. The wound healing process. *Dermatol Clin* 1993, 11(4):629–640.

Silver IA. The physiology of wound healing. *J Wound Care* 1994, 3(2):106–109.

Nutritional Factors in Wound Healing

Wound healing is a complex, integrated cascade of local cellular and systemic events that culminate in tissue repair. As described in Chapter 1, the synthesis and use of metabolic substrates, hypothalamic–pituitary hormone signalling and the production of cytokines and growth factors by different cell species are all intrinsic to different stages of the healing process. Nutrients provide the substrates for body metabolism and also influence its rate and direction via hormone signalling and enzyme activity. At a local level, nutrients are not only vital substrates for tissue metabolism, they also provide specific fuels for macrophages, fibroblasts and lymphocytes during the process of healing. In addition, they form the raw components from which new tissues are synthesized.

Potentially, nutrients can influence all aspects of healing but what evidence is there to suggest that they do? This is a challenging question with no facile answers because it requires critical appraisal of the evidence from wide-ranging in vitro and in vivo studies, notably isolated tissue preparations, animal and clinical investigations. Difficulties inherent in reaching the conclusion that malnutrition impairs wound healing and that repletion improves the healing process can be appreciated by considering just a few of the problems associated with such nutritional studies.

- Multiple factors, non-nutritional and nutritional, can operate in research subjects to affect nutritional status and the process of healing. Separating out specific nutritional factors from others can pose significant problems for study design and ethics (Meguid *et al.* 1990; Buzby & Mullen, 1984).
- Evidence derived from studies of wound healing in malnourished, stressed animals cannot necessarily be directly extrapolated to man. Species-dependent differences can exist in relation to tissue histology, endocrine function and metabolic and behavioural responses to fasting (Albina *et al.* 1994).
- Outcome measures used to describe wound healing in studies of nutrient depletion or repletion can be subjective, that is, 'wound sepsis' may be defined according to variable criteria and 'delayed healing' may result in either perfectly adequate or poor wound outcomes (Levenson *et al.* 1957, cited by Albina, op. cit.).
- 'Biological priority' of a healing wound can ensure healing occurs in many cases, despite the presence of an inadequate nutrient intake (Moore, 1959).

Despite these difficulties, several scientific investigations have, in recent years, established a crucial role for specific nutrients in the healing of different types of wound. Understanding of wound metabolism and the modulation of tissue repair has expanded considerably and has important implications for nutritional support. In addition, advances in enteral and parenteral nutrition have proved life-saving for many; this is not only the case for individuals who have sustained acute and severe injuries but is also evident in patients presenting with complex, chronic wounds.

MALNUTRITION: DEFINITIONS; CAUSES; EFFECTS

Evidence that either protein–energy malnutrition (PEM) or particular nutrient deficiencies can impair the healing of chronic wounds is considered later in this chapter. Before this, it is relevant to consider approaches adopted in the definition of PEM, its aetiology and more widespread systemic effects.

Definitions

Protein–energy malnutrition is 'a change in body composition and physiology resulting from an absolute or relative deficiency of energy and protein' (Taylor & Goodinson-McLaren, 1992). Traditionally, malnutrition has been viewed as a spectrum of intermediate gradations of mixed disturbance, ranging between absolute energy deficiency (marasmus) at one extreme and absolute protein deficiency (kwashiorkor) at the other. Golden (1988), reviewing different theories underpinning the aetiology of marasmus and kwashiorkor, commented that marasmus can be regarded as PEM, with kwashiorkor occurring as a secondary event, superimposed by the presence of infection and toxicity caused by the ingestion of contaminated food in Third-world populations. Clinically, it is rare to be faced with pure forms of marasmus or kwashiorkor and the vast majority of malnourished patients have PEM to some degree. Differentiation of PEM into two subtypes was proposed by McClave *et al.* (1992), who found a stress induced-hypoalbuminaemic form to be present in 45% of an acute hospital population receiving nutritional support; a marasmic form of PEM characterized by adaptation to starvation was found in 25% of the same population. The presence of the hypoalbuminaemic form increased the mortality risk by a factor of 4 and nosocomial sepsis by a factor of 2.5 above that seen in its absence. A significant association between hypoalbuminaemia and unfavourable clinical outcomes has been noted in many other investigations (Detsky *et al.* 1987). The impact of PEM may be assessed in different ways as is described later in this chapter.

Incidence

The incidence of PEM in selected hospitalized populations has been reported variously as between 19% (Bastow *et al.* 1983) and 50% (Weinsier *et al.* 1979). Many of these patients may have become malnourished before admission. Potter *et al.* (1995) identified severe PEM in up to 26% of elderly patients admitted to hospital with medical problems. Malnutrition in elderly people in the community has been associated with several risk factors, notably depression, low income, cognitive impairment, polypharmacy, physical disability, chronic disease and living alone (Chandra *et al.* 1991).

Overall, it is estimated that up to 70% of the malnourished hospital population may have acquired the problem before admission but many sustain further deterioration of nutritional status thereafter and 30% develop PEM entirely iatrogenically, that is, during their hospital stay (Weinsier *et al.* 1979). Since PEM has been associated consistently with increased mortality, morbidity and longer hospital stay, the problem is significant (Meguid *et al.* op. cit.).

Causes

Protein–energy malnutrition has been attributed to four major factors: a reduced nutrient intake, reduced nutrient absorption and digestion, increased metabolic use, and an array of factors unrelated to disease. Any one or all of these four factors may contribute to the development of a malnourished state in an individual with a chronic wound and should be borne in mind during patient/client assessments.

Reduced nutrient intake

This may result from periods of protracted nil by mouth after surgery or trauma, the presence of dysphagia of obstructive or neurological origin, the presence of nausea, vomiting and anorexia resulting from chemotherapy, the chronic nausea and anorexia associated with cachexia, physical disability or weakness resulting in loss of feeding skills in elderly people, particularly after neurological injury, social and psychological effects of any illnesses that increase social isolation, impair social interaction at meal times or result in depression, withdrawal and loss of appetite (Ganger & Craig, 1990; Malec *et al.* 1990; Allan, 1995; Twycross, 1995; Alexander & Norton, 1995; Bruera & Fainsinger, 1995).

Decreased nutrient digestion and absorption

Any gastro-intestinal inflammatory condition, particularly if of a chronic nature, can profoundly decrease nutrient digestion and absorption, for example, Crohn's disease, ulcerative colitis, enteropathies and the cluster of disorders known collectively as 'mal-absorption syndromes'. AIDS is also associated with diarrhoea, malabsorption and other gastro-intestinal symptoms (Kotler *et al.* 1990). Acute toxicity of radiotherapy on the gut epithelium resulting in epithelial sloughing, mucositis, local haemorrhage or fistula formation can also exert drastic adverse effects on nutrient digestion and absorption as can the side effects of cytotoxic chemotherapy (Taylor & Goodinson-McLaren, op. cit.; Sykes, 1995; Welshby & Richardson, 1995).

Increased metabolic use of nutrients or altered nutrient disposal

After severe injury, trauma or sepsis, the resulting metabolic injury response is marked by a profound change in hormonal secretion by the hypothalamic–pituitary–adrenal axis in conjunction with increased activity of the autonomic nervous system. As a consequence, energy, nitrogen and micronutrient requirements increase significantly, reflecting a hyper-metabolic state but nutrient disposal is also altered (Gann & Lilley, 1984; Grimble, 1990). Although the metabolic injury response occurs in acute injury, trauma and after elective surgery and is more readily associated with the increased nutrient requirements of indi-viduals with acute wounds (burns, surgical incisions, orthopaedic injuries), it can also occur in response to profound sepsis associated with tissue damage, that is, a grade IV pressure sore complicated by sepsis (Bonnefoy *et al.* 1995). The implications of this for assessment of nutrient requirements are a crucial aspect of management as discussed more fully later in this chapter.

Non-disease-related factors

A number of surveys noted the potential negative effects of the lack of emphasis placed on nutrition in the education of healthcare professionals, the ineffective professional liaison and decision-making on nutritional support and the negative effects of providing inappropriate or inadequate support services (British Nutrition Foundation, 1983; Payne-James *et al.* 1990; Kings Fund Centre, 1992). The recent development of nutritional-support teams has made a very positive contribution to the resolution of these problems as described in the final section of this chapter.

Systemic effects of malnutrition

Inadequate nutrient provision, intake, digestion and absorption can reduce the supply of metabolically available nutrients but in the short term, 'biological priority' of the healing wound may ensure that the process of healing proceeds. Protracted malnutrition, which has been correlated clinically with enhanced rates of wound complications, may reflect impairment of later stages of the healing response and more widespread effects of PEM on the immune system and vital organs (Barbul & Purtill, 1994; Redmond *et al.* 1991).

Effects of PEM on organ function and body systems can be wide ranging, with severity of effect related to magnitude and duration of starvation. Such effects have been observed in animal studies and trials involving healthy volunteers (Keys *et al.* 1950; Silberman, 1989). Figure 2.1 summarizes the key findings relating the systemic effects of PEM to impaired wound healing. In clinical studies, PEM is unlikely to be the only factor that affects organ function.

As is evident from Figure 2.1, once established, the effects of PEM on the gastro-intestinal tract can lead to a serious downward spiral of gradually increasing malnutrition.

ROLES OF SPECIFIC NUTRIENTS IN WOUND HEALING

Glucose

In a healing wound, glucose is a crucial energy substrate used in metabolism by leucocytes, macrophages and fibroblasts. In fibroblasts, it is also used to synthesize new tissue components, that is, proteoglycan polymers and hexoseamines. Efficient aerobic metabolism of glucose is critically dependent on adequate vascularization of the wound bed (neoangiogenesis, *see* Chapter 1) and physiological mechanisms regulating tissue perfusion and oxygen transport.

A characteristic feature of the stress–ebb phases of the metabolic response to injury is the hyperglycaemia induced by increased glucagon and adrenaline secretion, which accelerate hepatic glycogenolysis and decrease insulin secretion. Elevation of blood glucose concentration is thought to have evolved as an adaptive survival mechanism, designed to supply the wound with increased energy. The extent of the metabolic-injury response is dependent on injury severity; small wounds produce little effect on metabolism, but extensive injuries, for example, burns, can cause a significant rise in energy expenditure and hence energy requirements (Meyer *et al.* 1994). For example, the magnitude of glucose requirements after burns *circa* 40% was estimated to be 175 g, representing solely the amount used by the area of the injury (Wilmore, 1977).

Effects of impaired glucose metabolism on healing have been investigated in diabetic animal models by Goodson and Hunt (1977) and Barr and Joyce (1989). General observations were of diverse impaired aspects of healing, notably a decrease in the inflammatory response, fibroblast proliferation, epithelialization and collagen synthesis.

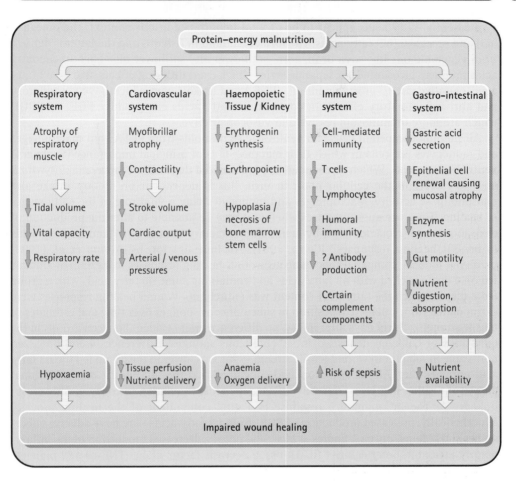

Figure 2.1 Selected systemic effects of protein–energy malnutrition on wound healing. (An up/down arrow implies increase/decrease in function/production.)

The latter could be reversed by vitamin C administration (Schneir *et al.* 1987). Vascular and neuropathic degeneration associated with diabetes mellitus and competitive inhibition by hyperglycaemia on vitamin C transport into fibroblasts and leucocytes may explain these observations in animal and clinical studies.

Polyunsaturated fatty acids

Considerable interest has recently been focused on the potential role of polyunsaturated fatty acids (PUFAs) in wound healing. Polyunsaturated fatty acids are intrinsic to cell-membrane structure and function and produce eicosanoids (prostaglandins, leukotrienes, thromboxanes), which exert profound physiological effects on cellular defence mechanisms, inflammatory responses and vascular tone (Suchner & Senftleben, 1994).

Two essential fatty acids appear to be of vital importance in this context: the omega-3 (n3) and omega-6 (n6) fatty acids. The former is found in fish oils and the latter is derived from vegetable oils like soya bean, corn, sunflower and safflower oils. Each of the fatty acids produces eicosanoids of separate series which exert differing effects, that is, n3 fatty acids can give rise to prostaglandin E_3 (PGE_3) and leukotrienes which have vasodilatory and anti-inflammatory effects. In contrast, n6 fatty acids can produce PGE_2 and PGI_2 which are more immunosuppressive and vasoconstrictive.

All immunocompetent cells can synthesize eicosanoids from PUFAs but macrophages and monocytes are cells in which their metabolism is of principal importance (Suchner & Senftleben, op. cit.). Which eicosanoids are synthesized depends on the availability of n3 and n6 PUFAs in the cellular pool; in turn, this is dependent on dietary intake and phospholipase activity. Macrophages and monocytes play a vital role in the early stages of healing. Thus, the question arises whether it may be possible to alter the production of eicosanoids by the macrophage, by manipulating dietary intakes of n3 and n6 fatty acids to benefit healing responses? (Cerra, 1991). An investigation by Albina et al. (1993) involving rodents, compared subcutaneous wound-healing responses in a group of animals fed on a diet enriched with n3 fatty acids and containing some n6 fatty acids with a group fed a diet in which the fatty-acid content was entirely n6. Wound healing responses were extrapolated from collagen deposition in subcutaneous sponges over time and estimates of tensile strength. Thirty days after injury, no differences were evident between groups in the quantities of collagen deposited in subcutaneous sponges. Differences were, however, noticeable in relation to wound tensile strength; this was lower in the group fed the n3 fatty acid-enriched diet. Albina et al. (op. cit.) concluded that the fibroplastic or maturational phases of healing had been adversely affected, possibly in relation to collagen fibre cross-linkage. As the inflammatory response is a vital component of the healing process, hypothetically, increased production of PGE_3 from n3 fatty acids may have adverse effects on healing (Albina, op. cit.). Endres et al. (1989) noted a decreased production of the inflammatory mediators interleukin-1 (IL-1), tissue necrosis factor-alpha (TNF-α) and platelet-aggregation factor in response to increased dietary n3 fatty acid intakes. The role of these cytokines is crucial in healing (see Chapter 1).

In contrast, clinical investigations by Gottslich et al. (1990) found that an enteral feed formula enriched with n3 fatty acids reduced the incidence of wound sepsis after burns. A hypothesis underlying this finding was that the eicosanoids derived from n3 fatty acids were less immunosuppressive than those derived from n6 fatty acids and that this may have accounted for the observed benefits in relation to sepsis. However, in this study, the enteral feed enriched with n3 fatty acids also contained other micronutrients that may have benefitted healing, thus the observed effects could not be exclusively attributed to n3 fatty acids. Clearly, further research is necessary to establish precisely which mixture ratios and doses of specific PUFAs produce favourable effects, under different pathophysiological conditions, before any definitive conclusions can be drawn.

A general dietary deficiency of PUFA per se has been noted to result in reduced eicosanoid synthesis, reduced leucocyte chemotaxis and reduced inflammatory responses (Suchner & Senftleben, op. cit.). In both animal models and clinical case studies, impaired healing responses have been observed in PUFA-deficiency states (Hulsey et al. 1980; Caldwell et al. 1972). Requirements for PUFA are increased following injury, a point which should be considered in the formulation of enteral and parenteral feeding regimens (Wolfram et al. 1978).

An array of immunological and systemic effects produced by different PUFAs may be of considerable future relevance to healing. These include:
- Increased graft survival (n6).
- Reduced incidence of sepsis in hypermetabolism (n3).
- Vasodilation (n3).
- Increased bleeding time (n3).

Amino acids

During the process of healing, amino acids are used to:
- Provide a metabolic fuel for macrophages, lymphocytes and fibroblasts.
- Synthesize acute-phase proteins that mediate the inflammatory response.
- Provide structural components for tissue repair, that is, collagen, elastin, actin, myosin, nucleoproteins and so on.

Dietary depletion–repletion studies showed that all essential and some non-essential amino acids (e.g. glutamine) are required for healing.
- Methionine and cysteine are essential for collagen formation and fibroblast proliferation (Williamson & Fromm, 1955).
- Histidine deficiency reduces wound-breaking strength which can be reversed by repletion (Fitzpatrick & Fisher, 1982).

The roles of two amino acids, arginine and glutamine, and are of particular interest in relation to healing.

Arginine

Considerable interest has focused on the role of arginine in wound healing after observations in both rodent and human studies. Early investigations by Seifter *et al.* (1978) demonstrated that rodents subjected to minor surgery and fed arginine-deficient diets developed significantly decreased wound-breaking strength and collagen accumulation (extrapolated from hydroxyproline deposition in subcutaneous polyvinyl sponge) in addition to greater weight loss and mortality in comparison with a control group fed a similar diet containing arginine. Subsequent studies replicated these findings and also demonstrated that the effects on wound healing in rodents were dependent on an intact hypothalamic–pituitary axis, suggesting that the underlying mechanisms could be hormonal (Barbul *et al.* 1983).

Later investigations in young, healthy human volunteers who ingested oral supplements of arginine ranging from 17–25 g daily over a period of 14 days, found that hydroxyproline deposition in subcutaneous polytetrafluoroethylene (PTFE) grafts increased in a dose-dependent manner (Barbul *et al.* 1990). Similar responses were observed in healthy elderly patients by Kirk *et al.* (1994). In this study, in addition to increased deposition of hydroxyproline into PTFE grafts in an arginine-supplemented group, a significant rise in serum insulin-like growth factor (IGF) was also observed when compared with a control group. Again, this was consistent with a role for arginine as a pituitary secretogogue.

A number of mechanisms have been postulated to explain the role of arginine in wound healing. Kirk and Barbul (1990) reviewed the evidence supporting the induction of growth hormone, prolactin, insulin and glucagon secretion by arginine, which could result in increased protein synthesis during healing and enhancement of immune function. Studies of experimental wounds suggested that arginine is converted by macrophages and neutrophils to citrulline and nitric oxide (NO). Fibroblasts subsequently convert citrulline to proline which is incorporated into collagen; this could explain the apparent enhancement of collagen synthesis by arginine (Kirk & Barbul, 1990). Nitric oxide is known to exert profound effects on the vascular endothelium but its relevance to local effects on wound healing remain speculative; vasodilation could, however, improve local delivery of oxygen and nutrients.

Glutamine

In acute injury, trauma and sepsis, both skeletal muscle and plasma glutamine concentrations decline in proportion to the severity of the injury (Roth *et al.* 1982). This efflux of glutamine may exert a number of beneficial effects at the wound site.

- It is used very extensively as a metabolic fuel by macrophages, lymphocytes and fibroblasts, in preference to glucose.
- In fibroblasts it is metabolized to glutamate, a precursor of proline and therefore, collagen.
- It is a precursor of purine and pyrimidine synthesis.
- Administered parenterally it reduces glutamine efflux from muscle, an anti-catabolic effect which may prevent wasting in hypermetabolic states.
- Beneficial general effects on recovery have been shown in humans after bone-marrow transplant.
- No effects on healing of colonic anastomoses in rodents were demonstrated by McCauley *et al.* (1991).

Micronutrients

A number of vitamins and trace elements are known to play important roles in wound healing, many acting as co-factors for enzymes involved in the synthesis of new tissue components. A summary of mechanisms underpinning effects on healing, together with evidence from animal and clinical studies, symptoms of deficiency, at-risk groups, and daily requirements for micronutrient intakes by different routes is given in Tables 2.1a–f. This is not intended to be a comprehensive summary and is focused solely on zinc, copper, iron and vitamins A, C and E, for which the research literature is relatively abundant.

Human studies

Chronic venous leg ulceration

Underlying venous disease accounts for the greater proportion (*circa* 67–76%) of total incidence figures reported for chronic leg ulceration. The incidence rises markedly with increasing age (Fletcher, 1991). Considerable interest has focused on the contribution of nutritional factors in their aetiology and treatment. What is the evidence supporting a possible role for macronutrient and micronutrient deficiency states in their aetiology?

Lewis *et al.* (1992) and Lewis and Harding (1993) conducted small-scale community dietary surveys in elderly individuals suffering from chronic leg ulceration. Anthropometric data, 5-day food diaries and social factors relevant to a dietary history were recorded.

Table 2.1a.
Micronutrients and wound healing: Zinc

Wound healing effects/ mechanisms	Evidence from animal/clinical studies	Clinical biochemistry (normal ranges)	Symptoms of deficiency/ at-risk groups	Suggested daily requirements oral/ § enteral/* parenteral
• Deficiency impairs healing; reversed by repletion • Component of >70 metallo-enzymes concerned with protein synthesis (e.g. RNA/DNA polymerase) • Deficiency decreases fibroblast proliferation, collagen synthesis, epithelialization • Inhibitory actions on Gram-positive bacteria • Conflicting evidence on role in healing in humans	• Clinical studies in leg ulcers (Halböok & Lanner, 1972; Agren, 1990) • Beneficial effects on healing of pilonidal sinuses in humans (Pories *et al.* 1967) • Enhanced healing after burns, surgery, in humans (Faure *et al.* 1991; Han, 1990) • Conflicting evidence (Haley, 1972; Sandstead *et al.* 1982)	• Normal: serum zinc 80–165 µg dl^{-1} • Serum level may not reflect whole body zinc status	• Eczematous dermatitis • Diarrhoea • Depression • Alopecia • Ataxia • Impaired taste • Mouth ulcers High-risk groups for deficiency • Protein–energy malnutrition • Long-term total parenteral nutrition • Malabsorption syndromes • Gut fistulae (increased loss) • Diarrhoea • Hyperzincuria (>4 mg/day) in hypoalbuminaemia, severe injury, chronic sepsis	§ 230 µmol * 100 µmol

Sources:

Clinical biochemistry: Taylor & Goodinson-McLaren, 1992; Dickerson, 1988; Lindeman, 1985.

Oral/enteral/parenteral: Food and Nutrition Board, 1980; American Medical Association, 1974; Baker & Lemoyne, 1987; Tayor & Goodinson-McLaren, 1992.

NB The values cited do not indicate special requirements to be taken into account in catabolic states, pregnancy, lactation, etc. The values cited refer to adults only. Readers are referred to the expert literature for requirements appropriate to specific medical conditions.

Table 2.1b.
Micronutrients and wound healing: Copper

Wound healing effects/ mechanisms	Evidence from animal/clinical studies	Clinical biochemistry (normal ranges)	Symptoms of deficiency/ at–risk groups	Suggested daily requirements oral/ § enteral/* parenteral
• Essential co-factor for lysyl oxidase which catalyzes cross linkage of lysyl residues in collagen • Essential for bone repair; supplements may enhance fracture healing • Copper deficient individuals cannot use stored iron because of impaired ferroxidase activity	• Clinical/ animal studies (Lindemann, 1984; Levenson & Demetriou, 1992) • Studies on bone repair (Dolwett & Sorensen, 1988)	• Serum copper 75– 150 µg/dl^{-1}	• Anaemia • Neutropenia, leucopenia • Bone demineralization High risk of deficiency • Protein–energy malnutrition • Long-term total parenteral nutrition • Enteropathies • Burns • Malabsorption	§ 30–45 µmol * 20 µmol

See footnote in Table 2.1a.

Mean 24-hour intakes of energy, protein and micronutrients were calculated and compared with reference values recommended for healthy individuals of the same age and sex (Department of Health, 1991). Findings were that mean 24-hour energy, iron, vitamin C and zinc intakes fell below the reference nutrient intake (RNI) and that the quality of protein consumed was poor. Nutrient intakes were affected by poor mobility, isolation and poor income (Lewis & Harding, 1993). In both surveys, many individuals were found to be obese on the basis of their body-mass index. These findings are in agreement with other larger scale community surveys of dietary intakes in elderly populations which suggest that many elderly people are malnourished (Chandra *et al*. op. cit.).

Valuable though these surveys are, low dietary intakes measured over a short period do not provide firm evidence that deficiency states exist. However, as illustrated in Tables 2.1a, 2.1c and 2.1e, zinc, iron and vitamin C play a crucial role in healing and low

Table 2.1c.
Micronutrients and wound healing: Iron

Wound healing effects/ mechanisms	Evidence from animal/clinical studies	Clinical biochemistry (normal ranges)	Symptoms of deficiency/ at-risk groups	Suggested daily requirements oral/ § enteral/* parenteral
• Deficiency impairs healing because of impaired oxygen delivery, reduced activity of lysyl and prolyl hydroxylases in collagen synthesis (co-factor); enhanced risks of sepsis due to impaired bacteriocidal activity of leucocytes	• Heughan *et al.* 1974 • Review by Levenson & Demetriou, 1992	Serum iron: Men 14–31 μmol/l Women 11–30 μmol/l Serum transferrin 2.5–3.0 g/l Haemoglobin: Men 13.5–17.5 g/l Women 11.5–15.5 g/l	• Hypochronic, microcytic iron deficiency anaemia • Glossitis • Cheilosis • Dysphagia • Paraesthesia • Gastric atrophy At-risk groups • Protein–energy malnutrition • Blood loss	Men § 180 μmol * 20 μmol Women § 320 μmol * 20 μmol

See footnote in Table 2.1a.

intakes over any time period are not likely to improve recovery. Similarly, low protein and energy intakes in the long term are unlikely to optimize tissue repair; a low serum albumin concentration can result in peripheral oedema which could impair diffusion of oxygen and nutrients to the area of ulceration. Further large-scale, longitudinal, dietary surveys which account for weekly and seasonal variations in nutrient intake and also include a range of assessments (i.e. serum concentrations of zinc, vitamin C and iron) are necessary. It may then be possible to link deficient dietary intakes with specific deficiency states and quantify the relative contribution of nutritional factors to the aetiology of venous ulceration, albeit retrospectively.

Nevertheless, the findings of Lewis & Harding (op. cit.) in relation to dietary zinc intakes are interesting, in view of research evidence concerning zinc deficiency and supplementation in the healing of chronic venous ulcers. Potentially, zinc can exert far-

Table 2.1d. Micronutrients and wound healing: Vitamin A				
Wound healing effects/ mechanisms	Evidence from animal/clinical studies	Clinical biochemistry (normal ranges)	Symptoms of deficiency/ at-risk groups	Suggested daily requirements oral/ § enteral/* parenteral
• Essential co-factor for enzymes involved in collagen cross linkage • Supports epithelialization • Beneficial immune effects on lymphocyte proliferation, natural killer cell activity • Moderates cell differentiation and controls growth factors and receptors • Reverses inhibitory actions of steroids on healing • Enhances tendon healing	Enhances wound-breaking strength (rodent studies, Levenson & Demetriou, 1992) Epithelial and immunity studies in animals (Olson, 1988; Hayashi et al. 1989; Kuroiwa, 1990; Smith et al. 1986) Anti-steroid actions in animals and humans (Hunt et al. 1960; Phillips et al. 1992) In vitro tendon studies (Greenwald, 1990)	Serum retinol >40 µg/dl Plasma retinol >20 µg/dl Serum vitamin A >0.7–1.7 µmol/l	• Night blindness Conjunctival dryness • Hyperkeratosis Bitots' spots • Abnormal taste, smell, balance At-risk groups • Protein–energy malnutrition • Alcoholism • Malabsorption • Cirrhosis • Burns	§* 1000 µg (supplements may be needed after burns but caution on risks of toxicity with high doses)

See footnote in Table 2.1a.

reaching effects on healing through its role as a co-factor in enzyme systems concerned with protein synthesis, trophic effects on the immune system and inhibitory actions on bacterial growth. In an investigation by Halböok and Lanner (1972), oral zinc supplementation was found to accelerate the healing of chronic venous ulcers in a group of patients with low serum-zinc concentrations, that is, with evidence of deficiency. No benefits were reported in patients whose serum-zinc concentrations were normal. Later

Table 2.1e.
Micronutrients and wound healing: Vitamin C

Wound healing effects/ mechanisms	Evidence from animal/clinical studies	Clinical biochemistry (normal ranges)	Symptoms of deficiency/ at-risk groups	Daily requirements oral/§ enteral/ * parenteral
• Depletion increases wound dehiscence, decreases tensile strength, impairs neoangiogenesis • Co-factor for prolyl and lysyl hydroxylase; deficiency impairs collagen synthesis • Limits tissue damage by breaking the chain of free-radical formation • Beneficial effects on immunity by increasing T cell numbers and complement synthesis; potentially reduces sepsis	Depletion of healing effects demonstrated in clinical studies (Hunt, 1940; Crandon *et al.* 1940; Schilling, 1976) Immune benefits in clinical studies by Penn & Purkins, 1991 Increases healing of surgical wounds in animal studies (Vaxman *et al.* 1990)	Serum ascorbic acid >0.3 mg/dl	• Scurvy • Adult syndrome of scurvy-fatigue, weakness, gingival loss, purpura, bleeding At-risk groups • Protein–energy malnutrition • Burns, stress, sepsis	§ 60 mg * 100 mg

See footnote in Table 2.1a.

investigations by Agren (1990) demonstrated benefits of topically applied zinc oxide in a double blind trial confined to individuals who had a low serum-zinc concentration. Epithelialization was higher and sepsis lower in the zinc oxide-treated group, for whom topical application was assumed to have corrected a local zinc deficit in tissue.

The extent to which low dietary intakes of zinc and abnormalities in zinc metabolism and distribution may variably contribute to local tissue deficits, which impair the healing

Table 2.1f.
Micronutrients and wound healing: Vitamin E

Wound healing effects/ mechanisms	Evidence from animal/clinical studies	Clinical biochemistry (normal ranges)	Symptoms of deficiency/ at-risk groups	Daily requirements oral/§ enteral/ * parenteral
• Prevents tissue damage by blocking lipid peroxidation in membranes by free radicals • Variable effects on healing reported: detrimental, zero or enhanced • Excessive vitamin E levels may impair healing; can antagonize beneficial effects of vitamin A on healing ? Mechanism	Animal studies on beneficial effects in free-radical formation (Powell, 1990; Sokrut et al. 1991; Yoshikawa, 1991) Detrimental effects in vitro on tendon healing (Greenwald, 1990) Zero effect on scar formation in humans (Jenkins et al. 1986) Beneficial effects on gravitational ulcers in humans (Lee,1953)	Plasma tocopherol lower limit is 5 µg ml or 0.8 mg/g lipid Varies with total plasma lipid levels	• Erythrocyte abnormalities • ? Ataxic neurological syndromes • Deficiency states rare in clinical setting • Deficiency symptoms likely if dietary intakes sustained at <3 mg/day	§/* 10 mg

See footnote in Table 2.1a.

of venous ulcers, remains an interesting topic of debate and speculation (Ackerman *et al.* 1990). Further large-scale investigations are necessary to identify the range of prevalence and specific micronutrient deficiency states, which exist in elderly populations with chronic venous ulcers, as a preliminary to confirming the benefits of vitamin or trace element repletion on healing. When micronutrient deficiency arises from an inadequate diet general PEM may be present. Nutritional interventions to support healing may then require attention to the diet in its entirety, in the light of individual requirements and underlying pathologies.

Pressure sores

Evidence concerning the role of nutritional factors in the aetiology and treatment of pressure sores is sparse in the research literature. Investigations fall into two main categories: those suggesting associations between indices of nutritional status and the presence or development of pressure sores and studies demonstrating the benefits of nutritional support and the importance of accurate assessment of requirements.

Pinchkofsky-Devin and Kaminski (1986) conducted a cross-sectional survey of elderly nursing home residents. Malnutrition was found to be present in 59% of the sample and was categorized as mild, moderate or severe on the basis of serum-protein concentrations, skin anergy and total lymphocyte count. Pressure sores (grades I–IV) were present in 7.3% of the sample; all patients with pressure sores were in the severely malnourished category. Severity of malnutrition, based solely on the serum albumin concentration, showed a strong negative correlation (r – 0.96) with pressure sore severity, that is, the more severe the sore, the lower the serum albumin concentration and vice versa.

A large cross-sectional survey of a hospitalized population found the prevalence of pressure sores to be 4.7% and a further 12.3% of patients to be at risk of sore development because of their restricted mobility (Allman *et al.* 1986). A range of variables, including hypoalbuminaemia and decreased body weight, were significantly associated with the presence of a sore. Prospective studies in the 'at risk' group confirmed that hypoalbuminaemia was a significant, independent predictor of sore development. Rationales for these findings were that a low body weight would increase pressure on bony prominence and hence vulnerability to sore development. Hypoalbuminaemia can result in interstitial oedema because of a fall in the colloid osmotic pressure of plasma. In turn, oedema could impair nutrient and oxygen delivery to tissue, increasing susceptibility to the temporary effects of pressure-induced ischaemia. Oedematous tissue is also more friable and vulnerable to shearing forces.

A later study by Ek (1987) also confirmed the importance of low serum-albumin concentrations and restricted mobility as features associated with the presence of sores on admission to hospital but skin anergy was predictive of pressure sore development in individuals without sores on admission. However, a clustering of low serum albumin, skin anergy and poor food and fluid intakes were also noted to be present in patients who developed sores after hospital admission.

Further insights into the presence of symptoms that could impair food intake and indicators of nutritional status in elderly hospitalized patients, with and without pressure sores, was provided by a large scale point-prevalence study (Meaume *et al.* 1994). Patients who had sores differed significantly from those without sores in relation to lower serum pre-albumin concentrations, increased cachexia (25%) and lower independence in eating. Patients with sores had a greater number of medical problems, including chronic neurological diagnoses and infectious diseases; the latter were confirmed by the presence of significantly higher levels of C-reactive protein and transthyretin levels.

Although these studies suggest important associations between selected nutritional variables and the presence and development of pressure sores, several limitations affect interpretation.

- Many non-nutritional variables can decrease serum-albumin concentrations (trauma, sepsis) and result in skin anergy (stress, sepsis, cancer).
- Albumin and other plasma proteins may be lost in exudate from a grade III or IV

pressure sore.

- No data in food intakes are included in these studies; it is therefore difficult to draw conclusions about dietary adequacy.
- Association between variables does not necessarily imply causation.
- Cross-sectional studies may identify factors particularly associated with the chronicity of the underlying disease.

Prospective studies by Ek (1992) and Ek *et al.* (1991) found both serum albumin and food intake to be predictive of pressure sore development. In a randomly selected subgroup of patients, provided with nutritional (oral) support, fewer patients, in comparison with a group of patients receiving a standard hospital diet, developed-pressure sores and evidence of improved healing was obtained.

The importance of monitoring nutritional status in individuals receiving nutritional support and making appropriate adjustments in energy and protein intakes was highlighted by Breslow *et al.* (1991). Investigations into a small number of elderly patients with and without pressure sores, receiving nasogastric feeding, found that energy and protein intakes were higher in the group of patients with sores. All regimens were dietician or physician prescribed using predictive equations for energy; adjustment factors for illness severity were also incorporated. Intakes were judged to be adequate in relation to clinical guidelines and protein intakes met recommended daily allowance (RDA) values. Despite this, patients with pressure sores had a lower body weight and lower serum-albumin and haemoglobin concentrations. Explanations for this were that this group were catabolic because of sepsis and the presence of pressure sores, which had increased their energy and protein requirements. In addition, albumin may have been lost through sore exudate.

This valuable study highlights the fact that predictive equations applied to individuals only provide approximate guidelines to energy and protein requirements. Indirect calorimetry measurements would provide more accurate information, as would nitrogen balance studies. Other studies noted the presence of catabolic states in patients with severe pressures sores were associated with the production of cytokines (notably IL-6) by damaged tissue and impaired nutritional status (low body weight) (Bonnefoy *et al.* op. cit.).

Burns

Advances in excision techniques, skin grafting, use of artificial and cultured skin and fluid-replacement therapies have reduced the morbidity and mortality associated with severe thermal injury. The hypermetabolic-injury response that occurs can be marked by elusive healing, in which sepsis poses significant risks. Nutritional support of the hypermetabolic state is an essential part of ensuring effective healing (Meyer *et al.* op. cit.). The role of early enteral feeding is vital in blunting injury responses and in preventing mucosal atrophy of the gut which can result in bacterial translocation.

Gottslich *et al.* (op. cit.) investigated the differential effects of three dietary regimens on selective outcome variables, including wound sepsis, after thermal injury. The regimens comprised two proprietary enteral feeds and one 'in house' formulation designed specifically to meet enhanced nutrient requirements after burns. The latter contained high protein, low fat, restricted linoleic acid and was enriched with omega-3 fatty acids, arginine, cysteine, histidine, vitamins A and C and zinc. In a prospective randomized, blind, trial patients were allocated to one of three feeding groups, which were comparable in terms of variables such as age, percentage thermal injury and energy and protein intakes.

In relation to outcomes at 4 weeks, the group receiving the non-proprietary 'in-house' formulation feed demonstrated a significantly lower incidence of wound sepsis and improved enteral tolerance. The components of this feed, notably omega-3 fatty acids, appeared to exert beneficial effects on immune function and inflammation; arginine increases protein synthesis, notably collagen, and micronutrients can influence all stages of healing. However, interpretation of the findings of this study were limited by the observation that serum micronutrient concentrations did not differ significantly between the feeding groups (all received micronutrient supplements beyond the remit of the feeds) nor did changes in serum albumin and retinol-binding protein. Although no feeding group underwent muscle repletion during the period of study, the group receiving the 'in-house' formulation experienced less loss of lean body tissue (extrapolated from creatinine excretion).

Further trials are necessary to confirm the optimal formulation of dietary regimens required to promote healing in thermal injury.

Surgery and trauma

Many studies have attempted to evaluate the influence of recent food intake and perioperative enteral or parenteral nutrition on clinical outcomes, including wound healing rates, incidence of sepsis and development of chronic complications, for example enterocutaneous fistulae.

Windsor *et al.* (1988) investigated patients awaiting elective gut surgery and divided them into two groups on the basis of an adequate or inadequate food intake in the week before admission. A dietary recall method was used for this purpose. The groups did not differ in relation to major variables such as age, sex, surgical procedure and selected indices of nutritional status. In the 7-day period after surgery, the wound-healing response was assessed by measuring hydroxyproline deposition (an index of collagen synthesis) into PTFE tubing that had been inserted subcutaneously in the arm.

Significantly more hydroxyproline was deposited in the group of patients whose recent food intake had been adequate. It was concluded that the maintenance of labile protein reserves before surgery had benefitted the healing response. A number of limitations arise in considering hydroxyproline deposition as an index of healing; this is a measure of collagen deposition, not cross linkage. Furthermore, the events leading to deposition in a PTFE tube do not correspond to the complex physiological events that occur in a wound.

Later studies by Haydock and Hill (1987) using the same method, found that in surgical patients given total parenteral nutrition (TPN) for 7 days, pre-operatively, wound healing responses were improved. Pre-operative nutritional support conferred greater benefits on healing than post-operative support alone. Similar findings were evident in a later study by Schroeder *et al.* (1991).

The formation of an enterocutaneous fistula is a serious complication after gut surgery and is associated with anastomotic breakdown. It can lead to rapid fluid, electrolyte and nutrient loss through the enterocutaneous channel. Nutritional support is vital here to prevent deterioration in nutritional status, to promote healing and to promote spontaneous closure. Meguid *et al.* (op. cit.) reviewed the evidence that enteral and parenteral nutrition can improve clinical outcomes. Beneficial effects of using TPN were noted in several studies and also in studies combining TPN with somatostatin. However, heterogeneity of study populations and lack of controlled trial design hindered the interpretation of such findings.

Multiple trauma can result in complex injuries that can be slow to heal. A prospective, randomized clinical trial conducted by Brown *et al.* (1994) in major trauma patients with a functioning gastro-intestinal tract, evaluated two types of enteral feeding regimen on outcomes. One group of patients received a standard formulation, the other a special formulation. The latter formulation was supplemented with arginine, ß carotene, and α-linolenic acid. It had a higher calorie density and protein content than the standard formula and also contained protein hydrolysates. Both groups received enteral support for 5–10 days. Results demonstrated a significant reduction in sepsis (all causes including wound sepsis) and improved nitrogen balance in the group receiving the special formulation. This study was very small in size and illustrates some of the frustrations in separating wound sepsis from general sepsis in outcomes. Further large-scale studies are necessary to confirm the benefits of different types of feeding regimen on the healing process. Enteral nutrition (if the gut is functional) is preferable for the critically ill.

Effects of malnutrition on acute, postsurgical wound healing in animals

Investigations of the effects of dietary protein deprivation or depletion on the healing of colon anastomoses have been conducted extensively in rodents (Daly *et al.* 1972; Irvin & Hunt, 1974; Ward *et al.* 1982). Indices of healing included in these studies were anastomotic-bursting strength and hydroxyproline content of tissue biopsies. Preoperative dietary protein depletion of variable duration, ranging from 1 to 7 weeks between studies, resulted in a decline in indices of healing and also in nutritional status; this was marked by weight loss and a reduction in the serum albumin concentration. Beneficial effects of post-operative intravenous feeding with dextrose and amino acid regimens were also demonstrated in these studies, that is, improvements in anastomotic-bursting strength and nutritional status. Albina (op. cit.) has raised some important points relating to the interpretation of these findings. Firstly, if deprived of dietary protein, rodents respond by reducing their total food consumption, that is, they sustain energy and protein deprivation, not protein deprivation alone. Furthermore, as a result of their high basal metabolic rate, rodents have a poor tolerance to fasting or food deprivation and can develop severe PEM rapidly. The study of Irvin & Hunt. (op. cit.) in which rodents were fed on a protein-free diet for 7 weeks, resulting in up to 34% loss of their initial body weight, exemplifies this point.

A later study by Irvin (1978) found that severe, pre-operative PEM in rodents reduced the breaking strength of abdominal incisions but not the healing of colon anastomoses. In contrast, later studies by Delaney *et al.* (1990) in well-nourished rodents demonstrated the value of early post-operative feeding on the healing of colon anastomoses. Intravenous feeding, using a balanced regimen of nutrients (dextrose–lipid–amino acids) commenced on the first post-operative day resulted in improved anastomotic healing and nutritional status (body weight gain) in comparison with animals subjected to either delayed feeding of the same regimen until day 3 or to delayed feeding with an amino acid–deficient regimen. Delayed feeding impaired anastomotic healing but administration of a nutritionally imbalanced regimen exerted the most severe impairment.

In conclusion, studies in rodents provide some evidence that PEM can impair or delay the healing of acute, postsurgical wounds. The adverse effects of short-term post-operative fasting on healing in well-nourished rodents have not been as extensively replicated.

CONCLUSION

This chapter has reviewed some of the scientific literature relating to the roles of specific nutrients in healing and the findings of nutrient depletion and repletion studies investigating healing in animals and humans. Although some of the evidence is far from conclusive, directions for future research are becoming clear. This will increase our understanding of wound metabolism and the mechanisms that underpin local and systemic regulation of healing. It may then be possible to modulate these events to benefit healing, using particular combinations of nutrients ingested by an enteral diet or parenterally. Although intangible, at present, it will undoubtedly provide considerable food for thought in the future.

SELF-ASSESSMENT QUESTIONS AND ACTIVITIES

Case study

Mrs Andrews, a widow aged 85 years, is admitted to an elderly care unit after a home visit by her GP. This visit has been requested by an anxious neighbour who has become alarmed by her increasing isolation, withdrawal and frail appearance after the death of her husband a year ago. Admission assessments confirm that she is confused, disoriented, emaciated and unable to stand. Peripheral oedema is present, and her skin is very dry, pale, scaly with patches of keratosis and purpura. A large sacral pressure sore (grade IV) is present, discharging a foul-smelling exudate. Biochemical investigations reveal a serum albumin concentration of 19 g/l and her axillary temperature is 38.8°C.

1. *Identify the symptoms of protein–energy malnutrition.*
2. *Which features could be indicative of specific micronutrient deficiencies?*
3. *What risk factors may have precipitated malnutrition in this case?*
4. *From a nutritional perspective, identify the priorities in management.*
5. *List the baseline indicators of nutritional status that could be measured, giving your reasons.*
6. *Why is the serum albumin an unreliable indicator of nutritional status in this case?*
7. *Briefly indicate how Mrs Andrews' energy, nitrogen and micronutrient requirements may be determined.*
8. *Identify other healthcare professionals with whom you would need to liaise to ensure that effective nutritional support is provided.*

(a) Protein–energy malnutrition (PEM)

1. *Define the term protein–energy malnutrition (PEM).*
2. *List the possible causes of PEM for three patients currently within your care. What measures are being undertaken to correct the situation?*
3. *Summarize the effects of PEM on body systems in general and explain how wound healing may be impaired as a consequence.*

(b) Nutritional assessment

1. *Briefly describe the anthropometric and biochemical methods of nutritional assessment, indicating the strengths and weaknesses of each. Identify which approaches would be most appropriate to your practice, justifying your reasons.*
2. *Briefly describe how dietary energy and nitrogen requirements can be determined. In your sphere of clinical responsibility, identify the approaches which are used.*

(c) The role of macronutrients and micronutrients

1. *Compare and contrast the role of glucose, protein and fatty acids in wound healing.*
2. *Describe the mechanisms underlying the effects of vitamins A, C and E on wound healing. What features could indicate the presence of deficiency states?*

(d) The delivery and evaluation of nutritional support

Identify key stages in the delivery and evaluation of nutritional support. With reference to your practice, reflect on the scope of professional responsibilities for undertaking activities related to these stages.

Welshby PD, Richardson AM. Palliative aspects of adult acquired immune deficiency syndrome. In: Doyle D, Hanks GWC, Macdonald N, eds. *Oxford Textbook of Palliative Medicine.* Section 16. Oxford: Oxford University Press; 1995:735–758.

Williamson M, Fromm H. The incorporation of sulphur amino acids into the proteins of regenerating wound tissue. *J Biol Chem* 1955, 212:705–712.

Wilmore DW. Influence of burn wound on local and systemic responses to injury. *Ann Surg* 1977, 186:444–458.

Windsor J, Knight G, Hill G. Wound healing response in surgical patients: recent food intake is more important than nutritional status. *Br J Surg* 1988, 75:135–137.

Wolfram G, Eckert J, Walther B *et al.* Factors influencing essential fatty acid requirements in total parenteral nutrition. *J Parent Ent Nutr* 1978, 2:634.

Yoshikawa T. Vitamin E in gastric mucosal injury induced by reperfusion. *Am J Clin Nutr* 1991, 52:2105–2135.

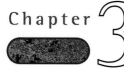
Wound Infection

DEFINITIONS AND THE USE OF LANGUAGE

According to the most recent figures (Emmerson *et al.* 1996) 'wound infection' in the UK and the Republic of Ireland accounts for 10.7% of all hospital-acquired infections (HAI) and 0.7% of 'community-acquired infections' (CAI), whereas 'skin infection' accounts for 9.6% of HAI and 15.4% of CAI. This apparent discrepancy highlights one of the most crucial issues in any discussion of wound infection: the problem of definition.

The wound-care literature contains literally hundreds of papers which, somewhere within their content, mention 'wound infection' and yet it is very clear that the loose use of this term has led to considerable confusion and has made comparison of publications extremely difficult. In fact, in most papers the authors tend not to give any definitions at all but include some bland statement such as 'a certain number of wounds being treated in the manner described "became infected" '. This leaves readers to draw their own conclusions regarding the significance of the results and, therefore, the relevance to their own practice.

In the case of the study cited above (Emmerson *et al.* op. cit.), a very precise set of definitions was used (Spencer, 1993). This enables a closer examination of the results and allows us to make intelligent observations about the problem of wound infection. Firstly, Emmerson uses the term 'wound' to refer specifically to 'a break in an epithelial surface that may be surgical or accidental' but he specifically excludes burns, ulceration or pressure sores. Conversely, 'skin infection' encompasses infected ulcers or pressure sores but excludes non-bacterial causes of skin inflammation. It can be seen, therefore, that the use of the term 'wound infection' may in fact be rather too broad and imprecise for everyday usage. It appears that infection of postoperative surgical wounds is of little significance in the community, whereas infected leg ulcers and pressure sores constitute an extremely large part of the workload of the primary healthcare team.

Recent US guidelines (Horan *et al.* 1992) also highlighted the difficulty of comparing results of infection studies and suggest that the term 'surgical-site infection' (SSI) be substituted for generic terms, such as wound infection, to define the location of the infection more precisely. Thus, they define infections as 'incisional-site SSIs' and 'organ/space SSIs' and these can be further classified as 'superficial' or 'deep' depending on the tissues involved. They have gone on further to develop a set of criteria that must be met in order for the site to be classified as 'infected'.

THE DIAGNOSIS OF WOUND INFECTION

Whatever term is being used to describe the site of an infection, the clinical problem is to decide whether or not a non-healing wound is infected. Although there are now a number of criteria that have been described and that can aid the clinician, there are some fundamental points that must first be understood. Possibly the most basic of these is that it is now widely accepted that the one piece of information that is not a necessary criterion in the diagnosis of infection is the findings of a microbiological swab processed by a laboratory. There are a number of reasons for this:

1. The presence of bacteria in a wound is not a sufficient condition to say that the wound is infected. All chronic wounds contain bacteria and, in general, cultures show the presence of more than one species (Gilchrist & Reed, 1989), often in very large numbers (Hutchinson, 1992).

2. The bacteria that are found often represent either secondary colonization or merely contamination, that is, they are not the pathogens actually causing the infection.

3. False negatives are not uncommon, that is, the bacteria causing the infection are not cultured. This may be especially so when the (actual) infection is caused by anaerobic bacteria, which are very difficult to sample with a routine cotton-tip swab and which will generally not be present on the surface of open lesions, where atmospheric oxygen is toxic to them. Specimens for anaerobic culture need careful collection and immediate processing if they are to be of any use and, as most chronic wounds are actually found in the community, swab results need to be interpreted with considerable caution.

Some authors advocate the use of quantitative bacteriology as the only precise means of defining wound infection (Robson & Heggers, 1984) and a rapid-slide method for detecting infection in surgical wounds has been described (Heggers & Robson, 1969). However, such methods all depend on the use of biopsy specimens and the immediate use of laboratory services. It is difficult to see this becoming of practical clinical use to practitioners, especially in community settings. There may also be some doubt about the applicability of such a system to the most common wounds that nurses have to deal with (that is, leg ulcers and pressure sores) for two reasons: firstly, it has been shown that bacterial counts can show considerable variation across the surface of an ulcer (Schneider *et al.* 1983) and there are no clear guidelines as to exactly where one should take the biopsy from; secondly, such cultures do not give any information about invasion, nor do they take into account the cause and extent of the wound in relation to the patient and the organism concerned (Thompson & Smith, 1994). It is known, for example, that some bacteria are considerably more virulent than others and that very small numbers may lead to catastrophic infections (Neal, 1994), whereas for certain species very large numbers appear to have no deleterious clinical effect at all (Hutchinson, op. cit.), (Table 3.1).

Infections in general have two effects:

1. They stop the wound from healing. Although the precise mechanisms are still not fully understood, they include:

- Prolongation of the inflammatory phase of healing.
- Depletion of the components of the complement cascade.
- Disruption of the normal clotting mechanisms.
- Disordered leucocyte function.
- Less efficient angiogenesis and formation of granulation tissue (Robson *et al.* 1990).

2. The body reacts to the abnormal presence of bacteria by producing a number of host reactions. The presence and detection of these host reactions allows a clinical diagnosis of wound infection to be made.

	Table 3.1. Common bacterial and fungal causes of skin infections (from Mims et al. 1993)	
Structure involved	Infection	Common cause
Keratinized epithelium	Ringworm	Dermatophyte fungi (Trichophyton, Epidermophyton and Microsporum)
Epidermis	Impetigo	Streptococcus pyogenes and/or Staphylococcus aureus
Dermis	Erysipelas	Streptococcus pyogenes
Hair follicles	Folliculitis Boils (furuncles) Carbuncles	Staphylococcus aureus
Subcutaneous fat	Cellulitis	Streptococcus pyogenes
Fascia	Necrotizing fasciitis	Anaerobes and microaerophiles, usually mixed infections
Muscle	Myonecrosis gangrene	Clostridium perfringens (and other clostridia)

The diagnosis of infection in surgical wounds

In the case of surgical wounds, the most commonly used definitions involve the presence of pus (Cruse & Foord, 1980) or purulent discharge, often associated with painful spreading erythema (Spencer, op. cit.). Indeed, all clinicians will be familiar with the classic signs of cellulitis: **heat, redness, swelling (oedema) and pain** (Figure 3.1), and in these situations, (perhaps in association with a pyrexia of greater than 38°C), the diagnosis of clinical infection is relatively easy. There is also very little debate about the treatment: drainage of the pus, either by the removal of all the stitches or by surgical excision if it is enclosed in an abscess cavity, prescription of appropriate systemic antibiotics, (which may be varied once culture results of the exudate are obtained) and possibly bed rest and elevation, especially when a limb is involved.

The diagnosis of infection in chronic, open wounds

In the case of the infected chronic wound, such as a leg ulcer or pressure sore, the situation is slightly more complicated. Wounds such as these are often (although not exclusively) found in elderly people, and it is not uncommon for elderly individuals to fail to mount a typical immune response as the immune system is often less efficient in this patient group (Gilchrist, 1993). Additionally, other patient groups may be at

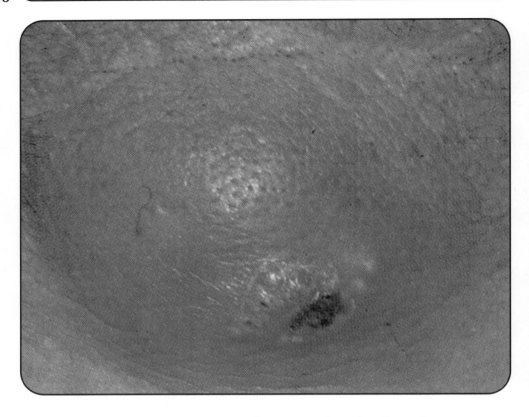

Figure 3.1   An infected sebaceous-gland cyst. The area is tender, red, swollen and warm. (Reproduced from Mills *et al.* 1988.)

higher risk of developing wound infection because of a reduced immune response resulting from systemic steroid therapy or because they are neutropenic (Cutting, 1994); as a result of their compromised immune response these patients do not demonstrate symptoms normally associated with a typical inflammatory response. Therefore, in the absence of classic cellulitis, the clinician will have to depend on other host reactions or clinical signs that may lead to the diagnosis being suspected.

These host reactions and clinical signs have been well described (Cutting & Harding, 1994) and include the following:

1. Presence of pus. This is a clear sign of infection in an acute surgical wound. Pus may also occur in a chronic wound, although it is not all that common, presumably because the open nature of most wounds allows it to drain from the wound surface (Figure 3.2). Another factor complicating this observation is that many hydrocolloid dressings dissolve to form an exudate not unlike pus in appearance and it may be difficult to tell the two apart.

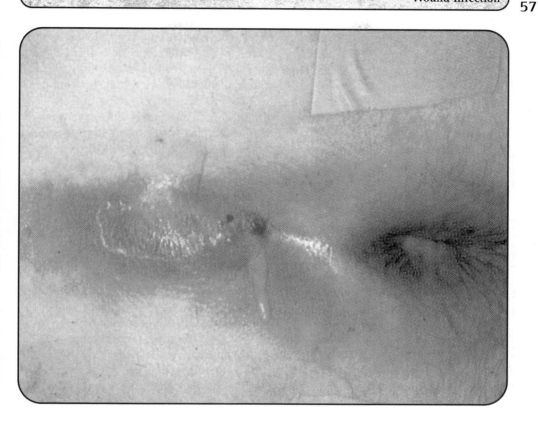

Figure 3.2 A painful pilonidal abscess with spreading erythema and discharging purulent material). (Reproduced from Mills *et al.* 1988.)

2. Increased wetness. Although there will be some exudate associated with most chronic wounds, normal granulation tissue is relatively dry and the sudden appearance of greatly increased amounts of exudate in a wound that was otherwise healing (and where adequate compression was already in place) may be an indicator of infection. This is because the underlying capillaries dilate as part of the normal inflammatory response, in order to allow white cells, in particular, to migrate to the source of the infection. In doing so, the capillaries become leaky and allow greater quantities of plasma to leak out as well. When a patient with a leg ulcer is seen for the first time there is often considerable difficulty in determining whether or not the wetness, generally seen in this situation, is due to infection or to the more likely causes of heart failure with an associated cardiac oedema or to oedema associated with uncontrolled venous hypertension. In the absence of any other symptoms, it would be usual practice to rule out heart failure clinically and, assuming that the ulceration is caused by venous disease, to apply

suitable compression to treat the problem rather than treating for clinical infection. Should the wetness persist, however, a course of antibiotics may be indicated.

3. Changes in pain. In general, a change in pain is an indicator that something untoward is occurring in a wound. Although this may be a sign that the wound has become infected, great care should be taken to first rule out other causes. Despite earlier suggestions that many chronic wounds are not painful, it is now clear that most chronic wounds are, in fact, associated with some degree of pain, albeit often manageable with simple analgesia (Cullum & Roe, 1995). The onset of a different, more acute, pain should alert the clinician to be on the lookout for a cause. The first candidate is not, in fact, infection but ischaemia and in chronic ulceration of the leg, the first test should be a repeat of the resting ankle pressure index (Cullum & Roe, op. cit.). If this is unchanged, then the use of systemic antibiotics may be indicated. In the absence of other symptoms, there are other wound-care situations in which an investigation for ischaemia will also be merited; in the case of pressure sores the clinician must be assured that a suitable pressure-relieving device is being used; in the case of rheumatoid disease, it must be established that the increase in pain is not an indicator of worsening disease or the presence of vasculitis. Naturally, ulceration with an underlying ischaemic cause (peripheral vascular disease or diabetes, for example) is itself especially prone to infection, often with anaerobes (Finegold, 1982). In this situation a prompt diagnosis must be made if serious consequences are to be avoided.

4. Change in the appearance of the granulation tissue. As well as increased wetness, infected granulation tissue often appears darker in colour and may be more friable, with a tendency to bleed more easily.

5. Odour. All wounds have some smell associated with them, however, the presence of any offensive odour may alert the clinician to the possibility of infection. Infections caused by anaerobic bacteria may produce an acrid or putrid smell, often because of the presence of necrotic tissue. It is often difficult to decide, however, whether or not the smell is caused by infection, or simply caused by colonization, which is most likely the situation in the case of fungating carcinomas which are often associated with a highly offensive odour.

It must be reiterated that all these signs and symptoms are associated with infection. The actual presence of bacteria does not equate with infection and, especially in the chronic wound healing by secondary intention, there is much evidence to show that the presence of bacteria does not stop wounds from healing (Gilchrist & Reed, op. cit.). Nevertheless, wounds do become infected and it may become necessary to take bacteriological samples for analysis by a laboratory.

BACTERIAL SAMPLING OF WOUNDS

There are a variety of methods with which to sample the bacterial flora of a wound (Stotts, 1995), some of which are summarized in Box 3.1. Some of these, such as biopsy, allow for the possibility of counting the number of bacteria present. Well-developed criteria suggest that, especially for surgical wound infections, a count of more than 10^5 bacteria per gram of tissue implies that the wound is, by definition, infected (Robson & Heggers, op. cit.).

> **Box 3.1.**
>
> Examples of methods for the bacterial sampling of wounds (from Morison, 1992)
>
> - Swab
> - Biopsy
> - Fine-needle aspiration
> - Colour imaging

Biopsy may also be the sampling method of choice when anaerobic bacteria are sought, as these are notoriously difficult to detect by routine swabbing (because atmospheric oxygen is toxic to them, causing problems of bacterial survival after sampling) (Swann, 1985). Recently, a method of sampling bacteria by detecting the odour they give off was described (Parry *et al.* 1995), on the other hand newer and more sophisticated methods of imaging and scanning are available for the detection and assessment of infection (Lazarus *et al.* 1994). However, such methods are at present either experimental or too cumbersome and expensive for general use, especially in the community where most chronic wounds are found. For the most part, sampling will continue to be by the time-honoured practice of using a cotton-tipped swab.

Local policies and practice for the collection of swabs vary considerably and there is really no consensus in the literature as to the 'correct' way to collect the specimens. A typical system was described by Lawrence (1993), who suggests that two swabs previously dipped in serum should be used. These should be rubbed across the surface of the wound in a zigzag manner while simultaneously rotating the swab between the finger and the thumb. The swabs are then placed in cooked meat medium or replaced in their container and sent to the laboratory for processing. Lawrence (op. cit.) claims that as long as the swabs are kept cool there will be no undue loss of bacteria for up to 48 hours. It is also claimed that such a system will allow for the detection of anaerobes, although it has been shown that by using other specialized techniques, greater yields of anaerobes can be obtained (Gilchrist & Reed, op. cit).

A number of studies showed that the repeated swabbing of chronic wounds does not yield any useful prognostic information (Eriksson *et al.* 1984; Hansson *et al.* 1995) as the bacterial flora are remarkably stable and it is not possible to relate their healing to the bacteria that are present (Blair *et al.* 1988). It would seem, therefore, that swabbing of wounds is probably only indicated in two situations:
1. As a baseline screening as part of the routine assessment of the wound when it is first seen.
2. When clinical infection is thought to be present.

In particular, there is a suggestion that ulcers should be routinely screened for group A *Streptococcus*, as this organism is especially virulent and smaller numbers may be needed to produce clinical infection, which may proceed very rapidly with severe results. In addition, there have been reports (Schraibman, 1990) that this bacterium may be associated with large, non-healing leg ulcers. It is advisable to seek first the advice of the local laboratory, as special media may be indicated. It is increasingly the case that many centres will not process wound swabs unless there is a clinical indication for doing so, as it has not been shown to be cost effective. Additionally, it is unlikely that specimens will be processed for anaerobes unless there is a specific indication for doing so.

Even when positive cultures have been obtained (in most cases not only will bacteria be found but it is also likely that more than one species will be present), considerable caution must be exercised in interpreting the results and it may be prudent to treat for anaerobes even without positive-culture evidence, as it has been shown that anaerobes are common in leg ulcers for example (Gilchrist & Reed, op. cit.).

It should also be remembered that bacterial infection may, in itself, be the cause of the wound being observed (as opposed to it being a complication of an existing wound) as in, for example, thrombophlebitis, where a blood culture is likely to reveal the causative organism, or a chronic wound associated with osteomyelitis, where tissue obtained during operative debridement will give more accurate findings than a swab culture from the wound site (Perry *et al.* 1991).

FACTORS ASSOCIATED WITH WOUND INFECTION

There is an increasing realization that wound care must focus on all aspects of the patient and not simply the skin defect that is the most visible manifestation of an extremely complicated process involving a wide variety of different cells, chemicals, hormones, antibodies and host factors, all of which play some part in the overall healing cascade (*see* Chapter 1). It is therefore important that these factors are recognized and, wherever possible, removed or alleviated.

Consequently, the emphasis must shift from making the first priority the choice of dressing to be used, to a situation in which most importance is placed on total patient assessment (and reassessment!) (*see* Chapter 4). To do this, the clinician must have an appreciation of the factors that are associated with an increased risk of the development of wound infection. It is not possible in all situations to do anything about such factors, for example, age (Gilchrist, op. cit.). What is important is that they are taken into consideration.

In the case of surgical wounds, possible risk factors have been well described (Bucknall, 1985; Sherertz *et al.* 1992; Leaper, 1995), and can be broadly divided into factors related to the host and factors related to the operation. In the case of the host, factors that have been established as being of most significance are the following:

- Age.
- Obesity.
- Prolonged hospital stay pre-operatively.
- The presence of infection at another site.
- Severity and number of concurrent diseases.

Other factors that may be important include: malnutrition, low serum albumin, cancer, diabetes mellitus and immunosuppressive therapy.

A number of operation-related factors have also been identified. One of the most significant is whether or not the patient has had a pre-operative shave with a razor, a factor highlighted by many studies. There appears to be little, if any, justification for the continued use of this practice, which is simply not justified from an infection-control point of view. The type of surgery being performed will clearly have an effect on the likelihood of infection. A number of studies classify surgery as clean, clean-contaminated or contaminated and have shown that the infection rates expected are different for each type. In addition, the duration of the surgery has a clear effect, as it allows a greater opportunity for bacterial contamination to occur. Interestingly, there is also evidence (Mishriki *et al.* 1990) that infection rates may be surgeon-related, although this may in part be related to the nature of the surgery being undertaken. There is a suggestion that experience and technique are also significant. For a more exhaustive list of other factors, the reader is referred to the literature.

In the case of chronic wounds, the risk factors are perhaps less well defined, although many of the same patient-related factors such as age, concurrent disease and so on can clearly play a part. However, the most significant factor in non-healing is likely to be incorrect identification of the underlying aetiology and related risk factors associated with non-healing, rather than infection, as described in Chapters 9–11.

It is important to realize that whatever associated risk factors are present, the fundamental issue in all patients is that resistance to bacterial invasion depends almost entirely on the efficiency of the host's natural defence mechanisms (Burke, 1980). Figure 3.3 illustrates some of the body's non-specific defence mechanisms. Intact skin is normally an excellent barrier (Box 3.2) but any defect of the skin is a breach of this defence mechanism. There are a number of other wound-related factors that may also impair this host resistance (Tobin, 1984):

- Presence of a foreign body in the wound, for example, pieces of discarded dressing, especially gauze and tulle, dirt, suture material, drains.
- The presence of dead tissue, as this may not only provide a nutrient source for bacteria but may also lead to a smaller number of bacteria being needed in the initial inoculum.
- Contused tissue.
- Tissue ischaemia.
- Previous or current irradiation.
- Presence of a haematoma.
- The use of vasoconstricting drugs.

These factors are discussed in more depth in Chapter 1.

TREATMENT OF INFECTED WOUNDS

Fundamentally, the treatment of infected wounds is simple: eradicate the causative organism by giving the appropriate antibiotic. Such a simple statement, however, belies the enormous complexities that occur in everyday practical wound care, many of which are covered elsewhere in this book; this chapter will cover only the general principles. There is, of course, a role for prophylactic antibiotics in some types of surgery (Bucknall, op. cit.), although their use in clean surgery, which does not include an implant, remains controversial.

Obviously, if clinical infection is present the use of an appropriate antibiotic is indicated but which one is the most appropriate and how should it be administered? The general answer is that most local centres now have clear guidelines based on knowledge

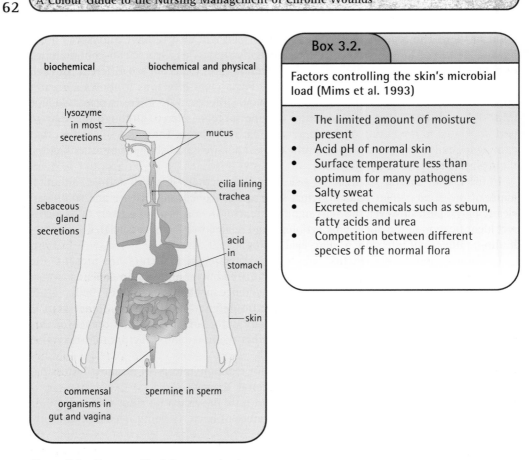

biochemical   biochemical and physical

lysozyme
in most
secretions
mucus

cilia lining
trachea

sebaceous
gland
secretions

acid
in
stomach

skin

commensal   spermine in sperm
organisms in
gut and vagina

Box 3.2.

Factors controlling the skin's microbial
load (Mims et al. 1993)

- The limited amount of moisture
  present
- Acid pH of normal skin
- Surface temperature less than
  optimum for many pathogens
- Salty sweat
- Excreted chemicals such as sebum,
  fatty acids and urea
- Competition between different
  species of the normal flora

Figure 3.3   Non-specific defence mechanisms.
(Reproduced from Roitt *et al.* 1996.)

of the sensitivity patterns of bacteria cultured locally and sometimes also based on economic factors and these should guide the clinician. In any case of doubt, the advice of the medical microbiology service should be sought, however, there are general principles that can be followed. In the case of surgical wounds, culture results from samples of pus will generally reveal the causative organism and an appropriate anti-biotic can then be prescribed. However, as discussed, this will often not be the case for wounds like leg ulcers and pressure sores, in which culture results may be misleading and in this situation care must be taken to cover *likely* bacteria as well as those present in the culture result (Finch, 1988).

In the case of chronic wounds it is important to remember that the presence of bacteria is the norm and it is now well accepted that wound sterility is not necessary in order for the wound to heal. This has been shown both in experimental wounds (Mertz & Eaglstein,

1984) and in clinical studies (Eriksson *et al.* op. cit.; Blair *et al.* op. cit.; Gilchrist & Reed, op. cit.). As a result of a study that showed no significant differences in either healing rates or bacterial flora when using prophylactic antibiotics, the use of such treatment is not advocated in this type of wound (Alinovi *et al.* 1986). There are some microbiologists who advocate the use of prophylactic antibiotics when group A *Streptococcus* is present because of the potential for harm, although there is neither general agreement nor any consensus about whether or not to treat *Pseudomonas aeruginosa* when it is present.

Of even greater controversy is the use of topical antimicrobial preparations. There are a number of reasons why the use of topical antimicrobials may be considered to be of no value in the treatment of chronic wounds (Selwyn, 1981):

- They may lead to local cell and tissue damage.
- They may lead to systemic toxicity.
- They may lead to the development of contact sensitivity and allergic reactions.
- They may cause disturbances in the normal skin ecology, leading to superinfection and the possibility of the development of antibiotic resistance.
- They may interact with other concurrent drug therapy, especially steroids.

The use of topical antibiotics has been advocated, especially in the case of burn wounds (Robson, 1991). However, an authoritative review concluded that 'Topical antibiotics are inappropriate for wounds and ulcers although they are widely promoted for this purpose. We know of no controlled trials ... showing their superiority' (Drug and Therapeutics Bulletin, 1991). An exception to this is the case of a malignant fungating lesion, for which the application of topical metronidazole is indicated for the control of the accompanying foul-smelling odour, generally associated with the presence of anaerobic bacteria (Editorial, 1990).

The use of topical antiseptic preparations such as the hypochlorites, chlorhexidine and iodine-based products has generated considerable debate in recent years and is covered in more detail in Chapter 5. However, evidence that wound fluid also contains cells and chemicals such as antibacterial proteins and live white blood cells, which are themselves part of an anti-infection mechanism (Hohn *et al.* 1977a,b) suggests that frequent repeated washing of the wound surface may be undesirable.

LOCAL WOUND CARE AND DRESSINGS

In an infected wound, the most important local measure is incision and drainage of the pus when it is enclosed, as in an abscess, or removal of all the skin sutures to allow drainage in the case of a postoperative wound that has become infected. In a wound healing by secondary intention or in a traumatic wound such as those seen in the Accident and Emergency Department, complete debridement of dead and necrotic tissue is the most important local measure (Haury *et al.* 1980). This is most effectively achieved by sharp debridement, that is, debridement using surgical instruments, sometimes under a local anaesthetic. However, a number of other methods have been described (McDonald & Nichter, 1994; Rodeheaver *et al.* 1994).

The choice of dressing for an infected wound is determined largely by the fact that, as described above, an infected wound is a wet wound. This means that dressings not designed to handle what can sometimes be considerable amounts of exudate will simply decompose or leak, leading to frequent dressing changes and patient distress and discomfort. Wounds do not heal while they are clinically infected, so the choice of wound dressing is determined by the necessity to control the symptoms, not to promote healing.

There is much research to show that the promotion of a moist-wound environment in itself leads to faster healing. However, it has been claimed that promotion of moisture in this way will lead to clinical infection (Bennett, 1982). A review of the literature would indicate that this is not the case (Gilchrist & Hutchinson, 1990) and there is much evidence to show that occlusion may have a role in reducing wound infection (Hutchinson & Lawrence, 1991). In addition, there is little evidence to support the traditional view that surgical wounds should not be allowed to get wet while the stitches are still in place (Gilchrist, 1990). A more detailed account of the principles behind dressing selection will be found in Chapter 6.

CONCLUSION

The diagnosis of wound infection is best achieved by close examination of possible risk factors, comprehensive patient assessment, identification of clinical signs of infection and rigorous attention to establishing correctly the aetiology of the wound.

Treatment is focused on debridement or drainage, restoration of an adequate blood supply, appropriate use of antibiotics and promotion of a moist-wound environment.

SELF-ASSESSMENT QUESTIONS AND ACTIVITIES

Case study

Mrs Jones is an 80-year-old widow who lives with her daughter in her own self-contained 'granny flat'. For the past 10 years she has been suffering from venous ulceration in her right leg, and she currently has an open ulcer about 10 cm² in area just above her medial malleolus. You have been treating this with a non-adherent dressing and an elastic compression bandage. Today when you visit her, she tells you that it has been very painful over the last week and you notice that there is exudate leaking through the bandage.

1. What questions would you ask Mrs Jones about her present condition?
2. What test would you wish to perform before you took any further action? How would you decide whether or not it was 'normal'?
3. The test is satisfactory. Should Mrs Jones see a doctor? What might the doctor do?
4. Would you take any form of specimen for the laboratory? If so, how? How would you store and transport it?
5. What treatment should Mrs Jones receive? For how long? How would it be administered?
6. What type of dressing might you choose to apply to the ulcer? Why?

Questions and activities

(a) Why does the presence of clinical infection in a wound delay wound healing?
(b) What signs and symptoms might lead you to suspect that a wound is infected?
(c) How common is infection in surgical wounds?
(d) Why might the swab result from a chronic wound be misleading?
(e) Identify a patient from your caseload who is being treated for a wound infection. How many associated risk factors can you identify applying to that patient?

REFERENCES

Alinovi A, Bassissi P, Pini M. Systemic administration of antibiotics in the management of venous ulcers. *J Am Acad Dermatol* 1986, 15(2):186–191.

Bennett R. The debatable benefit of occlusive dressings for wounds. *Dermatol Surg Oncol* 1982, 8:166–167.

Blair S, Backhouse C, Wright DD, Riddle E, McCollum CN. Do dressings influence the healing of chronic venous ulcers? *Phlebology* 1988, 3:129–134.

Bucknall T. Factors affecting the development of surgical wound infections: a surgeon's view. *J Hosp Infect* 1985, 6:1–8.

Burke J. The physiology of wound infection. In: Hunt T, ed. *Wound healing and wound infection.* New York: Appleton-Century Crofts; 1980:242–249.

Cruse P, Foord R. The epidemiology of wound infection: a 10-year prospective study of 62,939 wounds. *Surg*

Clin North Am 1980, 60:27–40.

Cullum N, Roe B, eds. Leg ulcers: nursing management. Harrow: Scutari Press; 1995.

Cutting K. Detecting infection. Nursing Times 1994, 90(50):60–62.

Cutting K, Harding K. Criteria for identifying wound infection. J Wound Care 1994, 3(4):198–201.

Drug and Therapeutics Bulletin. Local applications to wounds I. Cleansers, antibacterials, debriders. Drug Therapeu Bull 1991, 29(24):93–95.

Editorial. Management of smelly tumours. Lancet 1990, 335:141–142.

Emmerson A, Enstone J, Griffin M, Kelsey M, Smyth E. The second national prevalence survey of infection in hospitals – overview of the results. J Hosp Infect 1996, 32:175–190.

Eriksson G, Eklund A-E, Kallings L. The clinical significance of bacterial growth in leg ulcers. Scand J Infect Dis 1984, 16:175–180.

Finch R. Skin and soft-tissue infections. Lancet 1988, i:164–167.

Finegold S. Pathogenic anaerobes. Arch Int Med 1982, 142:1988–1992.

Gilchrist B. Washing and dressings after surgery. Nursing Times 1990, 86(50):71.

Gilchrist B. Wound infection in the elderly. J Ger Dermatol 1993, 1(3):130–131.

Gilchrist B, Hutchinson J. Does occlusion lead to infection? Nursing Times 1990, 86(15):70–71.

Gilchrist B, Reed C. The bacteriology of chronic venous ulcers treated with occlusive hydrocolloid dressings. Br J Dermatol 1989, 121:337–344.

Hansson C, Hoborn J, Moller A, Swanbeck G. The microbial flora in venous leg ulcers without clinical signs of infection. Acta Dermatol Venereol (Stockh) 1995, 75:24–30.

Haury B, Rodeheaver G, Vensko J, Edgerton M, Edlich R. Debridement: an essential component of traumatic wound care. In: Hunt T, ed. Wound healing and wound infection. New York: Appleton-Century Crofts; 1980:229–241.

Heggers J, Robson M. A rapid method of performing quantitative wound cultures. Mil Med 1969, 134:666–667.

Hohn D, Ponce B, Burton R, Hunt T. Antimicrobial systems of the surgical wound. I. A comparison of oxidative metabolism and microbiocidal capacity of phagocytes from wounds and from peripheral blood. Am J Surg 1977a 133(5):597–600,

Hohn D, Granelli S, Burton R, Hunt T. Antimicrobial systems of the surgical wound, II. Detection of antimicrobial protein in cell-free wound fluid. Am J Surg 1977b 133(5):601–606.

Horan T, Gaynes R, Martone W, Jarvis W, Emori T. CDC definitions of nosocomial surgical site infections, 1992: A modification of CDC definitions of surgical wound infections. Am J Infect Control 1992, 20(5):271.

Hutchinson J. Influence of occlusive dressings on wound microbiology – interim results of a multi-centre clinical trial of an occlusive hydrocolloid dressing. In: Harding K, Leaper D,Turner T, eds. Proceedings of the 1st European conference on advances in wound management. London: Macmillan; 1992:152–155.

Hutchinson J, Lawrence J. Wound infection under occlusive dressings. J Hosp Infect 1991,17:83–94.

Lawrence J. Wound infection. J Wound Care 1993,2(5):277–280.

Lazarus G, Cooper D, Knighton D, Margolis D, Pecoraro R, Rodeheaver G, Robson M. Definitions and guidelines for assessment of wounds and evaluation of healing. Arch Dermatol 1994, 130:489–493.

Leaper D. Risk factors for surgical infection. J Hosp Infect 1995, 30(suppl):127–139.

McDonald W, Nichter L. Debridement of bacterial and particulate-contaminated wounds. Ann Plast Surg 1994, 33:142–147.

Mertz P, Eaglstein W. The effect of a semiocclusive dressing on the microbial population in superficial wounds. Arch Surg 1984, 119:287–289.

Mills K, Morton R, Page G: A colour atlas of accidents and emergencies. London:Wolfe Medical Publications; 1988.

Mims CA, Playfair JHL, Roitt IM, et al. Medical microbiology. St Louis: Mosby; 1993.

Mishriki S, Law D, Jeffery P. Factors affecting the incidence of postoperative wound infection. J Hosp Infect 1990, 16:223–230.

Morison MJ: *A colour guide to the nursing management of wounds.* London: Mosby; 1992.

Neal M. Necrotising infections. *Nursing Times* 1994, 90(41):53–59.

Parry A, Chadwick P, Simon D, Oppenheim B, McCollum C. Leg ulcer odour detection identifies haemolytic streptococcal infection. *J Wound Care* 1995, 4(9):404–406.

Perry C, Pearson R, Miller G. Accuracy of cultures of material from swabbing of the superficial aspect of the wound and needle biopsy in the preoperative assessment of osteomyelitis. *J Bone Joint Surg* 1991, 73(5):745–749.

Robson M. Plastic surgery. In: Heggers J, Robson M, eds. *Quantitative bacteriology: its role in the armamentarium of the surgeon.* Florida: CRC Press; 1991:71–84.

Robson M, Heggers J. Quantitative bacteriology and inflammatory mediators in soft tissue. In: Hunt T, Heppenstall R, Pines E, Rovee D, eds. *Soft and hard tissue repair.* New York: Praeger Publications; 1984:483–507.

Robson M, Stenberg B, Heggers J. Wound healing alterations caused by infection. *Clin Plast Surg* 1990, 17(3):485–492.

Rodeheaver G, Baharestani M, Brabec M, Byrd H, Salzberg C, Scherer P, Vogelpohl T. Wound healing and wound management: focus on debridement. *Adv Wound Care* 1994, 7(1):22–36.

Roitt I, Brostoff J, Male D: *Immunology,* 4th ed. London: Mosby; 1996.

Schneider M, Vildozola C, Brooks S. Quantitative assessment of bacterial invasion of chronic ulcers. *Am J Surg* 1983, 145:260–262.

Schraibman I. The significance of haemolytic streptococci in chronic leg ulcers. *Ann R Coll Surg Eng* 1990, 72:123–124.

Selwyn S. The topical treatment of skin infections. In: Maibach H, Aly R, eds. *Skin microbiology. Relevance to clinical infection.* New York: Springer–Verlag; 1981:317–328.

Sherertz R, Garibaldi R, Marosok R, Mayhall C, Scheckler W, Berg R, Gaynes R, Jarvis W, Martone W, Lee J. Consensus paper on the surveillance of surgical wound infections. *Am J Infect Control* 1992, 20(5):263–270.

Spencer R. National prevalence survey of hospital acquired infections: definitions. *J Hosp Infect* 1993, 24:69–76.

Stotts N. Determination of bacterial burden in wounds. *Adv Wound Care* 1995, 8(8):46–52.

Swann A. Bacterial infection. *Care Sci Pract* 1985, 1:14–17.

Thompson P, Smith D. What is infection? In: Kerstein M, ed. A symposium: wound infection and occlusion — separating fact from fiction. *Am J Surg* 1994, 167(suppl.1A):7–11.

Tobin G. Closure of contaminated wounds. *Surg Clin North Am* 1984, 64(4):639–652.

Patient Assessment

This chapter explores the assessment process of patients with wounds. It builds on and applies the principles outlined in Chapters 1–3.

In all aspects of patient care, the findings from an ongoing process of assessment should form the basis for rational decision making. In the case of wound care, it is all too easy for the assessment process to focus on the wound itself, to the detriment of wider issues. Wound care has, for the most part, been researched at the individual, pathophysiological, organ-system level. Throughout this chapter it is suggested that it is essential that the emphasis be shifted from the wound towards assessment of the patient with a wound and to acknowledge the environmental and social factors that may influence the healing process.

As illustrated in Figure 4.1, individuals are seen as being members of families, which are in turn embedded within a local community, set in a wider society. The aim of assessment should therefore be to take a holistic approach to understanding the interaction of a multiplicity of variables on many different system levels. Although the focus of this chapter is predominantly at the level of the individual, there are many hints in the literature to suggest that society's view of health and healthcare and the attitudes of extended family, friends and healthcare professionals in the local community have an impact on the individual's experience of a wound; this is in addition to the nature of the wound itself. Failure to acknowledge the actual or potential impact of influences at all system levels on the individual's experience of a wound would be short-sighted and could lead to delayed wound healing. Figure 4.1 acknowledges the importance of healthcare professionals gaining some understanding of the unique context within which each individual's wound is to be managed.

The importance of using an organized approach to patient assessment has been described by Bale (1994). Assessment can be thought of at three levels:

- General patient assessment.
- Assessment of local wound conditions.
- Assessment of environmental and social conditions.

Patient assessment is considered in this chapter using this simple framework.

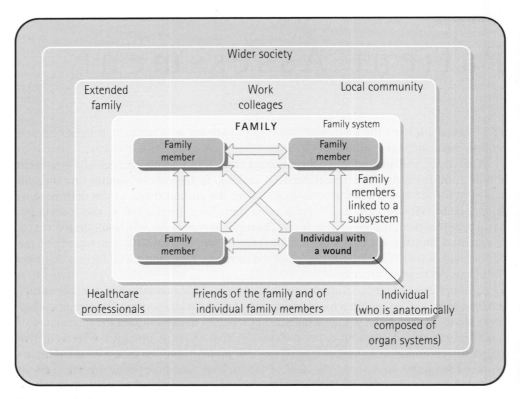

Figure 4.1   A conceptualization of the individual, embedded within a family, set in a local community and encompassed by a wider society. (Reproduced from Morison, 1996.)

GENERAL PATIENT ASSESSMENT

The starting point in the assessment process is the general assessment of the patient as a whole. This would include assessment of the following characteristics of the individual:
- Overall health and any disease processes that are ongoing.
- Mobility.
- Nutritional status.
- Sensory functioning.
- Cardiovascular status.
- Pain.
- Current medication.
- Anxiety, negative psychosocial factors.
- Understanding of the wound's aetiology and the associated treatment (*see* Chapter 8).

Further discussion of these factors and the mechanisms by which they affect the healing process is given in Chapter 1. Factors such as mobility, sensory functioning and cardio-vascular status are discussed in more depth in Chapters 9–11, in relation to wounds of specific aetiologies, such as pressure sores and leg ulcers. As a result of their particular significance to wound healing, nutritional status and pain are explored more fully below.

Nutritional status

Malnutrition is a very important cause of delayed wound healing. A number of indicators of protein–energy malnutrition (PEM) are discussed in Chapter 2 where the role of micronutrients is also discussed.

Malnutrition can be a problem for patients with chronic illnesses and especially for elderly people. The risk of malnutrition is present whether the patient is being cared for at home or in hospital (Torrance & Gobbi, 1994). In the hospital environment this is an ongoing problem (Dickerson, 1990). The importance of closely monitoring weight and other indicators of malnutrition is emphasized by Wood and Creamer (1996). It is of value for the team to work with the dietician if malnutrition is suspected.

Pain

Pain is a common and often underestimated problem for patients with wounds. Inadequately managed pain can lead to a vicious circle of sleep disturbance, irritability, anxiety, depression and increased pain (Seers, 1994).

Although undesirable and often preventable, acute pain after major surgery does at least have a positive physiological function, acting as a warning that particular care must be taken to prevent further trauma to the injured area. Pain after surgery is normally of a predictable finite duration, lessening over time as natural repair to damaged tissue proceeds. However, despite administration of analgesia one study found that patients' own assessment of postoperative pain was 60% of the maximum for the first day after the operation (Kuhnot et al. 1990). Seers (op. cit.) identified a gap between theory and practice in this field of pain management, finding that, although much information is available on assessment of pain and pain relief, adequate pain relief is not administered. In contrast, for a patient suffering with chronic pain, such as pain associated with carcinoma, or for a patient with severe peripheral vascular disease and an ischaemic ulcer in the lower limb, pain serves no useful functioning.

Pain is a complex phenomenon that is influenced only in part by the degree of tissue injury or disease. There are many accounts of soldiers having sustained very severe traumatic injury and yet reporting little or no pain, whereas at the other extreme there are patients who experience pain in the absence of any identifiable organic cause. Patients' perception of pain is influenced by factors such as the meaning of the pain to them (Waugh, 1990) which is influenced in turn by social and cultural factors, personality and current psychological status. Patients with pain caused by malignancy are faced with the possibility of imminent death. The uncertainty, fear, fatigue and depression that can accompany terminal illness lowers the patient's pain threshold, increasing perceived pain and the need for analgesia (Bond, 1984).

Pain is an individual response to a stimulus and is a different experience for all individuals. The most widely recognized definition of pain is that pain is 'whatever the patient says it is and exists wherever he says it does' (McCaffery & Beebe, 1989). With reference to paediatric nursing, children's pain has not been respected. It was only during the 1970s that the issue of pain in children was addressed and given serious consideration (Melfort, 1995).

Seers (op. cit.) has stressed the importance of comprehensively assessing pain as part of a nurse's routine assessment. Re-assessment and evaluation should also be undertaken at regular intervals. It follows that an assessment process for patients with wounds should also make an attempt to measure pain levels. A thorough assessment of pain should include:

1. Location of pain, documented by using a drawing of the human body.
2. Intensity of pain, documented by using a linear analogue scale.
3. Pattern of pain, document the type of pain, length of time present, when it starts, does anything make it better or worse.
4. Effect of pain, document changes in sleep patterns, loss of function, decreased socialization (Seers, op. cit.).

The assessment charts for closed wounds (Figure 4.2) and open wounds (Figure 4.3) encourage the nurse to record the site of any pain, its frequency and the patients' perception of its severity on a linear analogue scale of 0–10, with 0 meaning no pain and 10 the worst possible, as estimated by the individual.

Possible causes of pain at the wound site and at dressing changes are summarized in Box 4.1 which suggests factors that may require further assessment and the evaluation of practice.

More sophisticated methods for assessing and documenting pain and the factors that relieve it, suitable for patients with chronic, intractable wound pain, include the King's College Hospital Pain Clinic Chart, the McGill Pain Questionnaire and the London Hospital Pain Observation Chart. The use of these methods is reviewed by Latham (1990).

Assessing the cause of the wound

Identifying the immediate cause of a wound and, where possible, any underlying pathophysiology, is a prerequisite to planning appropriate care and to preventing recurrence in some wounds in the longer term. The following examples help to clarify this.

Pressure sores

The primary cause of most pressure sores is usually unrelieved pressure, often accompanied by friction and shearing forces (*see* Chapter 9). Sensory loss associated with a cerebrovascular accident, paraplegia or multiple sclerosis, may contribute to the development of a pressure sore and must be considered when planning immediate care and pressure sore prevention in the future.

Leg ulcers

The immediate cause may be minor traumatic injury but the underlying disease process may be a variety of aetiologies, the majority of ulcers being associated with chronic venous hypertension, poor arterial blood supply to the lower limb or both. The cause of the ulcer will determine the optimum treatment, as outlined in Chapter 10.

Diabetic foot ulcers

An accurate diagnosis of the cause of the wound is important. The immediate cause may have been ill-fitting footwear but the underlying cause may be peripheral neuropathy or vascular insufficiency. The use of orthotic shoes, vascular surgery and the care

Nature of operation _

Wound site _ Date of operation _ _ _ _ _ _ _ _ _ _ _ _

Method of closure _

Drains: (a) type _ _ _ _ _ _ _ _ _ _ _ _ _ _ _ _ _ _ _ (b) site _ _ _ _ _ _ _ _ _ _ _ _ _ _ _ _ _ _

SPECIAL INSTRUCTIONS FROM THE SURGEON _ .

_ _

General patient factors that may delay healing (e.g. obese, chronic chest infection) _ _ _ _ _ _ _ _

_ _

Allergies to wound care products _ .

Chart the following factors at *every* dressing change. If there is marked erythema, trace this and

note if erythema spreads.

Wound factors/Date				
1 **EXUDATE**				
a. amount: heavy/moderate/minimal/none				
b. type				
c. colour				
2 **ERYTHEMA OF SURROUNDING SKIN**				
a. around stitches only				
b. extending beyond a				
c. maximum distance from the wound edge (mm)				
3 **OEDEMA**				
Severe/moderate/minimal/none				
4 **HAEMATOMA**				
Severe/moderate/minimal/none				
5 **PAIN (SITE)**				
a. at wound itself				
b. elsewhere (specify)				
6 **PAIN (FREQUENCY)**				
Continuous/intermittent/only at dressing changes/none				
7 **PAIN (SEVERITY)**				
Patient's score (0-10)				
8 **ODOUR**				
Offensive/some/none				
9 **INFECTION**				
a. suspected				
b. wound swab sent				
c. confirmed (specify organism)				

WOUND ASSESSED BY: _

Figure 4.2   Assessment chart for surgically closed wounds. (Reproduced from Morison, 1992.)

Type of wound (e.g. pressure sore, venous leg ulcer) _

Location _ _ _ _ _ _ _ _ _ _ _ _ _ _ _ _ _ _ How long has wound been open? _ _ _ _ _ _ _ _ _

General Patient factors which may delay healing (e.g. malnourished, diabetes, chronic infection)

_ _

Allergies to wound care products _

Previous treatments tried (comment on success/problems) _

Special aids in current use (e.g. pressure relieving bed, compression bandage) _ _ _ _ _ _ _ _ _ _

_ _

TRACE THE WOUND WEEKLY, ANNOTATING TRACING WITH NATURE OF WOUND BED, ORIENTATION
OF WOUND, POSITION/EXTENT OF SINUSES AND UNDERMINING OF SURROUNDING SKIN.

All other parameters should be assessed at *every* dressing change and changes documented.

Wound factors/Date					
1	NATURE OF WOUND BED				
	a. healthy granulation				
	b. epithelialization				
	c. slough				
	d. black/brown eschar				
	e. other (specify)				
2	EXUDATE				
	a. colour				
	b. type				
	c. approximate amount				
3	ODOUR				
	Offensive/some/none				
4	PAIN (SITE)				
	a. at wound site				
	b. elsewhere (specify)				
5	PAIN (FREQUENCY)				
	Continuous/intermediate/only at dressing changes/none				
6	PAIN (SEVERITY)				
	Patient's score (0-10)				
7	WOUND MARGIN				
	a. colour				
	b. oedema?				
8	ERYTHEMA OF SURROUNDING SKIN				
	a. present				
	b. maximum distance from wound (mm)				
9	GENERAL CONDITION OF SURROUNDING SKIN				
	e.g. dry eczema				
10	INFECTION				
	a. suspected				
	b. wound swab sent				
	c. confirmed (specify organism)				

WOUND ASSESSED BY: _

Box 4.1.

Possible causes of pain at the wound site and at dressing changes
(based on Morison, 1992)
If the patient complains of pain at the wound site or experiences pain at dressing changes, the nurse should consider the following questions:

A. Pain at the wound site
1. Is the wound infected? Look for clinical and systemic signs of infection (*see* Chapter 3).
2. Is any overlying conforming or compression bandage too tightly applied? Has the bandage slipped? Are there tight bands of constriction overlying the wound or over any nearby bony prominence?
3. Is there underlying ischaemia? For example, in a patient with severe peripheral vascular disease even small open wounds can be very painful and there may be rest pain in the limb (*see* Chapter 10).

B. Pain at dressing changes
1. Is the dressing adhering, causing tissue trauma on removal? Even low-adherent dressings can adhere to the wound if they are left in place for too long, especially if exudate strikes through the dressing and then dries out. Fresh bleeding on removal of the dressing is an obvious sign of trauma.
2. If prescribed analgesia has been used, has it had sufficient time to become effective where it is anticipated that a dressing change may be painful? Consult your pharmacist if you are unsure how long an analgesic takes to become effective.
3. Is the most painless method of dressing removal being employed? Removal of adhesive dressings or the surgical tape used to hold it in place, can be very painful if removed against the lie of any hair present. Removing dressings and tapes in line with the hairs is virtually painless and releasing the adhesive bond of adhesive dressings facilitates easy removal. If a dressing has adhered to the wound bed, it should be gently soaked off, not ripped off 'quickly'.
4. Is a cleansing solution being used that could cause an irritant tissue response, for example, hypochlorite? (*see* Chapter 5)
5. Does the nurse lack empathy? Is the nurse underestimating the significance of the wound to the individual?
6. Is the most appropriate dressing type being used for this wound? Modern dressing materials provide a range of functions and provide a variety of wound environments (*see* Chapter 6). Choose the most appropriate for the wound.

of the diabetic foot clinic may all help in the treatment and prevention of further ulceration which, for diabetic patients, is a major cause of amputation (*see* Chapter 10). As is indicated in Chapter 10, management of diabetes and its side effects is at least as important as choosing the best wound dressing to promote healing.

← Figure 4.3 Open wound assessment chart. (Reproduced from Morison, 1992.)

Factitious wounds

A small percentage of patients will self-inflict injuries, the underlying problem here is not so much physical but psychological and all attempts to heal the injury are likely to fail if the patient's mental status is ignored. A variety of strategies can be employed to help the patient psychologically and to facilitate healing (Baragwanath *et al.* 1994). In this situation there is often poor prognosis with approximately 30% of patients having unhealed wounds in the long term.

If the cause of the wound or any underlying pathophysiology is ignored, treatment will only be directed at alleviating the symptoms of the problem. Even if the wound does heal there is a high probability that it will recur, whether the wound is a leg ulcer, a pressure sore or a self-inflicted injury.

ASSESSMENT OF LOCAL CONDITIONS AT THE WOUND SITE

After assessing the patient as a whole, including the immediate cause of the wound and any underlying pathophysiology, it is important to make an accurate assessment of the wound itself in order to:

- Identify any local wound characteristics that may delay healing, such as necrotic tissue, excess slough, infection or excess exudate (*see* Chapter 1).
- Document the local wound conditions as a baseline for future reference.

Accurate and ongoing wound assessment is essential to planning the most appropriate local wound management (*see* Chapters 5 and 6) and to evaluating its effectiveness. If frequent and thorough wound assessment is being undertaken, any abnormal changes in a previously healthy healing wound can be picked up quickly and appropriate therapeutic action taken. It is also important to be able to recognize when healing is progressing well, that is, to be able to recognize the clinical appearance of healthy granulation tissue and epithelium.

Clear and accurate documentation of the findings of assessment is essential because of the following:

- All members of the team of healthcare professionals caring for the patient need access to this information when deciding on a range of treatment options.
- Charting observations can help to develop the observational skills of students by highlighting the points that should be noticed.
- The documentation can be transferred between the hospital and community and vice versa, to help ensure continuity of care.
- It is a legal requirement to have this information clearly documented for purposes of accountability. There have already been a number of cases of patients with pressure sores suing health authorities for negligence when this information (or the lack of information) has been used as evidence.

Charting wound healing

There are several wound assessment charts available, two of which are featured in this chapter. They are intended to be an aid to the accurate recording of the most important parameters of wound assessment. The first chart (Figure 4.2) is for wound healing by primary intention, the parameters recorded give a good indication of whether the wound is healthy or unhealthy and whether healing is progressing well or with obvious delay. The second (Figure 4.3) is for wounds healing by secondary intention.

Surgically closed wounds

For sutured wounds, the early identification of postoperative wound infection is vital for prevention of the long-term complications associated with infection. Surgeons and surgical nurses spend much time and effort in the prevention of, and early detection of, wound infection and charting progress (Figure 4.2) can aid the early identification of complications.

Events in the operating theatre have an important bearing on whether a wound infection develops later. In a wound healing by primary intention, the first sign of infection may be spreading erythema, perhaps accompanied by pain, oedema and an elevated body temperature. Complete wound dehiscence can be dramatic and is a serious complication requiring immediate surgical intervention. Partial wound breakdown occurs when an isolated pocket of infection discharges through the suture line. This area of tissue breakdown usually occurs under the suture line but can occur, less typically, through the depth of the wound.

Open wounds

The wound assessment chart shown in Figure 4.3 is intended to be used for wounds healing by secondary intention. This will include surgically excised wounds such as drainage of abscesses, excised pilonidal sinuses that are left open and chronic open wounds such as pressure sores and leg ulcers.

Wound measurement techniques

Decrease in both surface area and volume of a wound are useful indicators of healing. There are a variety of methods of measuring wounds and these range from highly technical computerized systems to simple basic measurements. A number of these methods are outlined below. Some are costly and time-consuming and some can only cope with flat wounds. A number of factors have been identified as being particularly problematic:

- The definition of the wound's boundary, this is observer-dependent and so prone to inaccuracy.
- Wound flexibility; in wounds where there is undermining of the skin edge or the wound is large or deep; these wounds can be difficult to measure with precision and are capable of changing their appearance significantly according to the positioning of the patient.
- The natural curvature of the human body; currently measurement devices do not take this into account (Plassmann, 1995).

Area

Tracing One of the simplest and most popular methods of assessing the area of a wound is to trace the outline of the wound margin on to a clear plastic sheet using an indelible ink marker. In its simplest form a piece of plastic acetate sheeting can be used. To avoid the need to disinfect the tracing sheet, which has been in contact with the wound bed, a sheet of cling film can be used as the wound-contact layer and the acetate sheet placed on top of it. The cling film can then be discarded leaving the acetate sheet clean and uncontaminated. Commercially available plastic measuring sheets, working on these principles, are also useful for this purpose and some dressing manufacturers provide these for their customers. Plastic sheets with grids are used to calculate surface area. These tracings can be transferred to the nursing notes and annotated to include the nature of the wound bed, the extent of undermining of the surrounding skin and the position of the wound relative to other structures. An example of a simple annotated tracing is given in Figure 4.4. Tracings can be shown to patients, which is particularly important when the wound is positioned where it cannot be seen by the patient, as in the case of a sacral pressure sore or when the patient needs an extra incentive to participate fully in the treatment programme. It should be noted that when wound debridement is being undertaken, it is normal for the wound to enlarge as devitalized tissue is removed from the wound bed. This is why the state of the wound bed should also be documented in conjunction with size. As such a wound enlarges so that the percentage of devitalized tissue on the wound bed decreases. The calculation of wound area can be undertaken with wound tracings using a computer with a camera or hand-held scanner facility. This is a faster and more accurate method than using a planimeter or counting 1 cm squares (Plassmann, op. cit.).

Photography This has been attempted using a ruler next to the wound and taking the photograph from a standard distance. This method is time consuming and prone to inaccuracy and is currently not a popular method of assessing wound area. However, the use of photographs in the assessment process is discussed later in this section.

Volume

When a patient with a large cavity or undermining wound is being assessed, measurement of the wound area does not reflect healing from the depth of a wound. Large wounds and undermined areas are a common phenomenon in pressure sores and in this situation it is important to be able to evaluate a wound's progress on a regular basis with some degree of accuracy.

To date there is no single system that quickly, easily and cheaply assesses wound volume accurately. Some of the methods available include the following:

- Using two sterile probes. One probe is inserted into the deepest part of the wound, perpendicular to the wound surface and the other probe is placed across the wound surface. The maximum depth is then measured.
- A disposable ruler used to measure the maximum length, breadth and depth.
- The wound is occluded with a semipermeable film-dressing and sterile water or saline is injected to fill the wound. The volume can be calculated using the volume of saline needed to fill the wound.
- An alginate dental impression material was described by Resch *et al.* (1988). As when taking impressions in dentistry, the impression powder is mixed with water and pasted into the wound where it sets in minutes and provides a cast of the wound. Care is needed not to overfill or underfill the wound as this affects the volume measurement.
- Less widely available methods are ultrasonic surface scanners, stereo photography and structured light. Although more precise (Plassmann, op. cit.), they are expensive, difficult to use and need skill, technical knowledge and extensive training to use.

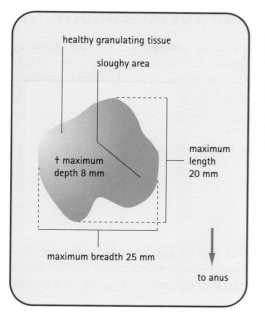

Figure 4.4 Example of a tracing of a sacral pressure sore. The maximum dimensions are included together with the nature of the wound bed. (Reproduced from Morison, 1992.)

Photography

The phrase 'a picture speaks a thousand words' certainly applies to wound assessment. The use of a Polaroid camera in conjunction with accurate assessment is an extremely useful form of documentation. Ideally, using the professional services of a medical photographer will produce the best quality photograph. However, this is not often possible, especially when caring for patients in the community. A number of factors will influence the success of the quality of the photograph:

- Standardization—where a series of photographs is to be taken over a period of time, the same camera, focal length and lighting need to be used. Having a ruler or measure in the frame also helps.
- Equipment—a medical Polaroid camera can be used or a 35 mm single-lens reflex is the camera of choice (Bellamy, 1995). A good quality colour film and a reputable film processor are needed.
- Control of patient—it can be difficult to position the patient in the same way for each photograph or even to get the patient into a suitable position which is comfortable.
- Lighting and background should be such that the wound can be seen clearly against an unobtrusive background. The ideal choice of colour for the background is mid-grey (Bellamy, op. cit.).

ASSESSMENT OF PHYSICAL AND SOCIAL CONDITIONS

Assessment of the patients' environmental and social conditions is now being recognized as an important part of the assessment process. Several issues are discussed in this section and those relevant to individual patients can be documented in their care plan. The following assessment issues will be considered:

- Physical environment.
- Ability and desire to self care.
- Altered body image.
- Consequences of the wound.
- Social problems.
- Healthcare systems.

Physical environment

The physical environment in which a patient is cared for can have an impact not only on the safety of that patient but also on the range of wound-care services that are available. Table 4.1 illustrates just how diverse the physical environment can be for a patient with a wound.

Ability/desire to self care

Many patients are willing and capable of being involved and, on occasion, in delivering their own wound care. Patients in conjunction with their nurse can become responsible for the following:

- Fluid and nutritional intake, especially when extra fluids and protein-rich foods may be recommended.
- Reporting the clinical signs of infection as they arise.
- Resting and gentle exercise.
- The hygiene of open granulating wounds and simple dressing changes.
- In children, the parents may take on these responsibilities on behalf of the child and give all the wound-related care to their child (Bale & Jones, 1996).
- Their physiotherapy (for patients with leg ulceration) and pressure-relieving techniques (for patients with pressure sores).
  Empowering patients to care for their wounds is important to patients who have a variety of commitments:
- Small children to care for, elderly relatives or handicapped relatives.
- Patients who wish to return to work or school and do not wish to have the services of the district or practice nurse.
- Patients who do not wish to be restricted by healthcare professionals calling at their homes or who are particularly independent.

The safety of the individual should be a primary consideration and the patients' wishes to become involved in their care will depend on their individual circumstances and their level of capability and understanding (Bale, op. cit.). Support needs to be available in the event of its being required, even for the most capable and independent individual.

Table 4.1.
Physical environment (from Davies et al. 1992)

Environment and carers	Implications	Indications and examples
Teaching hospital Specialist units and teams	Maximum expertise and facilities Constant availability Maximum cost Maximum disruption of patient's lifestyle	**Wounds requiring specialist management** Major wounds Minor wounds associated with other major problems Wounds with complications
District hospital General surgical and medical teams	High level of expertise and facilities Constant availability Visiting specialists	**Wounds requiring hospital facilities** Major wounds Minor wounds associated with other health problems Wounds with complications
Cottage hospital Supervised by GP General nursing care	Constant nursing and domestic care Intermittent advice	**Wounds not requiring full hospital facilities** Patients recovering from major wounds Minor wounds with other health problems
Nursing home Variable nursing experience GP visits	Domestic care Intermittent nursing care Intermittent advice	**Wounds not requiring hospital facilities** Less severe wounds in patients with additional problems
Residential care Community nurse visits GP visits	Domestic care Intermittent nursing care Intermittent advice Cost effective	**Wounds not requiring hospital facilities** Minor wounds in elderly or disabled patients
Sheltered housing Community nurse visits	Supervised own domestic care Intermittent care and advice	**Wounds not requiring hospital facilities** Minor wounds in elderly or disabled patients

Table 4.1 continues over....

Environment and carers	Implications	Indications and examples
Table 4.1 (continued) **Physical environment**		
GP's surgery Surgery nurse Nurse practitioner GP	Cost effective Minimal disruption to lifestyle Patient visits, facilities and carers	**Wounds not requiring hospital facilities** Minor wounds in mobile patients Postoperative wounds Healing major wounds
Patient's home Community nurse visits GP visits	Cost effective Little disruption to lifestyle Few facilities Intermittent advice and care or self-care	**Wounds not requiring hospital facilities** Minor or healing wounds in patients with limited mobility
At work Occupational nursing and medical specialists	Cost effective Specialist knowledge of work environment	**Wounds not requiring hospital facilities** First Aid for accidents at work Minor wounds in patients continuing to work
Site of accident Bystander or no care Paramedic/ambulance team Mobile hospital team or GP	Few facilities Variable expertise in First Aid	**Immediate treatment** Any accidental injury

Altered body image

The concept of body image can be defined as our own individual mental image of ourselves. Any change in physical appearance, no matter how big or small, can affect body image. Altered body image can be a problem with the following (Rodgers, 1994):

- Any type of surgical procedure, the suture line and resultant scar can be difficult to come to terms with.
- After mastectomy or breast surgery of any type, mastectomy in particular is associated with the 'loss' of a body part.
- After formation of a stoma, this can be devastating for the individual. When it is associated with cancer the problem could be worse.
- Traumatic injuries resulting in multiple or extensive scarring.
- Burns where scarring is extensive or highly visible or when complications occur with contractures and hypertrophic scarring.

Consequences of the wound

The cause of a wound has a direct bearing on the patient's feeling about it and its consequences. A young, otherwise fit woman who requires a Caesarean section for the safe delivery of her child is likely to suffer short-term discomfort but the degree of discomfort is lessened by its association with a happy event, the birth of a baby. Often the wound is planned and the long-term consequences are generally not serious.

In contrast, a young, otherwise fit man who loses a leg after a motor cycle accident not only suffers considerable physical pain in the short term but also has to face the long-term effects of physical disability with perhaps loss of job, loss of self-esteem, altered body image, altered social relationships and restricted recreational opportunities. All of these can be overcome and much depends on the individual's ability and determination to return to normality. In this case, the nature of the problem is related not only to the type of wound and its site but also to the person's level of support and personal philosophy.

The short and long-term consequences of the wound can have a significant effect on the individual patient. The short and long-term rehabilitation of patients, both physical and psychological, requires planning and sensitivity. Sympathetic counselling, involving the patient and his or her family, is an integral part of patient care from the outset (*see* Chapter 8).

Social problems

Problems associated with the wound can be due to a number of factors:
- Lack of income because of inability to work. This is a problem for the self-employed and casual workers, not all patients have a protected salary or insurance scheme.
- The requirement to purchase dressings and other products either on FP 10 or directly from the chemist. For patients with a restricted income because of sickness the added burden of such purchases (which may be a considerable weekly sum) causes added financial difficulties.
- Inability to care for themselves and be independent because of the wound or associated surgery or disease progress. This may range from needing help with cooking and cleaning to needing help, 24 hours a day, with all aspects of personal care. Such patients may require residential or nursing-home care for a period of time or may live with a more able relative or friend.

Healthcare system

In the UK, healthcare is provided free to all individuals at the point of delivery and generally is provided according to the individual's needs. An increasing number of individuals are opting to purchase private health insurance schemes. However, other countries have different systems which vary from Third-world countries, where resources are scarce and so services poor, to the USA, Australia and Canada where very basic care is available to all but where many individuals have a private health insurance scheme.

The impact of the healthcare system in the UK is that there are differences in the availability to patients of dressings, appliances and services depending on whether they are treated in hospital or in the community. Hospitals generally have a greater range of products and services available to patients than is the case when they are being cared for in the community. When treated in the community many patients are restricted to the products available on FP10 and prescribed by the general practitioner and equipment and other services provided by the Community Healthcare Trust.

SELF-ASSESSMENT QUESTIONS AND ACTIVITIES

Identify three patients currently within your care who have a wound. For each:

(a) Note the general patient factors that may be affecting the healing process, such as concurrent illness, reduced mobility and nutritional status (see also Chapters 1 and 2).

(b) Review the methods that you have used to measure and chart local conditions at the wound site itself. Are there any ways in which your methods could be improved on? If you do decide that change is required who needs to be involved and how would you set about it? (see also Chapter 12 for guidance here).

(c) List the consequences of the wound for the individual. Have you asked the patient what the issues are for him/her? (see also Chapter 13 which discusses issues relating to quality of life and its measurement). How and where would you document the patient's perception of the consequences of the wound?

(d) With the help of Box 4.1, identify the type of facility where you work and the possible implications of this for the patient's care. If you are not working in a specialist unit, could it be that the patient might benefit from a specialist assessment to determine the underlying cause of the wound? . Does the patient need a specialist referral within your own unit, for example, to the dietician (see Chapter 2) or to a dermatologist (see Chapter 7).

REFERENCES

Bale S. Wound healing in nursing practice. In: Alexander MF, Fawcett JN, Runciman PJ, eds. *The Adult*. Edinburgh: Churchill Livingstone; 1994.

Bale S, Jones V. Caring for children with wounds. *J Wound Care* 1996, **5**(4):177–180.

Baragwanath P, Shutler S, Harding KG. The management of a patient with factitious wounds. *J Wound Care* 1994, **3**(6):286–287.

Bellamy K. Photography in wound assessment. *J Wound Care* 1995, **4**(7):313–316.

Bond MR. *Pain: its nature, analysis and treatment.* Edinburgh: Churchill Livingstone; 1984.

Davies MH, Dinley P, Harden R *et al. The wound programme.* Dundee: Centre for Medical Education; 1992.

Dickerson JWT. Hospital induced malnutrition: prevention and treatment. In: Horne EM, ed. *The staff nurse's survival guide.* London: Austen Cornish; 1990:175–178.

Kuhnot S, Cooke K, Collins M, Jones JM, Hucklow JC. Perceptions of pain relief after surgery. *BMJ* 1990, **300**:1687–1690.

Latham J. Assessment, observation and measurement of pain. In: Horne EM, ed. *The Staff Nurse's Survival Guide.* London: Austen Cornish; 1990:179–185.

McCaffery M, Beebe A. *Pain. Clinical manual for nursing practice.* St Louis: Mosby; 1989.

Melfont M. Strategies to reduce childrens' perception of pain. *Nursing Times* 1995, **91**(2):34–35.

Morison M. *A colour guide to the nursing management of wounds.* London: Wolfe; 1992.

Morison M. *Family perspectives in bed wetting in young people.* Aldershot: Avebury; 1996.

Plassmann P. Measuring wounds. *J Wound Care* 1995, **4**(6):269–272.

Resch CS, Kerner E, Robson MC *et al.* Pressure sore volume measurement, a technique to document and record wound healing. *Am Geriatr Soc* 1988, **36**:444–446.

Rodgers SE. The patient facing surgery. In: Alexander MF, Fawcett JN, Runciman PJ, eds. *The Adult.* Edinburgh: Churchill Livingstone; 1994.

Seers K. *Pain. Nursing Practice Textbook.* In: Alexander MF, Fawcett JN, Runciman PJ, eds. *The Adult.* Edinburgh: Churchill Livingstone; 1994.

Torrance C, Gobbi H. Nutrition in nursing. In: Alexander MF, Fawcett JN, Runciman PJ, eds. *The Adult.* Edinburgh: Churchill Livingstone; 1994.

Waugh L. Psychological aspects of cancer pain. In: Horne EM, ed. *The staff nurse's survival guide.* London: Austen Cornish; 1990:194–201.

Wood S, Creamer H. Malnutrition in hospitals. *Nursing Times* 1996, **92**(26):67–70.

FURTHER READING

Brunner LS, Suddarth DS. *The Lippincott manual of medical surgical nursing*, 2nd ed. London: Harper and Row; 1990.

Morton PC. *The health assessment in nursing.* Pennsylvania: Springhouse; 1990.

Wound Cleansing

Wounds have been cleansed, using a variety of techniques, since the beginning of time in an attempt actively to promote healing. Throughout history, humans have applied a wide range of topical treatments to wounds ranging from the use of boiling oil, honey and diluted wine to sea water. In the clinical situation, the principles of wound cleansing have often been misinterpreted and poorly understood, resulting in the inappropriate and often ritualistic use of cleansing solutions. In the past, many practices have concentrated on drying out the surface of wounds and the removal of exudate, despite evidence provided by Hohn *et al.* (1977) that wound exudate contains active anti-microbial substances that naturally cleanse the wound bed. Evaluation of the effectiveness of commonly used wound-cleansing agents is long overdue because evidence to support claims of improved healing rates is generally lacking.

This chapter begins by briefly considering the body's own mechanisms of wound cleansing as a natural physiological response to injury. The purpose of wound cleansing by healthcare professionals is discussed and methods of cleansing are described. Factors affecting the selection of an appropriate method are discussed.

WOUND CLEANSING AS A NATURALLY OCCURRING PHYSIOLOGICAL RESPONSE TO INJURY

The physiology of wound healing is considered in detail in Chapter 1. Some mechanisms of relevance to wound cleansing are highlighted here.

The inflammatory phase of healing is part of the protective response to injury. During this phase the body's natural response is to cleanse the wound bed by reducing bacterial counts at the wound's surface as well as by debriding devitalized tissue. Phagocytic neutrophils are attracted to the wounded area immediately after injury and provide initial protection against invading micro-organisms. Macrophages are responsible for the release of tumour necrosis growth factors which initiate the breakdown of any cellular debris, fibrin, blood clots and necrotic tissue present at the surface of the wound. The presence of necrotic tissue in a wound will always actively prolong the inflammatory response and thus delay healing.

One of the main functions of lymphocytes and macrophages during the destructive phase of healing is to cleanse the wound bed by digesting bacteria and releasing proteolytic enzymes to destroy foreign bodies and cellular debris. This process is hindered if the migration of lymphocytes across the surface of the wound is interrupted by the presence of dehydrated eschar or devitalized tissue. Wound exudate production is increased during the inflammatory phase of healing as the permeability of blood capillaries increases, causing protein-rich fluid to seep into the interstitial spaces. This increased production of fluid facilitates wound cleansing as it washes across the surface of the wound and provides the optimal, moist, local environment required to maximize healing (Alvarez, 1988). The indiscriminate use of antiseptic agents is known to have detrimental effects on wound healing as they upset the delicate balance of the body's normal physiological cleansing process.

THE PURPOSE OF WOUND CLEANSING

Much confusion still surrounds the clinical indications for wound cleansing. The routine cleansing of clean granulating wounds with antiseptic solutions is a practice that still persists in some clinical areas today. Acute and chronic wounds may require cleansing for a variety of reasons. The primary objective of wound cleansing is to remove organic and inorganic debris before the application of a wound dressing, thus maintaining an optimum environment at the wound site for healing.

Additional reasons for cleansing a wound may include:

- To rehydrate the surface of a wound in order to provide a moist environment.
- To keep the skin surrounding the wound clean and free from excessive moisture.
- To facilitate wound assessment so that the size and extent of the wound can be visualized.
- To minimize wound trauma when removing adherent dressing materials.
- To promote patient comfort.

It is important to achieve the correct balance between the beneficial effects of wound cleansing, as indicated above, and the potential harmful effects of unnecessarily disturbing the delicate equilibrium that naturally exists at the wound surface.

METHODS OF CLEANSING WOUNDS

In the past, wound cleansing has been associated with ritualistic practice and many myths still surround this practice today. Advances in wound-care technology have, in recent years, provided practitioners with alternative methods of cleansing wounds that do not necessarily involve the use of traditional cleansing solutions. Advances in dressing technology, in recent years, have been responsible for the widespread acceptance of dressings as an alternative method of safe, effective wound cleansing.

Removing stale exudate and loose debris

The relative merits of different methods of cleansing wounds of stale exudate and loose debris are still fiercely debated and are discussed below.

Wound swabbing techniques

Thomlinson (1987) was able to demonstrate that no one method of swabbing wounds was significantly more effective at reducing bacterial counts at the wound's surface than another. Swabbing from clean to dirty areas, top to bottom or inside to outside merely resulted in the redistribution of bacteria across the surface of the wound. Swabbing the wound surface may mechanically dislodge loose, devitalized tissue but it does not actively remove pathogens from the wound. Vigorous cleansing using a swab has the additional detrimental effect of causing further tissue trauma particularly to epithelializing cells. This may be uncomfortable for the patient and may actively prolong the inflammatory response. If foreign bodies are present in the wound, swabbing may only serve to drive them deeper into the tissues where they can act as a focus of infection.

Traditional wound swabbing materials, such as cotton wool or gauze, are known to shed fine, fibrous particles onto the surface of the wound which can be responsible for foreign body reactions, a prolonged inflammatory response and an increased risk of wound infection (Wood, 1976). The Surgical Materials Testing Laboratory (1992) recommended non-woven swabs or non-filamented cotton wool as more appropriate for use in wound-cleansing procedures, as they shed fewer fibres than traditional gauze swabs.

The use of forceps or sterile gloves remains contentious and as long as the principles of asepsis are applied this issue should depend on personal preference. It is the practice of hand-washing between attending to different patients that minimizes the risk of cross-infection rather than the rigid adherence to an aseptic technique (Lawrence, 1993). From a practical point of view, it can be difficult to apply some of the new generation of dressing products using forceps, especially those that have an adhesive backing or are presented as a gel.

Wound irrigation

Wound irrigation can be performed using a variety of methods including syringes, spray canisters, semi-rigid ampoules or showering. Irrigation under pressure is an effective method of cleansing wounds that are infected or heavily contaminated (Marquez, 1995).

High pressure irrigation using a 30 ml syringe and a 18–20 gauge needle lowers the infection rates in contaminated wounds (Chisholm, 1992). Optimal pressures for effective wound irrigation are reported as being 10–15 pounds per square inch. Evidence suggests that achieving the correct pressure is more important than the type of cleansing solution chosen (Ferguson, 1990). High-pressure wound irrigation is usually achieved using syringes and needles. Care is required to avoid the risk of needle-stick injuries in both patient and carer. Consideration should also be given to the possibility of splash-back and the dissemination of micro-organisms into the surrounding tissues and possible contamination of the practitioner. The adoption of universal precautions is necessary to minimize the risks of cross-infection with hepatitis B virus or with human immuno-deficiency virus (HIV).

The availability of sterile saline in semi-rigid ampoules and pressurized canisters allows practitioners to irrigate wounds without the risk of needle-stick injuries. Advantages of using pressurized canisters when compared with the use of traditional methods of irrigation include speed, ease of use and cost effectiveness. Disadvantages include reliability of the canisters and difficulty in warming the contents to a consistent ambient temperature. Research has been undertaken to assess the risk of cross-infection of multi-use canisters. Lawrence and Lilly (1994) concluded that these canisters were safe for use in both hospitals and the community provided normal, sensible precautions are observed. However, irrigation at high pressure can cause damage to delicate granulation and epithelial tissue and may cause discomfort for some patients. The use of lower pressures is recommended for the irrigation of clean granulating wounds and the use of higher pressures should be reserved for infected wounds.

Hydrotherapy is popular in the USA where wound soaking and water agitation is reported to soften and loosen blood coagulants and remove gross contaminants (Marquez, op. cit.). Whirlpools with added antibacterial agents are used to help reduce wound infection.

When cleansing acute traumatic wounds it is particularly important to remove dirt and soil from the wound bed which provides the necessary conditions for the multiplication of micro-organisms (Rodeheaver, 1974). If insufficient care is taken to do this, there is the increased risk of avoidable infection and of long-term disfiguration (Figure 5.1).

Showering and bathing

It is becoming increasingly common practice for chronic wounds, such as leg ulcers, to be cleansed in the bath, shower or in a bowl of lukewarm tap water (Morison & Moffatt, 1994). As well as cleansing the wound and the surrounding skin, this practice can be of great psychological benefit to the patient. Patients with wounds in areas that are likely to be heavily contaminated with bacteria, such as perineal wounds, sacral pressure sores, pilonidal sinuses or rectal abscesses, will greatly benefit from being given the opportunity to allow adherent dressings to soak free. Bathing also facilitates thorough cleansing of these wounds and allows the patient to attend to their own personal hygiene needs. Care should be taken not to soak wounds for long periods of time, as open tissue has a tendency to absorb water which increases the amount of exudate produced over the next few days and often necessitates more frequent dressing changes. Chrinz *et al.* (1989) were able to show that allowing surgical patients to

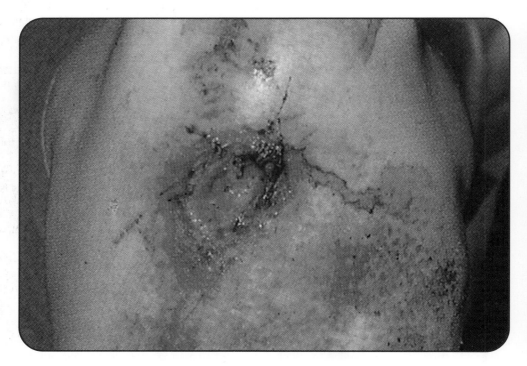

Figure 5.1 It is important to cleanse this dirty, superficial abrasion of all contaminants in order to prevent the tattooing effect caused by retained dirt. (Reproduced from Mills *et al.* 1984.)

remove dressings and shower on the first postoperative day did not increase wound infection rates. However, bathing facilities are not always available in patients' homes and some cultures and religions prohibit bathing in non-running water.

Removal of necrotic tissue and slough

There are several methods of debriding wounds contaminated by necrotic tissue and slough. The methods may be used in a variety of different clinical circumstances. The choice of an appropriate method of debriding is a complex one that can sometimes provoke controversy. In brief, the main treatment options include the following:

- Surgical excision.
- Hydrogel dressings.
- Hydrocolloid dressings.
- Alginate dressings.
- Polysaccharide pastes.
- Enzymatic treatments.

Further discussion of these options is to be found in Thomas (1994) and in Chapter 6.

SELECTING AN APPROPRIATE METHOD OF WOUND DEBRIDEMENT

There are a variety of different methods that can be used successfully to debride wounds. Selection of a particular method of wound debridement should be carefully considered and is dependent on the factors listed in Box 5.1.

Box 5.1.

Factors influencing the choice of debridement method

- The type of injury and potential contamination
- The wound aetiology
- The location of the wound
- The extent of tissue damage and type of tissue involvement
- The size of the wound and extent of devitalized tissue
- The amount of exudate production
- Time available
- Availability of resources, access to different methods
- User skill, knowledge base and professional accountability
- Cost-effectiveness
- The care environment: hospital or community
- The patient's wishes

The degree of contamination by micro-organisms, organic and inorganic debris is an important factor to be considered. Traumatic wounds differ from surgical or chronic wounds in a number of ways. They are often heavily contaminated by various combinations of dirt, oil, foreign bodies, bacteria, fungi or spores. This type of injury requires thorough cleansing and debridement of the wound and surrounding skin, which is best achieved using large volumes of saline or tap water.

Decontamination of traumatic wounds should be carried out quickly, as the organic and inorganic components of soil have detrimental effects on exposed tissue, providing the necessary conditions for the multiplication of micro-organisms (Rodeheaver, op. cit.). After thorough wound cleansing, surgical debridement is often required in order to facilitate the removal of devitalized tissue and foreign bodies. This can be performed under local or general anaesthetic depending on the extent of contamination and tissue damage. All traumatic wounds, however superficial, require careful exploration in order to exclude the possibility of even the smallest foreign body such as grit, splinters, glass or grease remaining within the wound where they are likely to delay healing by acting as foci for infection. The continued presence of grit in a wound may lead to the development of permanent 'tattooing' of the skin. The overall aim of surgical-wound debridement is to remove gross contaminants with the minimum of pain to the patient and trauma to the tissues. For minor traumatic wounds, asepsis is unnecessary until all gross contamination is removed.

The aetiology of the wound will influence the choice of different methods of debridement. It is well recognized that early surgical excision of devitalized tissue is usually the treatment of choice for a diabetic patient with a necrotic or sloughy foot ulcer because of the increased risk of infection associated with such wounds. Conservative methods of achieving debridement may not be appropriate in such circumstances because the slower removal of necrotic tissue may potentiate the risk of localized infection and wound deterioration.

The location and size of the wound and the amount of devitalized tissue present all influence selection of debridement methods. Smaller areas of slough or necrotic tissue can be quickly and safely removed using interactive dressing products such as hydrogels, hydrocolloids, alginates, polysaccharide pastes or enzymatic preparations (*see* Chapter 6). However, surgical debridement remains the quickest method of removing large necrotic areas. Care needs to be taken to determine the extent and type of tissue present in the wound. The presence of tendon, muscle or bone necessitates specialist referral before the decision to debride further is taken. Surgical management may be necessary, although conservative treatment in some circumstances may be a more appropriate option. Conservative treatment generally involves the use of dressings capable of facilitating autolytic wound debridement while preventing dehydration of the exposed tissues. Autolysis describes the body's natural ability of breaking down and liquefying devitalized tissue which is enhanced by the use of moisture-retentive dressings. The maintenance of a moist wound surface helps to promote rehydration of slough and necrotic tissue, while allowing leucocytes and enzymes present in exudate to break down avascular tissue (Alvarez, op. cit.).

The amount of exudate produced by the wound is also an important consideration when deciding which method of debridement is most suitable. Wet, viscous slough in a wound can be difficult to remove surgically at the bedside when compared with the removal of a hard, dry eschar. The use of alginate dressings, in the management of highly exuding, sloughy wounds, is effective, because they are capable of both absorbing excess fluid and debriding moist slough. It should be noted that alginates are unsuitable for debriding hard, dry, necrotic tissue as they require moisture in order to be effective. Enzymatic preparations are another useful method of removing necrotic tissue as they are able to penetrate softer, devitalized tissue quickly. The use of hydrogels and hydro-colloids may not be such an appropriate method for debriding highly exuding wounds because of their restricted ability to absorb large amounts of fluid; these methods are better suited to debriding wounds that produce less exudate. The use of dressing products to debride wounds is discussed in greater detail in Chapter 6.

In addition to the clinical factors already discussed, there are other practical considerations to be taken into account when debriding a wound.

The availability of resources is often determined by the care environment. Access to members of the multidisciplinary team who possess the appropriate technical skills to enable them safely surgically to debride a wound are usually more limited in the community setting; in such instances, the use of more conservative debridement methods may be a more realistic alternative. However, the length of time taken to achieve debridement is an important variable when considering the overall cost-effectiveness of treatment.

The patient's wishes should at all times be taken into consideration when deciding how best to manage a sloughy or necrotic wound as co-operation with treatment obviously influences the final outcome (*see* Chapter 8).

Methods of debridement to be used with caution

The following methods should be used with caution:
- Wet-to-dry saline soaks.
- Antiseptic solutions and creams.

Wet-to-dry saline soaks

The use of wet-to-dry saline soaks to achieve wound debridement remains common practice in some clinical environments (Bryant, 1992). This method of achieving debridement uses saline-soaked gauze which dries out on the wound surface facilitating the mechanical removal of devitalized tissue at dressing change. This technique is usually painful for the patient and carries the additional risk of damaging healthy tissue on removal. Frequent dressing changes are usually required and in practice this technique can encourage the tight packing of wound cavities which compromises capillary blood flow, causing additional patient discomfort and prolonging wound closure.

Antiseptic solutions and creams

Since the introduction of topical antiseptics by Lister in the 1860s, a wide range of anti-microbial agents has been used in an attempt to prevent and treat wound infections. For many years it has been established practice to rely on the use of antiseptic agents for both the cleansing and debriding of wounds. During the past 25 years, much conflicting research has emerged regarding the effectiveness of antiseptics on open wounds.

Interpretation of findings is difficult, as sample sizes are often small, methodologies incomparable and many studies have been conducted using either animal models or *in vitro* and *in vivo* techniques. The significance of these results for human tissue and the implications for clinical practice are still unclear and are fiercely debated (Rodeheaver, 1988; Moore, 1992).

Once the wound becomes clinically infected bacteria can cause local inflammation, delay wound contraction, reduce wound-tensile strength and may be leucocytotoxic. Criteria for judging whether the wound is clinically infected are given in Chapter 3. When considering using antiseptics it is important to balance the potential cytotoxicity of the bacteria against the potential cytotoxicity of antiseptics. Problems associated with the use of hydrogen peroxide and sodium hypochlorites (e.g. Eusol), have meant that in recent years the continued use of antiseptics for the routine cleansing of wounds has been widely questioned by practitioners.

Table 5.1 summarizes experimental and practice-based evidence that collectively indicates the potential damage that antiseptics may have on healthy tissue. Currently, the literature reveals a lack of consensual findings but the evidence presented indicates that the use of these antiseptics for wound management should be confined to specific clinical indications and should always be discussed within the multidisciplinary team, so that all those responsible for either prescribing or using a particular antiseptic are aware of the consequences of their actions. In addition to facilitating best practice, proof that such a discussion has taken place may be important should the individual practitioner be required to defend his or her actions against an accusation of negligence (Moore, op. cit.).

This brief review of commonly used antiseptics demonstrates the hazards associated with their indiscriminate use. The hazards of some less frequently encountered antiseptic solutions such as silver nitrate, mercurochrome and potassium permanganate were noted by Morison (1990). The general disadvantages of antiseptics are listed in Box 5.2. If antiseptics are used, careful consideration should be taken to ensure that their beneficial effects are maximized and that side effects are limited. In most instances, the principle of allowing sufficient contact time between the antiseptic and the wound surface is ignored in clinical practice. These practical constraints challenge the validity of the continued use of antiseptics for the routine management of wounds.

If, after all other alternative treatment options have been considered and rejected, the use of an antiseptic is considered to be the only appropriate course of action for the management of a particular wound, the principles listed in Box 5.3 should be followed to minimize the likelihood of any unwanted effects.

Table 5.1.
Some antiseptic solutions commonly used in wound management:
actions and possible adverse effects

Antiseptic	Action	Adverse effects reported
Hypochlorite solutions (e.g. Eusol)	Effective against Gram-positive and negative bacteria, some spores and viruses	Cell toxicity Reduced capillary blood flow Toxicity to granulation tissue Prolonged inflammatory response Skin irritation, discomfort and pain Localized oedema (Moore, 1992)
Hydrogen peroxide	Mechanical cleansing action, reacts with catalase in wounds, releasing oxygen which removes some contaminants	Toxicity to fibroblasts (Linweaver *et al.* 1985) Irrigation into closed cavities can cause air emboli and surgical emphysema (Sleigh & Linter, 1985) Effects are short lived Causes pain on contact Irritates surrounding skin (Morgan, 1993)
Acetic acid	Effective against *Pseudomonas aeruginosa* in superficial wounds as a result of altering the pH of the wound	Efficacy is short lived, requiring twice daily dressings Can cause overgrowth of *Staphylococcus aureus* and *Proteus spp.* (Sloss *et al.* 1993) Causes severe stinging on contact with wound (Morgan, 1993)
Povidone iodine	Has the broadest spectrum of any antiseptic	Extensive reviews suggest use should be avoided in larger, open wounds because of the delay in wound healing and iodine toxicity May increase infection rates in contaminated wounds (Rodeheaver, 1988).
Cetrimide	Broad-spectrum antiseptic	Marked fibroblast toxicity (Morgan, 1993) Can cause skin sensitivities Less effective against *Pseudomonas spp.*

Box 5.2.

Some disadvantages of antiseptics in general

Clinical disadvantages:
- Most are rapidly de-activated by the presence of organic material within wounds such as pus, slough, necrotic tissue (Rodeheaver, 1988; Morgan, 1993)
- Antiseptics do not penetrate into tissue or exudate (Rodeheaver, 1988)
- At low concentrations antiseptics only act as an irrigant solution, at high concentrations they can reduce bacterial counts, but can damage tissues (Thomas, 1990)
- Antiseptics require sufficient contact-time to be effective (Zamora, 1986)
- Many studies question the cytotoxicity of commonly available antiseptics (Linweaver et al. 1985; Rodeheaver, 1988)
- Bacteria are becoming increasingly resistant to antiseptics (Russel, 1986)
- Some antiseptics are known to cause allergic contact dermatitis (Bajaja & Gupta, 1986)
- Use of certain antiseptics, such as the hypochlorites, raises issues relating to professional accountability
- There are other more effective cleansing agents available today

Practical disadvantages:
- Chemical instability, resulting in a limited shelf-life
- Use can be associated with leakage and skin maceration
- Leakage may stain the patient's skin, clothes and bedding
- Effective use of antiseptics requires frequent dressing changes
- Use of antiseptics makes dressing changes more time consuming.
- Use of antiseptics can increase patient pain and discomfort
- They are not cost-effective when additional resources are considered

Box 5.3.

Some principles for minimizing unwanted effects when using antiseptics

- Cognizance should be taken of the contra-indications, precautions and warnings relating to each antiseptic considered for use, on an individual case-by-case basis
- Careful consideration should be given to the appropriateness of the antiseptic selected, in relation to local problems at the wound site, including the nature of pathogens, when the wound is clinically infected (see Chapter 3)
- Antiseptics should only be used for limited periods of time (usually no more than 3–5 days) and their use should be reviewed at regular intervals
- After cleansing with an antiseptic, the wound area should be liberally flushed with saline to minimize potential cell toxicity
- Antiseptics should not be used once the wound bed is clean and granulating

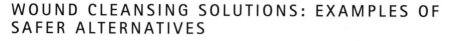
WOUND CLEANSING SOLUTIONS: EXAMPLES OF SAFER ALTERNATIVES

The characteristics of an ideal wound-cleansing solution can be summarized as:
- Non-toxic to human tissues.
- Remains effective in the presence of organic material, for example, blood, slough, necrotic tissue.
- Able to reduce the number of micro-organisms.
- Does not cause sensitivity reactions.
- Is widely available.
- Is cost-effective.
- Is stable and has a long shelf life.

An isotonic saline solution

For wounds that are not grossly contaminated, an isotonic 0.9% saline solution, applied at room temperature, is currently the cleansing agent of choice. There are no reports of any adverse effects on healing tissue, it is easy to use, inexpensive, widely available and as such fulfils the requirements of an ideal cleansing solution.

Water

For similar reasons, the use of tap water for wound cleansing is becoming an acceptable alternative for the cleansing of both acute traumatic soft-tissue wounds (Angeras & Brandbard, 1992) and chronic wounds such as leg ulcers (Cullum, 1994). Water has been used for centuries by all civilizations without any reported detrimental effects and has always been used in first-aid situations to cleanse wounds. Any fears concerning bacterial contamination of non-sterile water supplies and subsequent effects on wounds appear to be unfounded so long as the water comes from a properly treated supply. Microbiologists recommended the running of tap water for a few minutes before wound cleansing to flush out any potentially high levels of bacteria. However, bacterial cultures grown from wounds cleansed with tap water were never detected in the source of tap water used to cleanse the wound (Angeras & Brandbard, op. cit.). Immersion of ulcerated legs in water can also be used to moisturize the surrounding skin and to prevent dryness. Emollients can be added to lukewarm water. For many patients this practice is particularly soothing and can improve morale. Open wounds should, however, only be soaked in water for a short period of time as water is hypotonic and causes cells within the tissues to swell and eventually rupture because of the effect of osmotic pressure.

The continuing trend of early postoperative discharge and the increased use of day-surgery units inevitably means that patients can be back in their own homes within hours of surgery. The management of patients' wounds within their home environment has to be more appropriate to the philosophy of self-care and should make use of readily available resources such as tap water or normal saline.

TEMPERATURE OF CLEANSING SOLUTIONS

The temperature of a wound directly affects the rate of healing. Lock (1979) demonstrated that phagocytic and mitotic cellular activity are significantly decreased at temperatures below 28°C. The application of cool cleansing solutions can theoretically have similar local effects. It can take as long as 40 minutes for a wound to regain its original temperature after cleansing and up to 3 hours for mitotic division and leucocytic activity to return to normal (Myers, 1982). Theoretically, cleansing solutions should therefore be stored at room temperature or warmed, if cold, by immersing sachets in warm water.

BIOSURGERY

In recent years, sterile fly larvae have been used successfully in the debridement of wounds. Thomas *et al.* (1996) reviewed the literature on the use of maggots, especially in battle wounds. They reported that maggots were used in both the American Civil War and in World War I on grossly infected and contaminated wounds. Through the 1930s and 1940s maggots were successfully used to treat patients with osteomyelitis, abscesses, burns and fungating carcinomas. Thomas *et al.* (op. cit.) has successfully bred sterile larvae which can be placed directly on to the wound bed with an occlusive dressing protecting the skin surrounding the wound. A fine nylon mesh holds the maggots in place and an absorbent pad is applied to absorb exudate and liquified devitalized tissue; the maggots can remain active for 3 days.

Morgan (1995) suggested advantages of maggot therapy:
- They usually consume only necrotic tissue, slough and bacteria.
- They can be used topically.
- They are not reliant on a good peripheral blood supply.

Morgan cites the disadvantages of maggot therapy as:
- Aesthetic (social disapproval, disgust, revulsion and alarm, although their use in practice may be more offensive in the minds of healthcare professionals than in patients, who appreciate the attainment of a clean wound bed).
- Local pruritus may accompany their use.
- The requirement for sterile maggots, which may not be readily available.
- Problems where there is excess exudate, resulting in the maggots drowning or going elsewhere because of oxygen deficiency if the dressing becomes detached.

Thomas *et al.* (op. cit.) also suggest that some caution is needed with maggot therapy:
- Larvae produce very powerful enzymes that can damage or irritate healthy tissues if too many larvae are used or are left in place for too long.
- Where exposed blood vessels are present, large numbers of larvae should not be used.

SUMMARY

There are many undesirable consequences of wound cleansing. Removal of exudate may reduce the healing potential of the wound because exudate has bactericidal properties that help to cleanse the wound naturally during the inflammatory stage of healing. In practice, newly formed epithelial cells are difficult to distinguish from slough and fibrous tissue and are often removed accidentally in an attempt to cleanse the wound bed when the wound is roughly handled. Small areas of slough are not thought to impair wound healing significantly and can be safely ignored. The application of cold cleansing lotions can significantly impair the rate of healing by slowing down the rate at which mitotic cellular division occurs. This effect will be exacerbated if dressing changes are performed frequently and the wound is routinely cleansed on each occasion. The application of many cleansing solutions such as antiseptics may have undesirable side effects making their continued use questionable. Various cleansing techniques such as swabbing and the use of high-pressure irrigation can cause additional mechanical trauma to the delicate tissues within the wound.

For these reasons, it is not usually necessary to cleanse a patient's wound at every dressing change. The decision to cleanse a wound should be carefully considered after a detailed assessment of the patient's circumstances and the condition of the wound has been made. There are some valid justifications for wound cleansing. If after careful consideration the decision to cleanse is made, thought should then be given to the most appropriate method of achieving this and, as a matter of principle, the cleansing solution with the least toxic effects should be selected.

SELF-ASSESSMENT QUESTIONS AND ACTIVITIES

(a) *List all of the wound-cleansing agents that are currently used in your clinical setting. Describe the indications for their use, together with their advantages and disadvantages.*

(b) *Name a cleansing solution that you are sometimes asked to use in your own clinical area that research suggests is ineffective or hazardous. Summarize the arguments that you would put forward to other members of the multi-disciplinary team to support the discontinuation of this solution.*

(c) *Describe which methods of debridement you would consider to be appropriate to manage the following wounds:*

1. *A small, hard, dry, black necrotic pressure sore on a patient's heel (Figure 5.2)*

2. *An extensive, highly exuding, venous leg ulcer (Figure 5.3)*

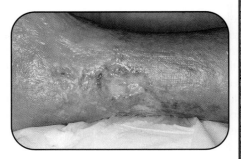

Figure 5.3

3. *A deep traumatic wound to the thigh caused by a road traffic accident (Figure 5.4.)*

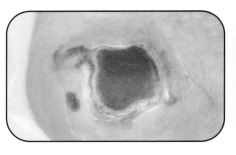

Figure 5.2

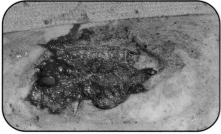

Figure 5.4 (Reproduced courtesy of Peter D Asmussen, Beiersdorf Medical, Hamburg.)

REFERENCES

Alvarez O. Moist environment for healing: matching the dressing to the wound. *Ostomy/Wound Management* 1988,:64–83.

Angeras AD, Brandbard A: Comparison between sterile saline and tap water for the cleansing of acute traumatic soft tissue wounds. *Eur J Surg* 1992, **158**(33):347–350.

Bajaja AK, Gupta SC. Contact hypersensitivity to topical antibacterial agents. *Int J Dermatol* 1986, **25**:103–105.

Bryant RA. *Acute and chronic wounds.* St Louis, Mosby Year Book; 1992.

Chisholm C. Wound evaluation and cleansing. *Emerg Clin North Am* 1992, **10**(4):665–672.

Chrinz H, Vibits H, Cordtz T *et al.* Need for surgical wound dressing. *Br J Surg* 1989, **76**(2):204–205.

Cullum N. *The nursing management of leg ulcers in the community: a critical review of the research.* London: HMSO; 1994.

Ferguson A. A systematic approach to trauma relief. The management of the A&E wound. *Prof Nurse* 1990, **6**(2):82–90.

Hohn D, Ponce B, Burton R, Hunt T. Antimicrobial systems of the surgical wound. *Am J Surg* 1977, **133**(5):597–600.

Lawrence JC. Wound infection. *J Wound Care* 1993, **2**(5):277–280.

Lawrence JC, Lilly HA. A novel presentation of saline for wound irrigation. *J Wound Care* 1994, **3**(7):334–337.

Linweaver W *et al.* Topical antimicrobial toxicity. *Arch Surg* 1985, **120**:267–271.

Lock P. *The effects of temperature on mitotic activity at the edge of experimental wounds.* Kent: Lock Laboratories; 1979.

Marquez RR. Wound debridement and hydrotherapy in wound management. In: Gogia PP, ed. *Clinical wound management.* Thorofare, NJ: Slack Inc; 1995.

Mills K, Morton R, Page G: *A colour atlas of accidents and emergencies.* London: Wolfe Medical Publication; 1984.

Moore D. Hypochlorites: a review of the evidence. *J Wound Care* 1992, **1**(4):44–52.

Morgan D. Is there still a role for antiseptics? *J Tissue Viability* 1993, **3**(3):80–84.

Morgan D. Myiasis: the rise and fall of maggot therapy. *J Tissue Viability* 1995, **5**(2):43–51.

Morison M. Wound cleansing: which solution? *Nursing Standard* 1990, **4**(52)(Supplement):4–6.

Morison M, Moffatt C. *A colour guide to the assessment and management of leg ulcers.* London: Mosby; 1994.

Myers J. Modern plastic surgical dressings. *Health Soc Serv J* 1982, 336–337.

Rodeheaver G. Identification of the wound infection potentiating factors in soil. *Am J Surg* 1974, **128**:8.

Rodeheaver G. Controversies in topical wound management. *Ostomy/Wound Management* 1988, **18**:58–68.

Russel AD. Bacterial resistance to antiseptics and disinfectants. *J Hosp Infect* 1986, **7**(21):213–225.

Sleigh JW, Linter SPK. Hazards of hydrogen peroxide. *BMJ* 1985, **291**:1706.

Sloss JM, Cumberland N, Milner SM. Acetic acid used for the elimination of *Pseudomonas aeruginosa* from burn and soft tissue wounds. *J Roy Army Med Corps* 1993, **139**:49–51.

Surgical Materials Testing Laboratory. *The Dressing Times, Surgical Materials Testing Laboratory Leaflet.* 1992, **5**(2):3.

Thomas S. *Wound management and dressings.* London: The Pharmaceutical Press; 1990.

Thomas S. Wound cleansing agents. *J Wound Care* 1994, **3**(7):325–328.

Thomas S, Jones M, Shulter S, Jones S. Using larvae in modern wound management. *J Wound Care* 1996, **5**(2):60–69.

Thomlinson D. To clean or not to clean? *Nursing Times* 1987, **83**(9):71–74.

Wood RAB. Disintegration of cellulose dressings in open granulating wounds. *BMJ* 1976, **1**:1444–1445.

Zamora J. Chemical and microbiological characteristics and toxicity of povidone-iodine solutions. *Am J Surg* 1986, **117**:181–186.

FURTHER READING

Goldenheim PD. An appraisal of povidone-iodine and wound healing. *Postgrad Med J* 1993, 69(Suppl. 3):97–105.

Morgan DA. *Formulary of wound management products – a guide for health care staff,* 6th ed. Haslemere: Euromed Publications; 1994.

Chapter 6

Wound Dressings

This chapter is concerned with priorities in the local management of open wounds such as leg ulcers, pressure sores and fungating wounds. Local wound management should only be considered once a full patient assessment has been undertaken. A comprehensive overview of three levels of patient assessment can be found in Chapter 4. More specific issues relating to the management of pressure sores, leg ulcers and other chronic wounds are considered in Chapters 9–11.

PRIORITIES IN LOCAL WOUND MANAGEMENT

The aim of local wound management is to provide the optimum environment for the natural healing processes to take place.

The cellular events involved in wound healing and their implications for practice are summarized in Chapter 1. An understanding of the physiological processes involved is a prerequisite to a true understanding of the principles of local wound management.

Priorities in local wound management are essentially the same, whatever the wound:

- Controlling bleeding (haemostasis).
- Removing foreign bodies which could act as foci for infection.
- Removing devitalized tissue, thick slough and pus.
- Providing optimum temperature, humidity and pH for the cells involved in the healing processes.
- Promoting the formation of granulation tissue and epithelialization.
- Protecting the wound from further trauma and from the entry of pathogenic micro-organisms.

The aims are to protect the individual from further physiological damage, to remove actual and potential causes of delayed healing whenever possible and to create an optimum local environment for vascular and connective tissue reconstruction and epithelialization. This is usually facilitated by covering an open wound with an appropriate dressing.

THE IDEAL DRESSING MATERIAL

When skin is damaged, a dressing material is usually used as a substitute to fulfil the functions of unbroken skin, as outlined in Chapter 7 and summarized in Table 7.1. A dressing can prevent contamination of the area by potentially pathogenic organisms and can protect the underlying tissues from further damage. Pharmacists have evaluated the physical properties of dressing materials and described the theoretical functions that an ideal material might provide, as summarized in Boxes 6.1 and 6.2. A synthesis of the characteristics of the ideal wound dressing is given in Box 6.3.

THE PROBLEM OF DRESSING SELECTION

A wide variety of wound-contact materials are currently available and provide a range of physical properties. One area in which many healthcare professionals experience difficulty is in choosing the most appropriate product to best meet the needs of their patients. As yet, no one material is suitable for all wound situations. The aim is to select

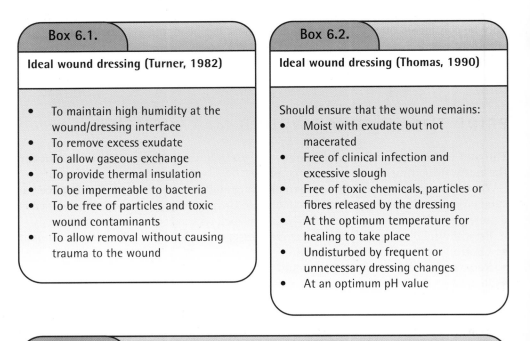

Box 6.1.

Ideal wound dressing (Turner, 1982)

- To maintain high humidity at the wound/dressing interface
- To remove excess exudate
- To allow gaseous exchange
- To provide thermal insulation
- To be impermeable to bacteria
- To be free of particles and toxic wound contaminants
- To allow removal without causing trauma to the wound

Box 6.2.

Ideal wound dressing (Thomas, 1990)

Should ensure that the wound remains:
- Moist with exudate but not macerated
- Free of clinical infection and excessive slough
- Free of toxic chemicals, particles or fibres released by the dressing
- At the optimum temperature for healing to take place
- Undisturbed by frequent or unnecessary dressing changes
- At an optimum pH value

Box 6.3.

Characteristics of the ideal wound dressing: a synthesis

- Non-adherent
- Impermeable to bacteria
- Capable of maintaining a high humidity at the wound site while removing excess exudate
- Thermally insulating
- Non-toxic and non-allergenic
- Comfortable and conformable
- Capable of protecting the wound from further trauma
- Requires infrequent dressing changes
- Cost-effective
- Long shelf-life
- Available both in hospital and the community

a wound-dressing material that is most suited to the individual's needs. This requires assessment not only of the local conditions at the wound site but also assessment of the patient's lifestyle and where and by whom the wound will be managed. Choosing a dressing requires detailed knowledge of the characteristics, uses, contra-indications and precautions for the wide range of dressing materials available, if the most appropriate dressing is to be selected. The problem of choice is complicated by several factors:

- Products that look alike and are grouped together by a broad generic term may have significantly different physical and chemical properties.
- Manufacturers may recommend different types of product for tackling the same clinical problem, for example, hydrocolloid dressings, hydrogels and enzymatic agents are all recommended as effective debriding agents, yet their relative effectiveness in specific clinical situations is not always known.
- The effect of therapeutic traditions, strongly held by practitioners in positions of influence, can make it difficult for others caring for patients, in the same domain, to use new products.
- There is often blurring of responsibility and accountability for wound management between nursing, medical and paramedical staff.
- The economics of wound management are complex. Many modern dressings have a high unit cost but require infrequent dressing changes. They can therefore be more cost-effective and convenient for the patient than traditional dressings when the total costs are balanced against the benefits. A number of recent clinical trials incorporated an evaluation of cost-effectiveness within the study design.
- New products and reformulations of existing products are coming on to the market all the time.

Developing a wound-management policy

There is an increasingly popular trend among health authorities in the UK towards quality assurance in wound management through implementing wound-management policies. This has been undertaken in an attempt to overcome some of the problems, outlined above, of dressing selection. Ways of developing a policy are described by Morgan (1990a,b). This is usually undertaken by the local Drugs and Therapeutics Committee, who may set up a working party to advise them. The working party should consist of representatives from all members of the healthcare team who have a responsibility for wound management.

The working party may be charged with drawing up a list of products to be routinely stocked by pharmacies, monitoring product use and developing a continuing education programme to keep all those involved in prescribing up-to-date with new products and the latest research findings. Thomas (1990, 1994a) reviewed the main categories of wound dressings and their uses. These books are useful for reference when drawing up a policy.

The responsibility of individual prescribers

Whether or not a hospital or unit has a list of recommended wound-care products and guidance on their use, the individual prescriber still has the final responsibility when it comes to selecting a dressing.

Before using any wound-care product for the first time, ALWAYS consult the manufacturer's recommendations, contra-indications, precautions and warnings.

As this information can change it is worth re-reading the manufacturer's instructions at frequent intervals. If there is still any doubt about the suitability of a dressing product it is prudent to refrain from using it until the advice of the pharmacist or the manufacturer has been obtained.

In the UK, there is a difference between availability of dressing materials depending on whether the patient is receiving care in hospital or in the community. Hospital trusts can choose from a wide range of products. Patients being cared for in the community are generally restricted by the products available on the drug tariff. The dressing materials listed on the drug tariff continue to increase but even when a dressing is available the range of sizes may be restricted, causing problems for community patients with large or extensive wounds.

CREATING THE OPTIMUM LOCAL ENVIRONMENT FOR HEALING

A number of factors need to be considered in creating the optimum environment for healing. Wounds of all aetiologies may exhibit a number of different physical characteristics throughout the healing phase. Several of the most frequently encountered and difficult situations are explained in this section.

Achieving haemostasis

Controlling bleeding is the first priority in wound management but, outside the Accident and Emergency Department (A&E) or the GPs treatment room, this is rarely a problem encountered by healthcare professionals. Direct pressure and elevation of the affected part is often all that is required to arrest bleeding in the short term. Further management of wounds involving major blood loss is a medical responsibility. Overt arterial haemorrhage requires very urgent management that is second only in importance to the maintenance of the airway in a severely injured casualty. Further discussion of the management of major haemorrhage in traumatic wounds is outside the scope of this book.

This chapter is concerned with more unusual situations in which bleeding can occur in open wounds. Although a haemostatic primary wound dressing is useful to arrest minor bleeding, in these situations it is always important to determine the cause of the bleeding and to treat this also, as the following examples illustrate:

1. When granulation tissue becomes infected. Treatment may require the use of systemic antibiotics and/or local, medicated dressings (*see* Chapter 3).
2. When excessive granulation tissue is present. In order to encourage epithelialization this tissue may need to be cauterized with silver nitrate or have a compression dressing applied or be treated with a steroid cream.

3. In a newly created open surgical wound where blood vessels have not been properly cauterized. Depending on the severity of the bleeding the vessel may need to be cauterized in theatre or it may be possible to use a suture or silver nitrate at the bedside. After this an alginate dressing should assist haemostasis.

4. Malignant fungating tumours may contain areas of fragile tissue that bleed spontaneously. Although all patients with fungating tumours may experience this problem it is particularly commonly encountered in patients with fungating carcinoma of the breast. An alginate dressing may prove useful (Bale, 1994). Further discussion of the complex issues associated with the management of fungating wounds is to be found in Chapter 11.

Removal of foreign bodies

Foreign bodies can act as a focus for infection in a range of wound situations. They include skin sutures and wound drains. Other situations in which foreign bodies can cause problems include:

1. Suture material discovered at the base of a surgical-cavity wound. The loose suture material can be trimmed off flush with the wound bed. Granulation tissue will form around it. No attempt should be made to pull the suture out of the wound as it may be attached to deeper structures. A surgeon's opinion should be sought.

2. Old dressing material (including dressing fibres) found on the surface of a superficial wound or deep within a cavity wound when cleansing has not been adequate. This can act as a focus for infection, especially where fresh dressings are applied on top. Thorough wound cleansing or irrigation is needed to remove this debris (*see* Chapter 5).

3. Retained foreign bodies such as splinters of wood, metal or glass. These may only be visible on X-ray and may need to be surgically removed. This can often be achieved using a local anaesthetic. The problem is particularly significant for diabetic patients, with peripheral neuropathy, who may be unaware of the presence of the foreign body. The potentially catastrophic consequences of deep-seated infection developing are discussed in Chapter 10.

Removing dead and devitalized tissue

The presence of slough and necrotic tissue in a wound will delay or in some situations prevent healing (Dealey, 1994). By virtue of being non-viable, devitalized tissue can harbour and encourage the growth of bacteria, so promoting infection. Although any wound deprived of a blood supply will become necrotic, pressure sores are the most commonly encountered wound type to exhibit sloughy and necrotic tissue (Thomas & Fear, 1993). In this situation, the presence of devitalized tissue within a pressure sore often masks the true extent of the tissue that has been damaged.

There are several methods of achieving debridement of devitalized tissue as summarized in Table 6.1 and described in Chapter 5. The removal of dehydrated, hard, devitalized tissue is particularly challenging. Rehydration of the eschar should be attempted as a matter of priority. This can best be achieved by the use of either an amorphous hydrogel or a hydrocolloid dressing (Dealey, op. cit.). Within 5–7 days, some degree of rehydration should be expected provided the devitalized area is kept occluded. Sharp debridement may be undertaken at this stage if appropriate.

Managing local wound infection

Until healing is complete, all wounds are at risk of becoming infected. Once infected the normal wound-healing process is impaired and healing is usually delayed or on occasions prevented.

The problem of managing local wound infection is most commonly associated with patients with chronic wounds. As most chronic wounds are heavily colonized by bacteria it can be difficult to differentiate between infection which causes delayed healing and colonization which does not. The criteria to use when diagnosing wound infection are discussed in Chapter 3. It is recommended that diagnosis of infection be based on the full clinical picture rather than on the presence and numbers of organisms alone (Cooper & Lawrence, 1996).

Table 6.1.
Methods of achieving wound debridement

Method	Advantages	Disadvantages
Sharp debridement	Rapid, effective, may need no anaesthetic	Requires skill and knowledge; may need a general anaesthetic
Modern dressing materials	Gentle, easy to use, non-traumatic, readily available	Requires some skill to achieve success especially in maintaining a very moist environment
Enzymatic agents	May be effective	Expensive, requires skill to apply, little scientific support
Chemical agents	Readily available in some areas	May damage tissues and surrounding skin, not always effective
Biosurgery (maggots, larval therapy)	Research to date demonstrates efficacy	May not be aesthetically acceptable to all patients. A relatively new technology which is undergoing further evaluation
Hydrotherapy/high pressure wound irrigation	Non-invasive, can be used in between dressing changes with modern dressing materials. Portable systems allow use at the bedside if necessary	Both methods require specialist equipment, only widely available in USA

Deciding on therapy

Some factors to consider are summarized in Figure 6.1. In some circumstances systemic antibiotics may be prescribed, for example if the patient has a spreading infection, cellulitis, a life-threatening infection or is severely immunocompromised. Microbiological swab results are best used for identifying the antibiotic sensitivity of organisms before antibiotic therapy is prescribed where this is indicated.

When infection is localized, the use of topical antimicrobial agents may be appropriate. Dressings containing iodine and silver have a broad spectrum of activity. There is much debate surrounding the use of topical antiseptics in wound management. Experimental studies using animal models and tissue cultures have shown a range of antiseptic solutions to be toxic to healthy cells (Thomas, 1994a), although there is, as yet, no firm evidence to support these findings in the human chronic wound. In clean, healthy, healing chronic wounds the use of antiseptic preparations is best avoided (*see* Chapter 5). However, in the chronic wound, where local infection is difficult to treat systemically because of the poor penetration of antibiotics in the peripheral tissues, topical antiseptics can play an important role in management. Gross fungal infection of open wounds is unusual in the UK, except in very debilitated patients.

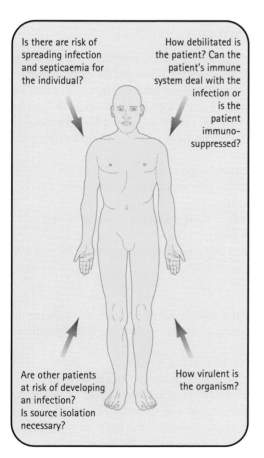

Figure 6.1 Deciding on therapy.

Is there are risk of spreading infection and septicaemia for the individual?

How debilitated is the patient? Can the patient's immune system deal with the infection or is the patient immuno-suppressed?

Are other patients at risk of developing an infection? Is source isolation necessary?

How virulent is the organism?

Coping with malodorous wounds

The presence of a malodorous wound can be very distressing for patients, leading to self-imposed social isolation, loss of appetite and depression. The best method of managing odour is to identify and treat the cause of the odour, rather than trying to mask it with odour-absorbing dressings. For patients in which anaerobic bacteria are causing malodour, topical metronidazole gel can be prescribed. Deep pressure sores containing necrotic, devitalized tissue and those with malignant fungating wounds are examples of such situations. Systemic treatment with metronidazole is very effective. When patients are unable to take oral antibiotics, suppositories may be better tolerated. In the interim, while waiting for the source of the infection to be treated, an activated charcoal dressing with silver can be an effective deodorizer, the silver in the dressing being bacteriostatic. When wounds are also exuding, an absorbent foam dressing with a charcoal backing may be used.

In addition to these measures, other simple remedies should not be forgotten:
1. Nursing the patient in a single room with the window open allowing fresh air to circulate.
2. Changing the dressing as frequently as needed.
3. Changing bed linen and clothing as soon as it becomes soiled by leaking exudate.

Coping with heavily exuding wounds

In any situation in which high levels of exudate are encountered, it is important to assess whether any underlying pathology, such as oedema related to congestive cardiac disease or hepatic impairment, is present and, where possible, to correct this, in conjunction with the management of the exudate at the wound site. High levels of exudate can be associated with extensive pressure sores, large surgical cavity wounds, infected extensive leg ulceration, burns and skin graft donor sites. When heavy exudate is not effectively controlled several problems are likely to occur:
1. The exudate may leak from around the dressing edge causing soiling of the patient's clothing and bedclothes, furniture, carpets and so on. This can be uncomfortable and distressing for the patient.
2. The margins of the wound and the surrounding tissues may be macerated and inflamed, leading to tissue breakdown and pain.
3. The wound itself may harbour an excessively high number of bacteria which could lead to wound infection.
4. Malodour may be a problem.

As the wound makes progress towards healing and reduces in size, the volume of exudate produced is likely to reduce but while high levels of exudate are being produced the following points should be considered:
1. Choose an appropriate dressing material for the level of exudate.
2. Use dressings that are large enough to fill the wound or cover the area. When several dressings are required to fill a large cavity consideration should be given as to how these will be retrieved. A retained dressing in a deep wound can lead to abscess formation and infection. Special arrangements with the hospital pharmacy may have to be negotiated to obtain the correct dressings for the patient when

patients are likely to be transferred from hospital into the community. When care is being given in the community, the full size range may not be generally available. Liaison with the hospital pharmacy or the community budget holder may be necessary to obtain the resources required.

3. Protect the skin surrounding the wound. This may be achieved by using a barrier cream or a proprietary skin preparation containing silicone.

4. Consider carefully the most appropriate secondary dressing to use. Layers of absorbent gauze and absorbent dressing pads prolong the life of the primary wound-contact layer. As these are relatively cheap, several layers can be used but they are bulky and may not be cosmetically acceptable to the patient in all situations. If secondary dressings are left in place for too long, they can also cause maceration and excoriation of the skin surrounding the wound.

5. Consider how the dressing is to be held in place. For limbs a light cotton, conformable bandage can effectively hold dressings in place without the need for surgical tape which may damage the skin. Semipermeable films can protect the dressings from contamination, for example, on the sacrum of an incontinent patient.

6. Change the dressing as frequently as required to prevent strike-through of exudate.

Managing heavily exuding wounds in difficult sites is frequently challenging and may require a multidisciplinary approach to providing the optimal care for the patient when the wound is associated with an underlying more general pathology.

USING DRESSING MATERIALS

This section describes some of the most frequently used dressings in the UK, their physical properties and the circumstances in which they are particularly useful. It is not intended to be a fully comprehensive list of all the dressing materials currently available, in all presentations.

Alginates

Since the 1880s when alginates were first described by a British chemist, these materials have been used for a wide variety of commercial uses, mainly as thickening and stabilizing agents for food products. Mixtures of alginates were used as styptics and haemostats in the late 1940s (Thomas, 1994a). Currently, alginate dressing materials are available in the UK in a number of presentations:

Sorbsan
This consists of pure calcium alginate and is available in a variety of forms ranging from small flat sheets to large sheets, packing rope and a thinner ribbon with flat sheets of varying absorptive capacities.

Kaltostat
This consists of a mixture of sodium and calcium salts of alginic acid in a ratio of 20:80 (Thomas, 1994a). This product also has a range of presentations, again ranging from small flat sheets to large sheets, packing and flat sheets with a range of absorptive capacities.

Tegagel

This consists of pure calcium alginate and here the fibres of the dressing are formed into an aperture fabric.

Alginates are extremely versatile and have, to a large extent, replaced gauze products in the management of a wide range of wound types. Alginates can be used dry to absorb wound exudate in conjunction with absorbent secondary dressings to increase their wear time. Alginate packing can be used to fill cavities and pack sinuses and can be gently irrigated from the wound surface without causing trauma to the healing tissues. For narrow cavities and sinuses the end of the alginate rope can be dipped into normal saline solution to assist packing the tract. The haemostatic Kaltostat can be used to help achieve haemostasis immediately postoperatively and also on fungating, eroding wounds where bleeding is a problem. In dry wound situations, the alginate dressings can be moistened with normal saline and used, in conjunction with a semipermeable film, to retain moisture at the wound bed.

Alginate dressings are useful in a wide range of wounds and their uses continue to be developed. Collagen has been added to an alginate dressing (Fibracol) and further developments are to be expected.

Foams

The foam range of dressing products is another versatile group, with absorbency and conformability being two of their particular properties. Variations in the manufacture of the foam alters the absorbency of the product, hence the diversity of products described.

Allevyn

This is a flat sheet dressing that consists of three layers. The wound-contact layer is a low-adherent aperture polyurethane net, with a hydrophilic polyurethane centre and a backing of moisture/vapour-permeable membrane. The adhesive version of this product needs no tape to hold it in place. This is an extremely absorbent dressing, capable of absorbing and retaining large amounts of exudate (Thomas, 1993).

Allevyn cavity wound dressing

This is an adaptation of Allevyn designed for the management of heavily exuding cavity wounds. Available in a range of shapes and sizes, this dressing consists of small chips of hydrophilic polyurethane foam surrounded by a membrane of perforated polyeretic film. One of several dressings can be used gently to pack the cavity. They can be held in place by a combination of absorbent padding and, depending on the level of exudate, with surgical tape or semipermeable film. For very heavily exuding cavities this dressing is invaluable.

CaviCare

CaviCare is a completely new formulation based on the original Silastic foam dressing.

An equal amount of base and catalyst are dispensed from two sachets. After being mixed together for 2 minutes the liquid is poured into the cavity wound where it quickly sets to form a soft, spongy stent, or mould, of the wound and its shape. This is a reusable dressing which should be removed twice daily for disinfection with 0.5% chlorhexidine.

After soaking in the antiseptic for 10 minutes all the disinfectant should be carefully rinsed from the dressing before removing excess water and replacing in the wound. Patients and their relatives find this an acceptable method of treating their healing wounds, especially when the patient wishes to return to normal activity and take responsibility for the care of their own wound without the help of a healthcare professional visiting on a daily basis. As the cavity wound heals a new foam stent will need to be made on average once a week. On a cautionary note, this dressing should not be used in narrow cavities or sinuses or where the wound undermines the skin and would prevent the dressing being easily removed. However, for cavities of even contour this is an extremely comfortable, conformable product which encourages patients to participate in their wound care.

Lyofoam
Lyofoam consists of a flat sheet of polyurethane foam that has been heat sealed on one side to form an absorbent surface. Lyofoam is freely permeable to gases and water vapour, allowing fluid to evaporate through the back of the dressing (Thomas, 1993). It is recommended for use on lightly to moderately exuding wounds of a variety of aetiologies, it is soft and conformable and can be held in place by surgical tapes or semi-permeable film.

Lyofoam C
This is used on malodorous wounds to absorb offensive exudate into the middle of the dressing. Lyofoam C consists of a layer of non-woven fabric that has been impregnated with activated carbon granules. This centre layer is sealed between a piece of Lyofoam and a backing layer (Thomas, 1993).

Lyofoam E
Lyofoam E is a polyurethane foam sheet which consists of a modified hydrophobic foam sheet with a wound-contact surface that is of low adherence and hydrophilic. The middle portion consists of a hydrophilic foam that absorbs and retains exudate and a foam backing that is moisture/vapour permeable. This product is designed to cope with moderate to heavily exuding flat wounds and can be held in place using either bandages or surgical tape, depending on the wound site.

Tielle
This is a hydropolymer dressing with four layers. The adhesive layer is attached to a waterproof, semipermeable backing. The central island of the dressing consists of an absorbent polyurethane foam with a non-woven absorbent layer. This multilayer dressing is very soft, comfortable and conformable and moulds easily to skin contours.

Spirosorb
Spirosorb is a polyurethane foam sheet that has been coated with a hydrophilic adhesive and has a backing of polyurethane film. It is soft and conformable and is recommended for lightly to moderately exuding flat wounds.

Hydrocolloids

This group of dressings was introduced in the 1980s after the great success of this material in the management of stomas. Although all the hydrocolloids vary in respect of their individual make-up, usually they consist of a semipermeable film coated with an absorbent mass of sodium carboxymethylcellulose in conjunction with a variety of other gel-forming agents, elastomers and adhesives (Thomas, 1992).

In sheet form, these materials are self-adhesive and conform to the periwound area providing an occlusive or semi-occlusive environment and are suitable for a wide range of wound aetiologies including burns, leg ulceration, pressure sores and traumatic injuries. The hydrocolloid material absorbs wound exudate and gels. Providing that a good margin around the wound edge has been left (approximately 5 cm) these dressings can stay in place for up to 7 days, depending on the rate of exudate production and absorptive capacity of the individual dressing. Before the dressing reaches its maximum absorption of exudate it should be changed, to avoid leakage of the gel. When the wound bed is sloughy or necrotic, hydrocolloid dressings provide occlusion and facilitate autolysis of the devitalized tissue from the wound bed.

Hydrogels

Amorphous hydrogels contain large amounts of water (80% or more) combined with a range of other materials, that is, hydrocolloid materials, alginate materials and starch-based polymers. The main application in which amorphous hydrogels have excelled is in the removal of sloughy and necrotic tissue from the wound bed of chronic wounds, especially pressure sores (Thomas, 1993). Although the precise action of these materials is not fully understood, they are thought to be effective because of their provision of a moist environment to the devitalized tissue. This encourages or facilitates autolysis of the devitalized tissue from the healthy wound bed. This action is faster and more effective when the wound is occluded by the use of a semipermeable film. For many practitioners the use of such gels has replaced traditional agents such as hypochlorites and enzymatic agents. The judicious use of surgical debridement using scissors or a scalpel to trim off loose devitalized tissue can further speed up the debridement process. Intrasite gel, Sterigel, Nugel and Granugel are all products in this group.

Low-adherent dressings

There are a wide range of products that belong in this category of dressing; only a few of the more commonly used products will be discussed. These dressings fall into the lower end of the price range and provide a relatively inexpensive wound-contact layer. They can be used alone for wounds producing little wound exudate or in combination with other products for specific purposes, as indicated by the manufacturer.

Tulles
Tulles were developed in the First World War by Lumiere (Thomas, 1994a,b) and consist of an open-weave cloth soaked in soft paraffin. Other agents have been incorporated into the paraffin, including antiseptics and antibiotics. When used in sufficient quantities and changed frequently they are unlikely to become stuck onto the wound bed and are useful for a range of traumatic injuries.

Multilayer dressings

These products combine a low-adherence dressing with an absorbent backing or middle in an attempt to be a low-adherent, absorbent product. Examples of such are; Melolin, Release and Telfa. These products can be used as primary dressings for wounds producing little exudate or as secondary dressings with a wide range of products including hydrogels and alginates. Problems have been described when such products are used as the primary dressing for leg ulcers and wounds producing viscous exudate (Thomas, 1994a).

Textile and porous materials
(NA dressing, Tricotex, Tegapore, Mepital)

These products are designed to have a low-adherence at the wound bed and facilitate transfer of exudate through the dressing on to an absorbent dressing. Such products can also be used with multilayer bandaging systems and with heavily exuding wounds for which absorbent pads are used. They are particularly useful for patients with fragile skin or patients who have experienced sensitivities to other more interactive dressings or adhesives.

Medicated dressings

For some patients the use or long-term use of systemic antibiotics is contra-indicated. The treatment of superficial, local wound infection for such patients with chronic wounds, especially leg ulceration and pressure sores, is therefore difficult. The careful use of a range of medicated dressings can successfully treat this group of patients. There is an increasing awareness of the important role that topical antimicrobial agents can play in the treatment of wound infection.

Iodine products

Inadine and Iodoflex deliver iodine directly to the wound bed. Although they are essentially very different products, the use of iodine is extremely effective at controlling bacteria on the surface of a wound. Some caution is needed, however, as these products should not be used on patients with a known allergy to iodine, thyroid diseases or very large wounds.

Silver-containing products

Arglaes is a semipermeable film dressing with slow controlled release of silver onto the wound area. Flamazine is a cream containing 1% silver sulphadiazine and can be applied to burns, traumatic injuries, leg ulcers and pressure sores. An absorbent material and retaining dressings need to be used in conjunction with this cream. Silver has a broad spectrum of action against Gram-negative and Gram-positive organisms and also yeasts and fungi.

Topical antibiotics

Metrotop gel is an amorphous hydrogel containing the antibiotic metronidazole (0.8%). It is extremely effective against anaerobic organisms and the odour produced by these bacteria, which are often very malodorous. Wounds that have a malodour problem due to anaerobic bacteria include fungating carcinomas and necrotic pressure sores. In these wound situations the odour disappears very quickly, often within a matter of 12 hours.

Relief from malodour is an important aspect of patient care and helps to reduce the social isolation caused by odour.

Film dressings

Modern polyurethane film dressings were developed in the early 1970s and since that time have been developed to perform many functions. The adhesives have been modified and are now much less likely to produce skin sensitivities. These films can give a range of fluid-handling capacities with a range of moisture/vapour transmission rates (MVTR), capable of holding or evaporating fluid. Films have a range of uses, from holding intravenous catheters in place (intravenous 3000 with a high MVTR of $3000 \, g/m^2/24$ hours) to covering suture lines (Tegaderm with a moderate MVTR of $730 \, g/m^2/24$ hours) (Thomas, 1996). Films with a moderate MVTR are also extremely useful as a primary wound contact material for low to moderately exuding superficial granulating or epithelializing wounds and also as a secondary dressing to hold other materials such as alginates, hydrogels and non-adhesive foam in place. As secondary dressings, films are very effective at holding the primary dressing in place and in containing wound exudate, while providing occlusion to allow the patient to bath and shower without risk of contaminating the wound. Films are comfortable and conformable, they can be cut into strips and used in sections for difficult to dress areas such as heels, elbows and the digits. Films can stay in place for several days at a time. Caution is needed, however, when removing films to minimize trauma to the skin surrounding the wound. Films are best removed by stretching the film to release the adhesive before removal; avoid pulling it off with a 180° peel (Thomas, 1996).

It is also possible to coat polyurethane films with hydrocolloid adhesives to produce a dressing with a low MVTR. Granuflex extra thin and Comfeel transparent dressings are included in this group.

Difficult areas to dress

Applying and retaining dressings can be particularly difficult in some areas of the body such as the axilla, the perineum and the perianal area. Applying and retaining dressings on babies and young children can be challenging, whatever the site. Some practical solutions in these circumstances are discussed below.

The axilla

Excessive amounts of surgical tape may be used in an attempt to stick the dressing to the area but this is not ideal. Other options are possible, these include:

- Making a vest out of retention net such as Netelast or cotton tubular bandage.
- In female patients, use a large dressing pad and the patient's bra to hold the dressing in place.
- Using a CaviCare stent with a thin strip of Netelast moulded into the stent at the time of pouring. This can be tied at the shoulder and avoids the need to use any tape.
- Using a hydrocolloid dressing or a semipermeable film as a means of holding the primary dressing in place.

The perineum

Access to this area can be difficult for dressing changes. Careful positioning of the patient can help, lying the patient on his or her side and asking a colleague or the patient to hold the buttock. It may be easier to use several pillows under the patient's hips with the patient lying prone. Time should be spent finding a comfortable position for the patient, which gives proper access to the wound. It is important to see all aspects of the wound in order to cleanse and dress the wound appropriately.

The perianal wound

The long-term management of perianal wounds can cause particular inconvenience for the patient. It is usually not possible for patients to change the dressing themselves. When in hospital the dressing can be changed after defecation. However, once the patient is discharged, dressing changes become more problematic. The district nurse can work with the patient in timing the dressing change at a time after defecation usually occurs.

Dressing wounds in babies and small children

By the very nature of their size, the retention of dressings for babies and small children can be extremely difficult. The use of semipermeable and occlusive dressings is invaluable in the prevention of contamination of wounds. Trauma at dressing changes can be avoided by involving the child and his or her parents and choosing dressing materials with care (Bale & Jones, 1996).

EVIDENCE–BASED PRACTICE: SYSTEMATIC REVIEWS

A series of systematic reviews looking at the effectiveness and cost-effectiveness of wound-care interventions, commissioned by the NHS Health Technology Assessment Programme, is being carried out at the University of York at the Centre for Reviews and Dissemination. The reviews will include:
- Debridement of chronic wounds.
- Topical and systemic antibiotics for treatment of chronic wounds.
- A review of dressings for chronic wounds.

These reviews will be available from the University of York and also from the Cochrane Library (telephone (+44) 1865 513902 for details of the Cochrane Library).

SELF-ASSESSMENT QUESTIONS AND ACTIVITIES

(a) *Select four dressings in common use in your clinical area. Draw up a profile for each dressing using the criteria for the ideal dressing summarized in Box 6.3.*

(b) *Do you have a local policy document for wound management that includes specific information on wound dressings? If not, list four advantages of developing such a policy and state which healthcare professionals would need to be involved.*

(c) *Select a patient currently or recently within your care with a heavily exuding wound.*

(1) *Is the exudate caused by any underlying pathology?*

(2) *How successful are you or were you in managing the practical and social consequences of this volume of exudate? If you have not been particularly successful so far, what do you plan to do next and who else might become involved?*

See also the Advanced Case Studies given at pp. 269–292, which include questions relating specifically to the selection of wound dressings, often in very challenging situations.

REFERENCES

Bale S, Jones V. Caring for children with wounds. *J Wound Care* 1996, **5**(4):177–180.

Bale S. Wound healing. In: Alexander MF, Fawcett JN, Runciman PJ, eds. *Nursing practice*. Edinburgh: Churchill Livingstone; 1994.

Cooper R, Lawrence JC. The prevalence of bacteria and implications for infection control. *J Wound Care* 1996, **5**(6):291–294.

Dealey C. *The care of wounds*. Oxford: Blackwell Scientific Publications; 1994.

Morgan DA. Development of a wound management policy: Part 1. *Pharm J* 1990a, **244**:295–297.

Morgan DA. Development of a wound management policy: Part 2. *Pharm J* 1990b, **244**:358–359.

Morison M, Moffatt C. *A colour guide to the assessment and management of leg ulcers*. London: Mosby; 1994.

Thomas S. Functions of a wound dressing. In: *Wound management and dressings*. London: The Pharmaceutical Press; 1990.

Thomas S. Hydrocolloids. *J Wound Care* 1992, **1**(2):27–30.

Thomas S. Foam dressings. *J Wound Care* 1993, **2**(3):153–156.

Thomas S. *Handbook of wound dressings*. London: *J Wound Care*; 1994a.

Thomas S. Low-adherent dressings. *J Wound Care* 1994b, **3**(1):27–30.

Thomas S. Vapour-permeable film dressings. *J Wound Care* 1996, **5**(6):271–274.

Thomas S, Fear M. Comparing 2 dressings for wound debridement. *J Wound Care* 1993, **2**(5):272–274.

Turner TD. Which dressing and why? *Nursing Times* 1982, **18**(29):Supp 1–3.

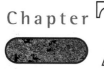
Dermatological Aspects of Wound Healing with special reference to the lower leg

The wounds most commonly encountered in a dermatology clinic are on the lower leg and the majority of these are associated with venous disease. A common complicating factor in the management of venous leg ulcers is the presence of eczema on the skin of the lower leg, found in approximately 60% of patients with a venous leg ulcer (Kulozic *et al.* 1988). The eczema may be a stasis eczema, an allergic contact dermatitis, an irritant dermatitis or be of mixed aetiology. The skin associated with venous insufficiency and affected by stasis eczema is particularly likely to develop reactions (contact dermatitis) to topical medicaments and bandages used to treat the ulcer (Kulozic *et al.* op. cit.; Paramsothy *et al.* 1988). An important aspect both in the prevention and management of leg ulcers is the maintenance of healthy skin around the ulcer; failure to do so may increase morbidity and delay healing. All patients should have their skin assessed at the first visit or on admission (if admitted to hospital). Although early interventions can prevent deterioration of the skin, they can only be implemented after thorough skin assessment, accurate diagnosis and after the implementation of an action plan. Therefore, it is essential that all the risk factors associated with the maintenance of skin integrity are carefully assessed, and all planned interventions are based on a clear rationale for the desired outcome as described in this chapter.

THE SKIN

The skin is the largest organ in the body and receives approximately one-third of the total blood supply to the body. The skin forms a barrier between the body and the external environment. As part of its function it provides protection from bacteria, prevention of moisture loss, temperature control and sensation. It produces vitamin D by the absorption of ultraviolet light and is capable of storing water and fat.

Structure of the skin

The skin is made up of two main layers: the epidermis and the dermis. The epidermis is itself composed of several layers. The outermost layer of the epidermis is called the stratum corneum (the horny or cornified layer), which consists of keratin and lipids. The skin continually repairs and regenerates itself with new epithelial cells that migrate upwards from the deeper basal cells of the epidermis, to replace the dead cells in the stratum corneum, a process that takes approximately 28 days. The thickness of the epidermis varies according to its function, being thick on the palms of the hands and soles of the feet and thin over the eyelids. The epidermis is supported by the dermis, which is thicker than the epidermis and composed of collagen, reticulum and elastin fibres which form a framework for the nerve endings, blood vessels, lymphatic capillaries, sweat glands, sebaceous glands and hair follicles (Figures 7.1 and 7.2). A layer of subcutaneous fatty tissue (the hypodermis) merges with the deepest layer of the dermis providing thermal insulation (Sneddon & Church, 1976). The functions of these layers are summarized in Table 7.1.

Loss of skin integrity

Loss of skin integrity can result from mechanical and chemical trauma and from various underlying pathologies.

Mechanical trauma may result from shear forces or result from the body being pulled over a surface causing friction. The sacrum and the heels are particularly vulnerable to this type of tissue injury, described in Chapter 9. In elderly patients, the skin overlying the shin may be atrophied and, therefore, be more vulnerable to trauma, especially if the patient suffers from rheumatoid arthritis (Chapter 10). Careful consideration must be

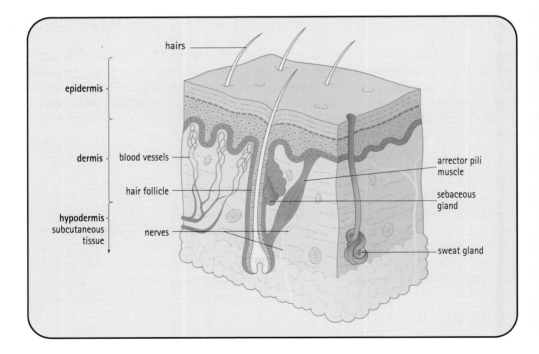

Figure 7.1   The structure of skin and its relationship to the hypodermis (subcutaneous tissue).

given to the choice of topical treatments applied to such thin vulnerable skin in order to prevent initial lacerations ending up as chronic leg ulcers.

Toxic chemicals used on the wound or surrounding skin may produce an irritant skin reaction, seen clinically as erythema or frank eczema. However, severe cutaneous damage that reaches down to dermal structures is termed a 'chemical burn'. Strong acids and alkalis are the major causes of chemical burns and severe tissue damage can result even after short exposure (Frosch, 1992).

Table 7.1. The structure and function of skin (reproduced courtesy of Professor Terrance Ryan)	
Structure	**Function**
Epidermis	
1 a Horny layer (stratum corneum)	Barrier, protection, armour of keratin and lipids
b Granular layer (stratum lucidum) (stratum granulosum)	Orderly death and organization of cell contents such as keratohyalin
c Prickle cell layer (stratum spinosum)	Initiates synthesis of keratohyalin, vitamin D, cytokines, etc.
d Basale cell layer (stratum basale)	Division and mobilization of cells, maintenance of contact with dermis
2 Melanocytes	Pigmentation
3 Langerhans cells	Allergen recognition and presentation
NB also differentiates into hair, nails, sweat glands, sebaceous glands	
Dermis	
4 Papillary layer	Generally supportive of epidermis. Dermal, epidermal adherence, supply of nutrition, exit of foreign or unwanted material
5 Reticular layer	Generally supportive in connective tissue, resists distorting forces, inflammatory response
6 Hypodermis (adipose tissue)	Storage of energy, dispersal of distorting forces, insulation, body shape control
NB mast cells, blood supply, lymphatic drainage, present at all dermal levels	NB a principal function is the 'look good feel good factor' of the skin, as an organ of communication. 1–6 play their part.

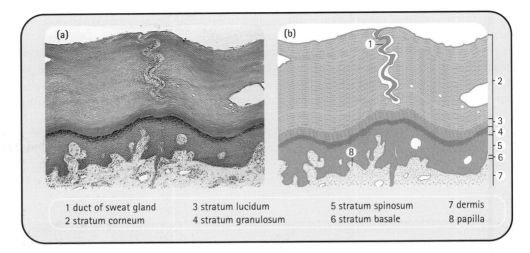

| 1 duct of sweat gland | 3 stratum lucidum | 5 stratum spinosum | 7 dermis |
| 2 stratum corneum | 4 stratum granulosum | 6 stratum basale | 8 papilla |

Figure 7.2 Photomicrograph of the epidermis and dermis (x 250) illustrating the skin's microscopic appearance. (©John D Cunningham/Visuals Unlimited.)

A number of pathophysiological diseases and disorders pose a risk to skin integrity. These include venous insufficiency, diabetes, vasculitis, infection, eczema, blistering diseases and skin diseases, summarized in Table 7.2.

Assessing the skin

When assessing the skin it is important to consider its colour, temperature, texture and integrity.

Colour
Inflammation produces a reddish skin tone, whereas pallor or bluish tones indicate poor vascularity. Brown staining around the gaiter area is indicative of venous disease (Figure 7.3). Normal skin colour varies from person to person and colour changes may be difficult to see in a dark-skinned person.

Temperature
Skin should feel warm to the touch, heat is usually associated with inflammation and cold with poor vascularization.

Texture
Is the skin dry or is there a moist condition? Hyperkeratosis (excessive dryness and scaling) is a chronic condition associated with venous disease. Weeping skin is often associated with an acute condition.

Integrity
Areas of broken skin should be noted and a risk-assessment undertaken to determine the patient's susceptibility to further tissue breakdown. Excessive moisture on the skin may result in maceration and possible skin erosion (Figure 7.4).

Table 7.2.
Factors associated with loss of skin integrity

Type	Cause	Examples
Mechanical trauma	Pressure	Over-night bandaging
	Shear	Insufficient support of a person in a bed or a chair
	Friction	Repeated rubbing of a skin
Chemical trauma	Irritants	Strong acids and alkalis, skin cleansers, antiseptics
Medical or physiological disorder	Eczema	Stasis ezcema, allergic contact dermatitis
	Endocrine dysfunction	Diabetes
	Vasculitis	Erythema nodosum, polyarteritis nodosum
	Venous insufficiency	Venous leg ulcer
	Bacterial infection	Impetigo, erysipelas, cellulitis
	Blistering diseases	Bullous pemphigoid
	Other dermatoses	Psoriasis
	Cutaneous infestations	Scabies
	Auto-immune diseases	Systemic lupus erythematosis
	Malignancy	Squamous cell and basal cell carcinoma
	Fungal infections	*Candida spp*

The factors listed in this table are either the direct cause of the tissue damage or
are exacerbating or contributing factors to skin breakdown.

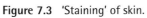
Figure 7.3 'Staining' of skin.

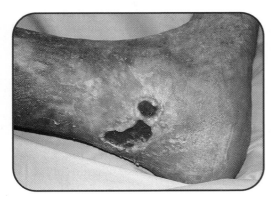

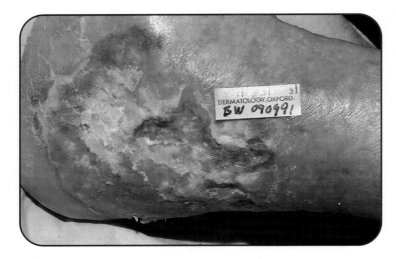

Figure 7.4
Maceration from
exudate.

Skin problems associated with wounds in the lower leg

Skin problems associated with wounds in the lower leg include:
- Eczema or dermatitis.
- Infection.
- Blisters or bullae.
- Pressure ulcers.

This chapter focuses mainly on the various forms of eczema together with the required treatment. The assessment and management of patients presenting with an infected wound or pressure ulcer are discussed in Chapters 3 and 9, respectively.

ECZEMA/DERMATITIS

The term eczema is used synonymously with the term dermatitis. Eczema is an inflammatory disorder of the skin characterized in the acute phase by itching, redness, exudation and vesiculation (Figure. 7.5) (Monk & Graham-Brown, 1992). In the chronic phase there is irritation and possibly some exudate but less than in the acute phase and there tends to be more scale. Eczema may arise from a variety of causes which may be either exogenous or endogenous in aetiology and in some cases a mixture of the two, such as when a contact eczema occurs in a patient with varicose eczema.
   Eczema falls into two groups, endogenous and exogenous.
- Endogenous eczema describes the type of eczema that is considered to be related to constitutional (internal) factors and includes atopic eczema, discoid eczema and varicose eczema.
- Exogenous eczema is used to describe the types of eczema that result from a reaction to an external stimulus and include irritant eczema and allergic contact eczema (Table 7.3).

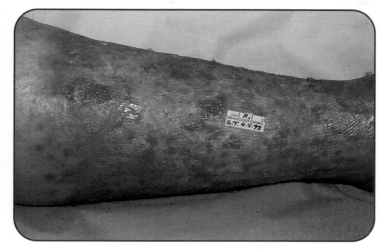

Figure 7.5   Eczema.

Table 7.3. Classification of eczema or dermatitis on the lower leg	
Endogenous eczema (related to internal factors)	Exogenous eczema (related to external factors)
Venous (stasis) eczema	Irritant-contact dermatitis
Atopic eczema	Allergic-contact dermatitis
Discoid eczema	

The clinical manifestations and treatment of various forms of endogenous and exogenous eczema are described, beginning with the endogenous forms.

Atopic eczema

This is an endogenous eczema that often occurs in people who have either hay fever or asthma or a combination of the two. Most patients exhibit raised immunoglobulin E (IgE) levels and specific IgE antibodies. The condition usually develops in early childhood but onset may be delayed until adult life (Hunter & Savin, 1983). Although the distribution and characteristics of atopic eczema vary, the skin tends to be dry and excoriated and general dryness of the skin may persist throughout life.

Management of atopic eczema

Management of general skin dryness is with regular use of emollients. Topical cortico-steroid preparations may be prescribed, the potency depending on the severity of the eczema and the area to be treated. Potent steroids are used only for a short period and should never be applied to the face. Medium and low-potency steroids are used for the face and for the treatment of mild eczema on the body. Steroids should be applied sparingly once or twice daily to the affected areas only (Colver & Savin, 1994).

Discoid eczema

This is characterized by well-defined coin-shaped scaly plaques. The condition may irritate the patient and in the acute phase, vesicles that exude serum may be evident (Fry & Cornell, 1985).

Management of discoid eczema

Treatment in the acute phase requires a potent topical corticosteroid preparation. If there is secondary bacterial infection a combined corticosteroid and antibiotic preparation may be prescribed. Antihistamines may be required to reduce itching (Monk & Graham-Brown, op. cit.).

Venous-stasis (varicose) eczema

Venous-stasis eczema is endogenous in aetiology, usually commencing on the inner aspect of the lower leg. It is thought to be caused by the skin changes that occur in venous insufficiency. Incompetence of the venous valves allows backflow of blood from the deep veins to the superficial veins resulting in a high ambulatory pressure in the superficial veins, which is then transmitted to the capillary circulation in the skin and subcutaneous tissues (*see* Chapter 10). The increased capillary pressure, which results from venous hypertension, causes haemosiderin deposition and lipodermatosclerosis (Burnand *et al.* 1982). This localized pathophysiology is thought to be conducive to tissue breakdown, venous-stasis eczema and induration.

Management of venous stasis eczema

Dry eczematous skin is managed with regular use of an emollient. Immersing the leg in warm tap water for 10–20 minutes, before application of the emollient, will soften and loosen skin scales. Emollients come in the form of creams and ointments. Creams are an emulsion of oil in water and take a semi-solid form. When applied to the skin most of the cream evaporates because of the high water content. However, creams contain emulsifiers and preservatives that may cause sensitivity problems in patients with a leg ulcer and where possible should be avoided. Ointments contain little or no water, are occlusive and rehydrate the skin. A simple cost-effective emollient that is unlikely to sensitize is a mixture of 50% white soft paraffin in 50% liquid paraffin.

Acute weeping eczema may be treated with a dilute solution of potassium permanganate (using only enough potassium permanganate for the solution to be a pale pink colour). The leg should be immersed in the solution daily for 10–15 minutes, followed by application of a topical corticosteroid ointment (Hunter & Savin, op. cit.). A paste bandage containing ichthammol is very effective in controlling this condition.

Venous insufficiency is treated by graduated compression therapy (*see* Chapter 10) and this has been shown to have an effect on the calf-muscle pump with a reduction in the degree of pigmentation and eczema over time (Struckman, 1986). Therefore, it is essential that any local skin treatment for venous-stasis eczema should be combined with adequate compression therapy.

Secondary infection is a complication of eczema that requires treatment with systemic antibiotics together with a topical corticosteroid ointment; if required, the corticosteroid ointment may also contain an antibiotic.

Failure to respond to treatment If, despite appropriate treatment, the eczema fails to respond, the condition may be a contact dermatitis and the patient should be investigated by patch testing to determine whether they have become sensitized to their current treatment.

Atopic, discoid and venous-stasis eczema are endogenous forms of eczema. Exogenous forms of eczema are described below. Contact dermatitis is an exogenous eczema caused by direct contact with external substances; the resulting reaction may be irritant or allergic in aetiology or a combination of the two.

Irritant-contact dermatitis

Frosch (op. cit.) describes irritant-contact dermatitis as a non-immunological inflammatory reaction of the skin to an external agent. Substances that produce inflammation of the epidermis by chemical disruption of the stratum corneum are described as 'irritants'. Irritants may affect the skin in different ways with the clinical spectrum ranging from slight scaling and redness to marked eczema (Frosch, op. cit.). The severity of the reaction will vary according to the skin area exposed, the method of exposure, the substance used and the concentration (Lahti, 1992). The patient may complain of pain, burning, stinging and itching. Regular skin contact with a mild irritant can result in 'hardening' of the skin, this results in the skin becoming hyperkeratotic (McOsker *et al.* 1967). Patients most at risk of an irritant-contact dermatitis are those in which the skin barrier function has been disturbed by an endogenous condition such as venous stasis eczema. Therefore, the application of medicaments around a leg ulcer or on eczematous skin may lead to the development of an irritant-contact dermatitis. Many preparations used in the care of chronic leg ulcers may be responsible for producing an irritant reaction and these may have a cumulative action. Itching can lead to scratching of the affected area, which may well result in loss of skin integrity and infection.

Management of irritant contact dermatitis

Wound exudate Prolonged exposure to wound exudate can irritate the skin and lead to maceration and loss of epithelium. A barrier preparation, such as zinc oxide paste, applied to the skin around the ulcer will protect the skin from wound exudate (Cherry *et al.* 1991). If the skin is already very wet the zinc oxide paste will need to be added to a small amount of a mixture of 50% white soft paraffin and 50% liquid paraffin (50:50 mixture) to aid application. Zinc oxide paste is a barrier preparation and therefore cannot be removed by washing. To remove the zinc oxide paste at dressing changes some 50:50 mixture should be massaged into the zinc oxide paste, to soften it, before gently wiping off with soft gauze.

Cleansers Wounds may be cleansed with warmed tap water or sterile normal saline as described in Chapter 5. Other skin-cleansing solutions, if used in strong concentrations or used repeatedly or excessively, may damage the stratum corneum (Frosch, op. cit.). The use of antiseptics should be avoided as they have been shown to cause irritant skin reactions when applied to damaged skin (Patti *et al.* 1990). Antiseptic toxicity was explored by Brennan *et al.* (1986) who suggested that antiseptics may adversely affect healing.

Dressings Careful consideration should be given to the type of dressing used for patients with eczema. Particular attention should also be given to the removal of dressings, to prevent further trauma, especially if the dressings have adhered to the wound and surrounding tissue. Healthcare professionals need to be aware of the fact that adhesive dressings can themselves cause irritation in some patients (Mallon & Powell, 1994). If this happens the adhesive dressing should be changed to a non-adherent dressing (*see* Chapter 6). The use of adhesive tapes to secure dressings and pads to the skin should be avoided on fragile or eczematous skin as removal may cause discomfort to the patient and trauma to the surrounding healthy tissue.

Bandages Bandages that have not been applied correctly may slip or rub, resulting in blisters on the skin and tissue breakdown (*see* Chapter 10). Rubber in elastic bandages is generally covered with cotton to prevent allergic reactions, however, if bandages or elastic tubular supports are applied directly to the skin of patients with venous ulcer-ation or venous-stasis eczema they are likely to cause irritation. Scratching of dry, irritated skin can lead to tissue breakdown and the occurrence of ulceration. Paste bandages often have a soothing effect when applied to itchy eczematous skin and those containing ichthammol are particularly effective in the treatment of eczema. Paste bandages can be applied under elastic bandages, described in Chapter 10.

Allergic-contact dermatitis

Allergic-contact dermatitis, also referred to as contact sensitivity, is a delayed, type IV, T-cell mediated hypersensitivity, induced by the reaction between an antigen and sensitized T lymphocytes (Baer, 1986). An allergen sensitizes through skin contact. On renewed contact with the allergen, the skin produces a reaction seen clinically as eczema (Scheper & von Blomberg, 1992). Sensitivity to topical applications is common in patients with venous leg ulcers. It has long been considered that the occlusive nature of leg ulcer treatments, on skin where the barrier function has been disturbed by maceration and eczema, may create the perfect environment for sensitization to occur (Stolze, 1966). Allergic contact dermatitis usually presents in the area in direct contact with the allergen (Figure 7.6) but if severe enough, can spread to become a generalized eczema. However, this is not always the case and it is possible for sensitivity to be only expressed as poor ulcer healing or persistent irritation (Fisher, 1971). Failure to recognize sensitivity was reported by Cameron (1990) who found that 23% of 52 patients with

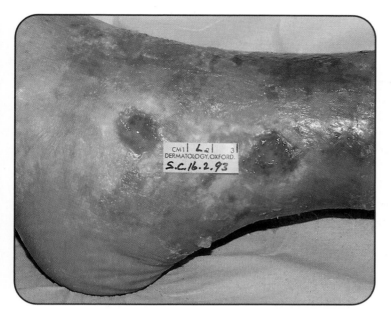

Figure 7.6 Allergic-contact dermatitis.

chronic venous leg ulcers were sensitized to their current treatment. Sensitization may occur after a short period of exposure to an allergen or after a long period of use.

The diagnosis of allergic-contact dermatitis is established by patch testing (Box 7.1) and this requires referral to a dermatologist. Patients with non-healing chronic leg ulcers should be considered for patch testing if they have eczema around the ulcer, a reaction to topical treatment or if they are failing to heal despite appropriate treatment.

Common leg ulcer allergens found in a wide range of wound-care products, such as emollients, medicaments, dressings and bandages, include the following:

- Topical antibiotics.
- Vehicles and emulsifiers.
- Preservatives and biocides.
- Rubber.
- Adhesives.
- Perfumes.

The common sources of these allergens are described in Box 7.2.

After patch testing, advice should be given to patients and carers on suitable skin treatments that do not contain any identified allergens. Patients should be strongly discouraged from using over-the-counter preparations because these may contain sensitizers.

Management of allergic-contact dermatitis

Referral to a dermatologist will be required to identify the allergen responsible. Initial treatment should consist of resting the affected limb and treating the eczema with a topical corticosteroid ointment. The potency of corticosteroids falls into four groups: (1) mild, (2) moderately potent, (3) potent and (4) very potent. The potency of the corticosteroid required will depend on the degree of eczema present on the limb. A potent

Box 7.1.

Patch testing

Diagnostic patch tests

The International Contact Dermatitis Research Group (ICDRG) guidelines determine the concentrations and suggest suitable vehicles for the purpose of patch testing (Wilkinson *et al*. 1970). The patch test substances are commercially prepared according to these guidelines. Patch testing can lead to false positive and false negative results if the correct concentrations are not used. Various test systems are available commercially. A commonly used system consists of hypoallergenic tape (Scanpor tape) with small aluminium discs attached (Finn chambers). These discs are filled with dilute concentrations of prepared allergens before patch testing.

Patch test procedure

Small amounts of the test substances are applied under occlusion to healthy skin on the patient's back. Any active eczema should be controlled as far as possible before patch testing. The test substances used are a standard series of allergens and extra allergens relative to the clinical problem. The optimum time points for the patch test procedure are considered to be 2 days exposure time, with examination of the area after removal of the tests, and a further examination 2 days later (Paramsothy *et al*. op.cit.).

Day 1 The test strips are applied and their location marked on the patient's back using a suitable skin marker. The test substances are left in place for 2 days.

Day 3 The test strips are removed and discarded. A generalized redness may be apparent after removal of the patch tests and therefore a minimum period of 30 minutes should be left between removal and examination of the area. The back is then examined for any erythema, oedema, induration and vesicle formation. The patient is required to keep the patch test site dry for a further 2 days.

Day 5 The back is again examined at the test site, as before, for any erythema, oedema, induration and vesicle formation. The responses are graded, as recommended by the ICDRG as no response (-), irritant reaction (IR), doubtful reaction (?+), weak reaction (+), strong oedematous or vesicular reaction (++) and extreme reaction (+++).

False positives A strong positive reaction to a patch test can sometimes influence the reactivity of adjacent patch test sites leading to false positive reactions, which may be seen clinically as an eczematous reaction over the whole area under the test strip or one strong positive reaction with all the other test sites showing a weak reaction. This phenomenon is referred to as the angry back syndrome (Mitchell, 1975). If this occurs, all the suspected allergens have to be tested individually to identify the true positives and negatives.

False negatives A patient may have negative patch tests if the inflammatory response has been suppressed by the use of an oral or topical corticosteroid preparation (Sukanto *et al*. 1981). In some instances, a skin reaction may be caused by a combination of ingredients that test negative when tested individually (Kellett *et al*. 1986).

Box 7.2.

Leg ulcer allergens

Topical antibiotics

Neomycin; framycetin; gentamicin The most commonly reported sensitizers in leg ulcer patients are neomycin and framycetin. Cross sensitivity occurs between neomycin, framycetin and gentamicin, therefore, an allergic reaction to one of the group means that they should all be avoided (Forstrom & Pirila, 1978; Rudzki *et al.* 1988). Sensitivity to neomycin may be masked in products in which the antibiotic is combined with a topical corticosteroid, the latter suppressing the sensitivity reaction.

Bacitracin and sodium fusidate A high incidence of sensitivity to bacitracin reported by Zaki *et al.* (1994) was thought to be the result of local prescribing practice. Sodium fusidate is considered to be a low sensitizer but there have been isolated reports of sensitivity when used to treat a leg ulcer (De Groot, 1982; Verbov, 1970).

Vehicles and emulsifiers

Lanolin (wool alcohols, Amerchol L 101, eucerin) Lanolin is contained in some barrier preparations, creams, bath additives and emollients, including baby products. Lanolin has long been recognized as one of the main sensitizers in patients with venous-stasis eczema and leg ulcers (Fisher *et al.* op. cit.; Malten & Kuiper, 1985; Kulozic *et al.* 1988; Wilson *et al.* 1991; Zaki *et al.* 1994). Therefore, it is not advisable to use any product containing lanolin on a patient with a leg ulcer.

Cetylstearyl alcohols This allergen is particularly difficult to avoid as it is found in creams, emulsifying ointment and some paste bandages (Cameron & Powell, 1992). The use of creams is popular among nurses and patients as they are less greasy than ointments.

Preservatives and biocides

Parabens (hydroxybenzoates) The parabens group possesses antibacterial and antifungal properties and are widely used as preservatives in topical medicaments, moisturizers and some paste bandages. Until recently, most of the paste bandages contained parabens (hydroxybenzoates) but changes in the formulation of some of the paste bandages and the introduction of a preservative-free paste bandage addressed this (Powell *et al.* 1994). Parabens are a significant sensitizer when used on leg ulcers (Dooms-Goosens *et al.* 1979; Kulozic *et al.* op. cit.; Cameron, op. cit. Wilson *et al.* op. cit.).

Chlorhexidine This was reported as a significant sensitizer in a Danish study (Knudsen & Avnstorp, 1991) and a recent UK study reported that 13% of 85 patients with chronic leg ulceration were sensitive to chlorhexidine (Zaki *et al.* op. cit.).

Quinoline mix (3% clioquinol and 3% chloquinadol) These have both antibacterial and antifungal activity and are commonly used in creams and ointments to treat skin conditions. They have been reported as significant sensitizers when used on leg ulcers (Paramsothy *et al.* op. cit.; Zaki *et al.* op. cit.).

(continued over)

Box 7.2 (continued)

Leg ulcer allergens (continued)

Rubber
Mercapto mix; thiuram mix; carba mix This is a group of chemicals used in the rubber industry. Rubber may be found in bandages, support hosiery, tubular elastic supports and latex gloves. Approximately 5%–8% of leg ulcer patients have been reported to have positive-patch tests to rubber allergens (Paramsothy *et al.* op. cit.; Cameron, op. cit.; Wilson *et al.* op. cit.). The rubber in bandages is usually covered in cotton to help prevent contact with the skin, although this may not be enough to prevent a skin reaction in a sensitized patient. Another potential source of rubber coming into contact with the skin around a leg ulcer is from the latex gloves worn by the carer. If a rubber allergy is suspected, the carer should wear vinyl gloves to treat the patient. A further source of rubber may come from compression hosiery, although most stockings available on drug tariff are rubber-free.

Adhesives
Colophony; ester of rosin Colophony and its derivatives can be found in the adhesive backing of plasters and in some tapes, bandages and dressings (Mallon & Powell, op. cit.).

Perfume
Fragrance mix; balsam of Peru These are markers for perfume sensitivity and are found in many over-the-counter preparations such as moisturisers, bath additives and baby products.

Others
Although the above-mentioned allergens are considered to be the main sensitizers in leg ulcer patients, other preparations used in the management of the skin have been reported as causing sensitivity and much will depend on local prescribing habits.

---

steroid (e.g. betamethasone 0.1% or beclomethasone dipropionate 0.025%) should be applied daily for a few days then the amount reduced over several days by gradually replacing the steroid ointment with a simple emollient such as 50% white soft paraffin in 50% liquid paraffin. For use on a chronic eczema, for which long-term maintenance therapy is required, a moderately potent corticosteroid ointment (e.g. clobetasone butyrate 0.05%) would be suitable (Cameron, 1995).

Failure to respond to treatment If the corticosteroid ointment is stopped suddenly, without first reducing the dose, there may be a rebound effect of the eczema. However, corticosteroids may themselves sometimes sensitize and this needs to be considered (Guin, 1984). The most commonly reported corticosteroid sensitizer among leg ulcer patients is hydrocortisone and for this reason it should be avoided in the treatment of leg ulcers (Dooms-Goosens *et al.* 1986). Detection of sensitivity can be difficult, because the anti-inflammatory effect of the corticosteroid may mask the allergy. It may be seen clinically only as a failure to heal or as a poor response to treatment. In such cases, further investigation is required including patch testing.

INFECTION

When its barrier function has been disturbed, skin is at greater risk of infection. However, there is a distinction between 'infection' and 'colonization'. Although the majority of chronic wounds often have microbial colonization of the tissue, few are infected (Schraibman, 1987). *Staphylococcus aureus* appears to be the most common pathogen found in venous leg ulcers (Eriksson *et al.* 1984; Trengrove *et al.* 1994; Hayes & Gill, 1995). However, the role of bacteria in contributing to impairment of the healing process, in wounds that are not clinically infected, remains controversial (*see* Chapter 3). Clinical infection is characterized by heat, swelling, pain, odour and erythema (Figure 3.1). A diffuse infection of the skin and subcutaneous tissue is referred to as cellulitis. Treatment of cellulitis is by use of systemic antibiotics; if sufficiently severe, the patient may require admission to hospital for intravenous antibiotics. The affected limb should be rested and supported. Compression bandages should be avoided during the acute phase and only light retention bandages used to hold dressings in place. In the case of recurrent infections, prevention may require treatment with long-term antibiotics (Jeffs, 1993).

Superficial mycoses affect the keratinous tissues of the skin and are sometimes seen on the skin around a leg ulcer. Correct diagnosis is required because clinical signs associated with a fungal infection in the skin around a leg ulcer are similar to eczema with red, scaly, macerated, irritated skin. There may also be pustules and skin erosions present. They can be tested for by mycological examination of skin scrapings for hyphae and their culture (Fry & Cornell, op. cit.). After identification, treatment is by appropriate antifungal preparations.

OTHER SKIN CONDITIONS THAT MAY BE ENCOUNTERED

Vasculitis

Vasculitis (inflammation of the blood vessels) leads to occlusion of the small vessels and tissue breakdown (*see* Chapter 10). Treatment of vasculitic ulcers is aimed at disease suppression for which corticosteroids and other immunosuppressives may be required. However, long-term steroidal therapy leaves patients with thin vulnerable skin that breaks down easily and is slow to heal (Hunter *et al.* 1989). The area on the front of the shin is particularly vulnerable.

Blisters or bullae

Blisters may result from external damage such as friction or tight bandaging pinching the skin. Protection of the skin with suitable padding, especially over the shin and around bony prominences in the ankle and foot, is essential before applying a compression bandage (*see* Chapter 10). Foam pads are commercially available for applying to concave areas such as below the malleolus. Blisters or bullae are also associated with oedema, eczema and the blistering disease 'bullous pemphigoid'.

The condition of bullous pemphigoid is an auto-immune disease that mainly affects the elderly population. The eruption presents as large tense blisters on an urticarial base which is often very itchy (Fry & Cornell, op. cit.). Treatment is with systemic or topical corticosteroids. Locally, the fluid is released by lightly using a scalpel blade to split the blister. Prescribed topical corticosteroids with antibiotics may be needed. The dressing should be non-adherent with a pad covering. No tapes should be used to hold the dressings in place, only a lightly applied gauze retention bandage or a length of tubular cotton. Great care is required in the removal of the dressings and it may be necessary to soak the dressings before removal.

Lymphoedema

Oedema represents a failure of the lymphatic system. In acute oedema, when the skin is taut and shiny, lymphorrhoea may occur in which fluid leaks out of the skin in the affected area. The affected limb becomes soaking wet with increased risk of infection. Treatment requires non-adherent sterile dressings to be applied together with compression bandaging (Veitch, 1993). Chronic venous hypertension and damage to the lymphatic vessels can result in gross thickening of the dermis with increased skin scale (Ryan, 1987). Treatment of this dry skin condition is by liberal application of emollients and massage.

Pressure ulcers on the heels

Heel ulcers can be caused by pressure due to immobility, tight shoes, medical appliances and/or friction (*see* Chapter 9). Pressure ulcers are caused when the external pressures on the heel exceed capillary closure pressures and the compromised blood flow results in localized tissue necrosis (Krasner, 1990). Skin is more resistant to pressure than underlying soft tissue and what may appear to be a stage I pressure ulcer may have underlying tissue necrosis (Colburn, 1990). In patients deemed to be at risk, early intervention is essential to prevent any tissue damage. Prevention consists of pressure relief, frequent changes of position, skin care and adequate nutrition (*see* Chapter 9). Particular attention should be given to the skin overlying any bony prominences. Moisturizing the skin with a simple emollient will help prevent any dryness and cracking. However, care must be taken when applying an emollient over a bony prominence as massage of these areas may cause tissue damage (Olson, 1989).

EVALUATION OF THE EFFECTIVENESS OF TREATMENT

Ongoing evaluation of the chosen treatment should always be undertaken as modifications may need to be made if conditions change. If, on evaluation, there has been little or no response to treatment, check that all appropriate interventions have been implemented. If, despite appropriate treatment, there is still no response, consider referral to a dermatology department for patch testing and further investigations.

SELF-ASSESSMENT QUESTIONS AND ACTIVITIES

Case study

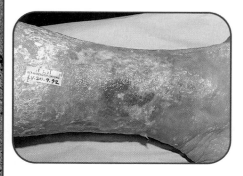

Mrs Brown has a heavily exuding venous ulcer, as illustrated in the photograph above. She is complaining of irritation over her shin and on examination you discover that her skin is very dry in this area, there are several small excoriated areas where she has been scratching and the bandage has adhered to her leg. You also note that her heel has become very red from resting her foot on a hard foot stool.

1. *How would you protect the area around her ulcer from the wound exudate?*
2. *List the emollients that you could use on her leg to relieve the dryness. Can any of these emollients themselves lead to an adverse tissue response?*
3. *Think about why Mrs Brown's skin might be so itchy and then list the interventions you could use to reduce the irritation.*
4. *Summarize the interventions that you would employ to prevent Mrs Brown's heel from breaking down (see Chapter 9 for further guidance).*
5. *List four circumstances that may cause you to consider referring Mrs Brown for a specialist opinion (see Chapter 10 for further guidance).*

Activities

(a) *Think about a patient that you know with a non-healing venous leg ulcer and explore whether their topical therapy contains any of the main leg ulcer allergens (summarized in Box 7.2).*

(b) *Consider the application of a topical corticosteroid preparation on a patient with a venous leg ulcer and discuss why it would be more appropriate to use a preparation in an ointment-base rather than a cream.*

(c) *Discuss the nursing interventions that would be required to prevent a rebound effect when treating a patient's eczematous condition with a potent corticosteroid preparation.*

REFERENCES

Baer RL. The mechanism of allergic contact hypersensitivity. In: Fisher AA, ed. *Contact Dermatitis*, 3rd ed. Philadelphia: Lea and Febiger; 1986.

Brennan SS, Foster ME, Leaper DJ. Antiseptic toxicity in wounds healing by secondary intention. *J Hosp Infect* 1986, **8**:263–267.

Burnand K, Whimster I, Naidoo A. Pericapillary fibrin in the ulcer bearing skin of the leg: the cause of lipodermatosclerosis and venous ulceration. *BMJ* 1982, **285**:1920–1922.

Cameron J. Patch testing for leg ulcer patients. *Nursing Times* 1990, **86** (25):63–64.

Cameron J. The importance of contact dermatitis in the management of leg ulcers. *J Tissue Viability* 1995, **5**(2):52–55.

Cameron J, Powell SM. Contact dermatitis: its importance in leg ulcer management. *Wound Management* 1992, **2**(3):12–13.

Cherry GW, Cameron J, Ryan TJ. *Leg ulcer blue print*. London: ConvaTec Ltd; 1991.

Colburn L. Early intervention for the prevention of pressure ulcers. In: Krasner D, ed. *Chronic wound care*. Pennsylvania: Health Management Publications; 1990.

Colver G, Savin JA. Eczema and dermatitis. In: Smith T, Simmons M, eds. *Understanding skin problems*. London: Family Doctor Publications Ltd; 1994:11–12.

De Groot AC. Contact allergy to sodium fusidate. *Contact Dermatitis* 1982, **8**:429.

Dooms-Goosens A, Degreef H, Parijs M, Kerkhofs L. A retrospective study of patch test results from 163 patients with stasis dermatitis or leg ulcers. I. Discussion of the patch test results and the sensitisation indices and determination of the relevancy of positive reactions. *Dermatologica* 1979, **159**(2): 93–100.

Dooms-Goosens A, Verschaeve H, Degreef H, van Berendoncks J. Contact allergy to hydrocortisone and tixocortol pivalate: problems in the detection of corticosteroid sensitivity. *Contact Dermatitis* 1986, **14**:94–102.

Eriksson G. The clinical significance of bacterial growth in venous leg ulcers – its clinical significance. *Scand J Infect Dis* 1984, **16**(2):175–180.

Fisher AA. Allergic contact dermatitis due to ingredients of vehicles. *Arch Dermatol* 1971, **104**:286–290.

Forstrom L, Pirila L. Cross sensitivity within the neomycin group of antibiotics. *Contact Dermatitis* 1978, **4**:312.

Frosch PJ. Cutaneous irritation. In: Rycroft RJG, Menne T, Frosch PJ, Benezra C, eds. *Text book of contact dermatitis*. Berlin: Springer-Verlag; 1992.

Fry L, Cornell MNP: Bacterial infections. In: Fry J, Lancaster-Smith MJ, eds. *Dermatology – (management of common skin diseases in family practice)*. Lancaster: MTP Press Ltd; 1985.

Guin JD. Contact sensitivity to topical corticosteroids. *J Am Acad Dermatol* 1984, **10**:773–782.

Hayes M, Gill C. Microbiology and immunology in patients with leg ulcers. *J Wound Care* 1995, **4**(3):129–133.

Hunter JAA, Savin JA. *Common diseases of the skin*. Oxford: Blackwell Scientific Publications; 1983.

Hunter JAA, Savin JA, Dahl MV. *Clinical dermatology*. Oxford: Blackwell Scientific Publications; 1989:119–121.

Jeffs E. The effect of acute inflammatory episodes. *J Tissue Viability* 1993, **3**:51–55.

Kellett JK, King CM, Beck MH. Compound allergy to medicaments. *Contact Dermatitis* 1986, **14**:45–48.

Knudsen BB, Avnstorp C. Chlorhexidine gluconate and acetate in patch testing. *Contact Dermatitis* 1991, **24**:45–49.

Krasner D. Pressure ulcers of the heels: how to decrease their occurrence in healthcare facilities. In: Krasner D, ed. *Chronic wound care*. Pennsylvania: Health Management Publications; 1990.

Kulozic M, Powell SM, Cherry G, Ryan TJ. Contact sensitivity in community based leg ulcer patients. *Clin Exp Dermatol* 1988, **13**:82–84.

Lahti A. Immediate contact reactions In: Rycroft RJG, Menne T, Frosch PJ, Benezra C, eds. *Textbook of contact dermatitis*. Berlin: Springer-Verlag; 1992.

Mallon E, Powell S: Allergic contact dermatitis from Granuflex hydrocolloid dressing. *Contact Dermatitis* 1994, **30:**110–111.

Malten KE, Kuiper JP. Contact allergic reactions in 100 selected patients with ulcus cruris. *VASA* 1985, **4**(14):340–345.

McOsker DE, Beck LW. Characteristics of accommodated (hardened) skin. *J Invest Dermatol* 1967, **48:**372–383.

Mitchell JC. The angry back syndrome: eczema creates eczema. *Contact Dermatitis* 1975, **1:**193.

Monk BE, Graham-Brown RAC: Eczema. In: Monk BE, Graham-Brown RAC, eds. *Skin disorders of the elderly.* Oxford: Blackwell Scientific Publications; 1992.

Olson B. Effects of massage for the prevention of pressure ulcers. *Decubitus* 1989, **2**(2):32–37.

Paramsothy Y, Collins M, Smith AG. Contact dermatitis in patients with leg ulcers. *Contact Dermatitis* 1988, **18:**30–36.

Patti J, Cazzaniga A, Marshall DA, Leyden JS, Mertz PM. An analysis of dermal irritation of several OTC first aid treatments. *Wounds* 1990, **2:**35–42.

Powell SM, Cameron J, Hofman D, Poore S, Cherry GW, Ryan TJ. Patch test study of a new medicated paste bandage in patients with chronic leg ulcers. In: Cherry GW, Leaper DJ, Lawrence JC, Milward P, eds. *Proceedings of 4th European Conference on Advances in Wound Management.* London: Macmillan; 1994:66–68.

Rudzki E, Zakrzewski Z, Rebadel P, Grzywa Z, Hudymowicz W. Cross reactions between aminoglycoside antibiotics. *Contact Dermatitis* 1988, **18:**314–316.

Ryan TJ: *Management of leg ulcers, 2nd ed.* Oxford: Oxford University Press; 1987.

Scheper RJ, von Blomberg M. Cellular mechanisms in allergic contact dermatitis. In: Rycroft RGJ, Menne T, Frosch PJ, Benezra C, eds. *Contact Dermatitis.* Berlin: Springer-Verlag; 1992:11–24.

Schraibman IG. The bacteriology of leg ulcers. *Phlebology* 1987, **2:**265–270.

Sneddon IB, Church RE. The functions and structure of the skin. In: Sneddon IB, Church RE, eds. *Practical dermatology.* London: Edward Arnold Ltd; 1976.

Stolze R. Dermatitis medicamentosa in eczema of the leg. *Acta Dermato-venereologica* 1966, **46:**54–61.

Struckman J. Compression stockings and their effect on the venous pump, a comparative study. *Phlebology* 1986, **1:**37–45.

Sukanto H, Nater JP, Bleumink E. Influence of topically applied corticosteroids on patch test reactions. *Contact Dermatitis* 1981, **7:**180–185.

Trengrove NJ, Stacey MC, McGechie D, Stingemore N, Mata S. Qualitative bacteriology and chronic leg ulcer healing. In: Cherry GW, Leaper DJ, Lawrence JC, Milward P, eds. *Proceedings of 4th European Conference on Advances in Wound Management.* London: Macmillan; 1994:142–144.

Veitch J. Skin problems in lymphoedema. *Wound Management* 1993, **4**(2):42–45.

Verbov JL. Sensitivity to sodium fusidate. *Contact Dermatitis Newsletter* 1970, **7:**150.

Wilkinson DS, Fregert S, Magnusson B, *et al.* Terminology of contact dermatitis. *Acta Dermato-venereologica* 1970, **50:**287–292.

Wilson CL, Cameron J, Powell SM, Cherry G, Ryan TJ. High incidence of contact dermatitis in leg ulcer patients–implications for management. *Clin Exp Dermatol* 1991, **16:**250–253.

Zaki I, Shall L, Dalziel KL. Bacitracin: a significant sensitiser in leg ulcer patients? *Contact Dermatitis* 1994, **31:**92–94.

FURTHER READING

Books and book chapters

Cameron J. Contact sensitivity and eczema in leg ulcer patients. In: Cullum N, Roe B, eds. *Leg ulcers: nursing management.* Harrow: Scutari Press; 1995:101–112.

Cox NH, Lawrence CM. *Diagnostic picture tests in clinical dermatology.* London: Mosby–Wolfe; 1995.

duVivier A. *Atlas of clinical dermatology.* London: Gower Medical Publishing; 1993.

Holgate ST, Church MK. Eczema and contact dermatitis: pathophysiology. In: Holgate ST, Church MK, eds. *Allergy.* London: Gower Medical Publishing; 1993a:23.1–23.10.

Holgate ST, Church MK. Eczema and contact dermatitis: diagnosis and treatment. In: Holgate ST, Church MK, eds. *Allergy.* London: Gower Medical Publishing; 1993b:24.1–24.10.

Leppard B, Ashton R. *Treatment in dermatology.* Oxford: Radcliffe Medical Press; 1993.

Wilkinson JD, Rycroft RJG. Contact dermatitis. In: Champion RH, Burton JL, Ebling FJG, eds. *Textbook of dermatology.* Oxford: Blackwell Scientific Publications; 1992:611–715.

Patient Education

Health education is based on the assumption that the health of individuals and communities can be affected positively (Coutts & Hardy, 1985). Health education approaches today acknowledge the importance of understanding people's beliefs, values and feelings. It is now recognized that many factors can intervene to modify the translation of beliefs into behaviour, including other competing beliefs and personal priorities (Stahlberg & Frey, 1994). The importance of understanding the social, political and economic context of health behaviour is also acknowledged (Butterfield, 1990).

In the past 3 decades there has been a paradigm shift in health promotion away from a 'top-down' biomedical approach, which assumes that health care professionals know what is 'best' for individuals, towards a human science paradigm, with its emphasis on partnership and empowerment of the individual, which respects the individual's rights to self determination and autonomy. As a consequence of this paradigm shift there are those, such as Lindsey and Hartrick (1996), who challenge the problem-solving approach of the nursing process, suggesting that such a top-down, nurse-focused approach is inconsistent with the concepts of mutuality, egalitarianism and shared responsibility that characterize a client-centred approach to health promotion.

In this chapter, a middle way is adopted which pragmatically acknowledges the value of a systematic approach to assessment, planning, implementation and evaluation of patient education in the healthcare setting, as suggested by Christensen and Kenney (1990) and yet seeks to move beyond this model by viewing clients as their own experts rather than as passive recipients of advice. In relation to patient education, healthcare professionals are regarded as facilitators, rather than as experts whose views should not be challenged. When such a client-centred approach is adopted, the process of patient education moves away from a focus on the individual's deficits towards focusing on and facilitating the client's potential for self help (Orem, 1991; Lindsey & Hartrick, op. cit.).

This chapter begins with a discussion of compliance in the context of client-centred care. This is followed by a brief review of theories of motivation and an overview of how to create a therapeutic environment for learning. The chapter ends with practical advice on patient education in the clinic or home setting, with particular reference to wound care.

COMPLIANCE

Compliance is defined in the Chambers Dictionary (1994), as:
'... *yielding; agreement, complaisance; assent; submission ... the degree to which patients follow medical advice ...*'

Compliance is seen as the extent to which an individual's behaviour coincides with the advice given.

A wide range of factors is now known to affect wound healing (*see* Figure 1.9). Many treatment regimes require active patient co-operation, for example, in the management of leg ulcers patients are encouraged to take regular exercise, to rest by sitting or lying with their ankles above the level of their heart, to eat sensibly and to avoid interfering with their bandages and dressings (*see* Chapter 10). In a study of leg ulcer care in the community, Roe and Luker (1992) found that 82% of community nurses viewed poor patient compliance as a constraint to practice. The assumption is that the advice of healthcare professionals is 'good' for the patient and that non-compliance is likely to delay healing.

In the Wirral study, in which nurses were asked to rate the level of compliance of each individual leg ulcer patient in their care, 56% of patients were regarded as very compliant, 33% as of average compliance and only 11% as poorly compliant (Cullum & Last, 1993). How can these differences in compliance be accounted for?

Research suggests that a number of factors can affect patient compliance:

- The extent to which the patient understands what it is they are to do.
- The patient's perception of the severity of their condition.
- The presence or absence of pain.
- The amount of change required in the patient's lifestyle.
- The actual amount of inconvenience involved, offset against the perceived benefit
- The complexity of the regimen that the patient is asked to undertake.

Encouraging patient compliance may be a very high priority for healthcare professionals, yet there is evidence that patients and healthcare professionals define compliance differently and have different treatment goals in mind (Roberson, 1992). Roberson suggests that patients often define compliance in terms of apparent good health and seek treatment approaches that are manageable and, in their view, effective. They may develop systems of self-management that are suited to their lifestyles, to their beliefs and to their own personal priorities. Roberson (op. cit.) suggests that many people who are labelled as non-compliant by healthcare professionals see themselves as 'doing a pretty good job'.

As Strauss *et al.* (1984) pointed out, people with chronic illnesses of whatever kind normally spend most of their time away from a medical environment and they must rely on their own judgement, wisdom and resources for managing their illness. Yet when patients do take responsibility for managing their illness or disability and choose to use methods that have not been recommended to them by healthcare professionals,or are not seen as conforming to what would be current medical advice, these individuals may be labelled as deviant, unreliable and uncooperative. Their efforts at self-help may be greeted with hostility and other negative sanctions may be applied to encourage them to step back into line with conventional wisdom. It is easy to see how tension can arise between a healthcare professional's desire to respect an individual's autonomy and the belief that compliance with medical advice is necessary for treatment to be successful and to prevent avoidable complications.

Hayes-Bautista (1976) found that modification of a treatment plan was a means whereby patients perceived themselves to be in control of a situation where they were dissatisfied with some aspects of the consequences of the plan originally given to them by professionals. Morison (1996) discovered that families evaluated the suggestions made by healthcare professionals and then based their actions on their own know-ledge, ideas and experiences, as well as those of wider family and friends. Some of the decisions taken by individuals may seem to professionals to be, at the least, unhelpful and sometimes potentially hazardous, yet the individual's failure to follow the advice of healthcare professionals may be a reflection of their low expectations of a successful outcome, should a prescribed treatment be followed, which may be based on a history of repeated failure with treatments tried.

For patients with leg ulcers, who may have been subjected to numerous treatment regimes over the years, it is not difficult to see how these individuals may become disillusioned and come to believe that healthcare professionals have little left in their therapeutic armamentarium that is likely to bring about the desired outcome of a healed ulcer. The patient's belief in the healthcare professional's ability to help them may be of pivotal importance in ensuring that simple advice, which should contribute to a positive therapeutic outcome, is adhered to.

An alternative approach, which involves listening to the client, participatory dialogue, exploration of the issues, identification of priorities, envisioning action and positive change, is discussed later in this chapter. Empowerment involves enhancing the individuals' sense of their own control over the situation (Gibson, 1991) and their own self efficacy. Perceived control and self efficacy are important contributory factors for motivation.

MOTIVATION

Patients with chronic non-healing wounds, such as leg ulcers and pressure sores, frequently appear to be apathetic and many seem to professionals to have little motivation to help themselves. A discussion of motivational theories, such as those of Ford (1992), Weiner (1992) and Skinner (1995), is beyond the scope of this chapter. However, a few points can be briefly made here. Ford (op. cit.) summarizes the requirements for goal achievement and a sense of competence as:

$$\text{Achievement/competence} = \frac{\text{motivation x skill}}{\text{biology}} \quad \text{x} \quad \text{responsive environment}$$

Ford (op. cit.) suggests that achievement is the result of a motivated, skilful and biologically capable person interacting with a responsive environment that facilitates or, at least, does not excessively impede progress towards a goal.

Healthcare professionals have an important role to play in providing a responsive and supportive environment for clients with wounds; this takes full account of the individual's beliefs, capabilities and access to resources. Individuals can be taught certain skills, for example, how correctly to apply compression hosiery (*see* Chapter 10) or how to reposition themselves in a bed or a chair if they are at risk of developing a pressure sore. The equation implies that the individual must have the biological capability to achieve the allotted task. In the case of illness or disability, this can be a major threat to goal achievement. For example, a patient with rheumatoid arthritis may have great difficulty in achieving competence in the application of compression hosiery (*see* Chapter 10). It may be that in such circumstances self-care is not fully possible and the help and training of a carer will be necessary.

Perceived control

In his book *Motivating humans: goals, emotions and personal agency* Ford (op. cit.) suggests that it is not enough to have a goal in mind and the objective skills and circumstances to achieve it. He suggests that people must also believe that they have the capabilities and opportunities needed to achieve their goals. Indeed, he suggests that such beliefs can be more fundamental than the actual skills and circumstances they represent, in the sense that they can motivate people to create opportunities and acquire capabilities that they do not yet possess.

It is the individuals' sense of control and perception of themselves as being capable of influencing the situation that may be of pivotal importance in determining whether or not treatments suggested by healthcare professionals are initiated and sustained (Morison, op. cit.).

Self-efficacy and the expectation of success

According to Bandura (1989) an individual's emotions and behaviour are a reflection of the interaction of a belief in self-efficacy and outcome expectancy. Effective action is most likely, according to Bandura (op. cit), when an individual has a positive judgement of his or her self-efficacy and a high expectation of a positive outcome. An individual who believes that his or her self-efficacy is low and that a positive outcome is unlikely is, by contrast, likely to be apathetic and resigned in a way that is reminiscent of many individuals with chronic wounds.

Part of the art of healing may well be to encourage in clients a sense of their own control which can lead to positive emotions such as optimism. Bandura (op. cit.) suggests that an individual's expectation of success in a given situation may be enough to create that success in that it can lead to prolonged engagement with a difficult task and can blunt the impact of minor failures.

CREATING A THERAPEUTIC ENVIRONMENT FOR LEARNING

Burnard (1995), Heron (1991), Perry (1993), Porritt (1990) and Tschudin (1991), among others, emphasize the importance of empathy between healthcare professionals and their clients as the basis for any therapeutic relationship. Empathy involves understanding clients' feelings about a situation from their perspective and communicating this understanding to them in a way that indicates awareness of and respect for them as individuals and acknowledges their specific needs.

In a therapeutic relationship patients are helped to understand where they are (the here and now) in relation to where they would like to be (the goal) (Figure 8.1). The healthcare professional encourages the client to explore the issues that are of importance to them, to identify priorities and to envisage a positive outcome after exploring a number of alternatives.

Therapeutic, client–centred communication

Effective, client-centred communication is a prerequisite for success. A number of the elements of a therapeutic client-centred approach are summarized in Box 8.1. The healthcare professional fosters reflection, drawing on the client's experiences and engages with the client in a process that reflects the professional's respect for the client as an individual. Actively listening to the client and picking up cues about the issues that are of immediate concern is both an art and a skill that improves with practice. The process of listening in itself communicates an interest in and respect for the individual.

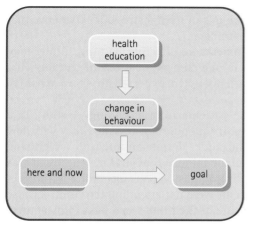

Figure 8.1
Education for change.
(Reproduced from
Morison, 1992.)

Box 8.1.

The basic elements of therapeutic, patient–centred communication (from Morison & Moffatt, 1994)

- Physical closeness: the nurse indicates to the patient a willingness to become involved
- Active listening: nurse communicates interest to the patient non-verbally
- Open-ended comments: the patient is allowed to determine the direction that the interaction should take
- Acknowledgement of the patient's comments as of value
- Restating/seeking clarification: the nurse confirms the accuracy of their own appraisal of the patient's problems, at the same time as demonstrating a desire to understand the problem from the patient's perspective
- Focusing and/or summarizing helps to clarify the most important issues for both parties
- Mutual decision making: deciding on goals and future actions together in a way which emphasizes the patient's involvement

Non-therapeutic communication

Learning is hindered by non-therapeutic communication. Some indicators of non-therapeutic communication are summarized in Box 8.2. They suggest a lack of interest in, and concern for, the individual and run contrary to the spirit of the process of empowerment in which the client, rather than the healthcare professional, is seen as 'centre stage'.

Barriers to effective learning

A number of barriers to effective learning are summarized in Table 8.1. These barriers include environmental factors, negative attitudes of healthcare professionals, physical factors associated with the individual's illness or disability, social factors, psychological factors and, in a practical sense, the form and way in which information is presented.

When the patient is in hospital, hospitalization is in itself a stressful experience that produces a less than ideal environment for learning.

Clinical settings are also often poor environments for effective learning. Clinics may be cramped with several patients being seen in one clinical area. Use of curtains does little to provide the privacy required by patients when expected to share sensitive information.

The clinical environment may deter some patients from attending. A study in a health authority with a very high ethnic minority population revealed that very few patients with leg ulceration were attending the clinics despite an intensive advertising campaign and working with the help of an ethnic minority facilitator. Initially, it was conjectured that a genetic link may be protecting against venous ulceration but further investigation showed that female Muslim patients were not attending the clinic because they feared treatment by male staff and exposure of their limbs in a busy clinical area. In the 'Riverside Project', a minority of patients and relatives admitted to finding it distressing to see other patients' limbs when curtains were inadvertently parted. Elderly

---

Box 8.2.

Indicators of non-therapeutic communication (from Morison and Moffatt, 1994)

- Maintaining a distance or walking away: the nurse suggests that he or she is unwilling to interact with the patient, or regards interaction as a low priority
- Failure to listen: the nurse places his or her needs above those of the patient and demonstrates a lack of interest and concern
- Changing the topic: indicates to the patient that the nurse is in control of what can and cannot be discussed and in so doing negates the concept of mutuality
- Peremptory reassurance: denies validity of patient's fears and feelings
- Being judgemental/giving advice: by imposing his or her own assessment of the situation the nurse is denying the patient's rights to have opinions and to make decisions

gentlemen were particularly concerned. Few were upset by the view of the ulcer but expressed concern about seeing an exposed limb in an elderly lady (Moffatt *et al.* 1992).

Although the clinic may provide effective peer support it does not necessarily provide a good environment for group health education. An attempt to carry out a health-education programme in a leg ulcer clinic using a series of videos in a separate

Table 8.1. Barriers to effective learning	
Environmental factors Noise Lack of privacy Lack of space and time Furniture used to create barriers Frequent disturbances	**Professional attitudes** Autocratic/power-orientated approach Lack of respect for patients Judgemental attitude Setting unrealistic goals Poor awareness of verbal, paraverbal and non-verbal communication Personality clashes Poor knowledge base
Physical factors Pain Tiredness General ill health Poor hearing Poor eyesight Hunger Thirst	**Social factors** Cultural taboos Poor housing Family commitments Loneliness Poverty Stigma Patient perceives professionals too busy Lacks ability to articulate questions Perceives professional as helper, not teacher
Psychological factors Anxiety Depression Apathy Lack of motivation Psychological dependency Regression Denial Fear Anger Hostility Embarrassment Low self-esteem Previous negative experiences Lack of trust Limited cognitive ability Poor memory Fear of prognosis	**Presentation of information** Inappropriate method of delivery Inappropriate level of information Too much information Poor sequencing of important messages Inappropriate portrayal of patient group Use of technical terms or jargon Wrong size print Inappropriate use of humour or cartoons

waiting room was found by Moffatt to be completely unsuccessful (personal communication). The patients did not watch the videos, preferring to chat with each other and drink tea. Attempts to organize peer support in a clinic situated within a wealthy area of London were similarly thwarted. Patients neither wanted nor perceived themselves as requiring such intervention, preferring to sit alone and not to communicate with other patients.

THE PATIENT EDUCATION PROCESS

As discussed in the introduction, the adoption of a client-centred approach to health promotion and patient education and the empowerment of the individual challenges the nature of the relationship between healthcare professional and clients. In essence, Labonte (1989) suggests that professionals need to learn to surrender their 'service provider need to control'.

Lindsey and Hartrick (op. cit.) pointed out the value-laden nature of the labels given to the four main phases of the nursing process: assessment, planning, implementation and evaluation, each of which implies action being taken by the nurse on behalf of the client. Hartrick *et al.* (1994) suggested an alternative framework:

- Listening to the client.
- Participatory dialogue.
- Pattern recognition.
- Envisioning action and positive change.

The professional is concerned with understanding the nature of the experience (e.g. of living with a leg ulcer or a pressure sore) from the individual's perspective and discovering how the patients manage the condition for themselves. Through a dialogue, the client is encouraged to explore issues and to become aware of factors that may be affecting his or her health in general and the specific condition which has brought him or her to the healthcare professional, which may be a chronic wound.

Through a process of critical reflection, the client is encouraged to identify patterns of behaviour which may be facilitating or hindering the potential for healing. During this process the client is encouraged to express not only his or her understanding of the situation, in the cognitive sense, but also his or her feelings about it.

The final process of envisioning action and positive change is about enabling the individual to identify priorities for action, to explore alternatives and to make informed health-related choices. Lindsey and Hartrick (op. cit.) described this not so much as a problem-solving process but rather a problem-posing process, as the client and healthcare professional move away from focusing on the client's deficits to focusing on the client's potential. This is a collaborative process in which the agenda is determined by the client. The nurse is clearly in a facilitative rather than an autocratic role. Such a process enhances the individual's sense of control and self-efficacy and in this sense can be a very powerful determinant of motivation.

Determining the most suitable strategy or strategies in a particular situation

In the domain of wound care, counselling may be a very important element. In her book *Helping the client: a creative practical guide* Heron (op. cit.) describes six major categories of counselling interventions:

1. Prescriptive intervention: seeks to direct the behaviour of the client.
2. Informative intervention: seeks to impart knowledge, information and meaning.
3. Confronting intervention: seeks to raise the client's consciousness of some limiting attitude or behaviour.
4. Cathartic intervention: seeks to enable the client to discharge pent-up emotions such as grief, fear and anger.
5. Catalytic intervention: seeks to elicit self-directed learning and problem solving in the client.
6. Supportive intervention: seeks to affirm the worth of the client as a person.

Although acknowledging the central importance of a client-centred approach, Heron (op. cit.) suggested that a number of different strategies may be required in particular situations. Of the interventions listed, the first three are clearly authoritative, with the practitioner taking some responsibility for or on behalf of the client, whereas the second three are described as facilitative because the practitioner is seeking to enable clients to become more autonomous in the ways described. Heron (op. cit) suggested that no one way is intrinsically better than another in all circumstances. The needs of the client, the nature of the client–practitioner relationship and the focus of the intervention will determine which types of intervention are likely to be of most value in a particular situation.

Imparting specific information and teaching practical skills

In the case of wound care there are many situations when it may be helpful to impart specific knowledge to the individual. By way of example, the individual who is diabetic and has developed a foot ulcer may need specific advice on foot care, diet and how to monitor his or her blood-sugar levels.

When specific information needs to be imparted, it can be very helpful to develop a teaching plan based on the perceived needs of the individual. Implementation involves using non-technical language that the patient can understand, at an appropriate time and in an appropriate place, bearing in mind the many barriers to effective learning (summarized in Box 8.2 and Table 8.1).

Basic principles of imparting information include the following:

- Organizing the material in a logical framework.
- Working from the known to the unknown.
- Giving the most important information first and giving this to the patient in a written form.
- Giving specific rather than general advice, which is relevant to the patient's particular situation.
- Maximizing patient involvement.
- Using a variety of teaching methods even within the same session.

- Continually ensuring the relevance of the material to the individual's needs by means of a participatory dialogue.
- Verifying at every stage that the teaching is understood.

Many patients with chronic wounds are elderly. It is important to be aware that short-term memory loss is common in elderly people and will affect their ability to remember information given to them and to maintain newly learned behaviour. Elderly people may require more time to learn new skills and although accuracy does not necessarily diminish, their time to learn may be rather slower. Rogers (1977) noted a number of issues associated with the elderly learner. These included a fear of looking foolish and a belief that they were too old to learn new information. Additionally, the patient's social, economic and cultural background may affect communication and the learning process.

It is important to recognize the fact that some patients may not at first wish to take an active part in the management of their wounds and they may not wish to receive information. Roe *et al.* (1995) found that 60% of leg ulcer patients did not want further information. This conflicts with many other chronic conditions for which there is a high demand for information (Cartwright, 1964).

If a patient is being taught a specific practical skill, for example, how to put on compression hosiery (*see* Chapter 10), then supervised practice will be required until the patient is and feels safely competent. Many elderly and infirm patients rely on help from relatives, friends and neighbours and they too should be actively involved in the teaching sessions.

Identifying those who are the principal carers and including them in any teaching sessions and in care planning is of fundamental importance in ensuring the success of a more directive teaching programme.

CONCLUSION

Ultimately, the success of patient education depends not on the extent to which the client adheres to the advice of healthcare professionals but on the extent to which the client is enabled to live life according to his or her own preferred lifestyle, while not unduly jeopardizing the chances that his or her wound will heal.

For many people with a chronic wound the problem may not resolve quickly. The healthcare professional may therefore require considerable patience, as well as empathy, in what may prove to be a long haul to complete healing. In some cases, as discussed in Chapter 11, the goal of healing may not be a realistic one and issues relating to quality of life may assume paramount importance. As described in Chapter 13, it is only in recent years that research has begun to explore the effect of wounds on the individual's quality of life (Franks *et al.* 1994). Clear evidence is presented in Chapter 13 to suggest that patients' experience of pain in association with chronic wounds has been greatly under-estimated by healthcare professionals and pain can hinder the learning process.

There is evidence to suggest that, far from creating a therapeutic environment, some healthcare professionals blame carers when chronic wounds, such as pressure sores, develop. A study involving the wives of patients with severe pressure sores revealed the way in which some wives perceived themselves as being blamed for causing the sores, in spite of having been provided with social and healthcare support. On admission of her husband to hospital, one wife reported that the surgeon had asked why she had not arranged for her husband to be admitted before and suggested that her negligence could lead to his death (Baharestani, 1996). Although such a professional reaction is clearly lacking in empathy it also highlights that, as a professional, it is all too easy to fail to recognize the differences in the knowledge of the professional and of lay people, whether they be patients or carers.

Clients are likely to enter into clinical relationships with preconceived ideas about the causes of their wounds and how to treat them. In many cases, these views may be at variance with the views of professionals. It is suggested that the difference between lay and professional viewpoints can lead to failures of intervention, especially when individuals regard the treatment suggestions of healthcare professionals to be ill-conceived. Failure of professionals to assess and take cognizance of the responsiveness, or otherwise, of the social environment in which their treatments are to be conducted may also lead to treatment failure, as discussed in Chapter 4. Understanding the individual's perspective enables a dialogue to be pursued in which account is taken of the reality of the individual's circumstances, including their beliefs, capabilities and access to resources. Such communication demonstrates a respect for the individual's rights to self-determination.

SELF-ASSESSMENT QUESTIONS AND ACTIVITIES

Case study

Mr Allan was referred to a hospital outpatient clinic with a leg ulcer that had been present for 18 years. His manner towards staff was described by them as both aggressive and demanding and some staff felt intimidated by the fact that he carried a knife in his back pocket. Mr Allan's aggressive outbursts led staff to request that another member of staff be present during dressing changes. Mr Allan resented this situation.

During discussion with the one nurse who seemed to have developed a close relationship with Mr Allan, it transpired that he felt very angry about the failures of many previous professional interventions. On further questioning, Mr Allan expressed doubts that his ulcer would ever heal.

He also had a number of social problems, including problems with a failing marriage. He said that he would like to look after the wound for himself but in the meantime, he was prepared to accept some supervision.

1. Identify the barriers to effective learning noted in the above example. You may like to refer to Table 8.1 as a guide.

2. Imagine that you are the manager responsible for this outpatient clinic. Outline some of the strategies that you might adopt to promote a therapeutic environment for Mr Allan, while at the same time addressing the issues of concern for many of the staff. Would you consider involving any other agencies, if so which ones?

3. What information would you consider it to be essential to impart to Mr Allan on his first visit to the outpatient clinic (see also Chapter 10). What strategies might you adopt to impart this information?

REFERENCES

Baharestani M. The lived experience of wives caring for their frail homebound elderly husbands with pressure ulcers: a phenomenological investigation (Abstract). *Ninth Annual Symposium on Advanced Wound Care*. Atlanta GA: Health Management Publications; 1996.

Bandura A. Human agency in social cognitive theory. *Am Psychol* 1989, **44**(9):1175–1184.

Burnard P. *Counselling*. Oxford: Butterworth-Heinemann; 1995.

Butterfield PG. Thinking upstream: nurturing a conceptual understanding of the societal context of health behaviour. *Adv Nurs Sci* 1990, **12**(2):1–8.

Cartwright A. *Human relations and hospital care*. London: Routledge and Kegan Paul; 1964.

Christensen PJ, Kenney JW. *The nursing process: application of conceptual models, 3rd ed*. Toronto: C V Mosby; 1990.

Coutts LC, Hardy LK. *Teaching for health: the nurse as health educator*. Edinburgh: Churchill Livingstone; 1985.

Cullum NA, Last S. The prevalence, characteristics and management of leg ulcers in a UK community. *2nd European Conference on Advances in Wound Management*. Harrogate; 1993. In: Cullum N, Roe B, eds. *Leg ulcers: nursing management*. London: Scutari Press; 1995.

Ford ME. *Motivating humans: goals, emotions, and personal agency beliefs*. London: Sage; 1992.

Franks PJ, Moffatt CJ, Connolly M, *et al*. Community leg ulcer clinics: effect on quality of life. *Phlebology* 1994, **9**:83–86.

Gibson CH. A concept analysis of empowerment. *J Adv Nurs* 1991, **16**:354–361.

Hartrick G, Lindsey E, Hills M. Family nursing assessment: meeting the challenge of health promotion. *J Adv Nurs* 1994, **20**:85–91.

Hayes-Bautista DE. Modifying the treatment: patient compliance, patient control and medical care. *Soc Sci Med* 1976, **10**:233–238. In: Roberson MHB. The meaning of compliance: patient perspectives. *Qual Health Res* 1992, **2**(1):7–26.

Heron J. *Helping the client: a creative practical guide*. London: Sage Publications; 1991.

Labonte R. Community and professional empowerment., *Can Nurse* 1989, **85**(3):23–28. In: Lindsey E, Hartrick G. Health–promoting nursing practice: the demise of the nursing process? *J Adv Nurs* 1996, **23**:106–112.

Lindsey E, Hartrick G. Health–promoting nursing practice: the demise of the nursing process? *J Adv Nurs* 1996, **23**:106–112.

Moffatt C, Franks PJ, Oldroyd M, *et al*. Community clinics for leg ulcers and impact on healing. *BMJ* 1992, **305**:1389–1392.

Morison MJ. *Family perspectives on bed wetting in young people*. Aldershot: Avebury; 1996.

Morison MJ: A colour guide to the nursing management of wounds. London: Mosby; 1992.

Morison MJ, Moffatt, CM: A colour guide to the assessment and management of leg ulcers. London: Mosby, 1994.

Orem DE. *Nursing: concepts of practice*. St Louis: Mosby Year Book; 1991.

Perry R. Empathy – still at the heart of therapy: the interplay of context and empathy. *Aust NZ J Fam Therapy* 1993, **14**(2):63–74.

Porritt L. *Interaction strategies: an introduction for health professionals, 2nd ed*. Edinburgh: Churchill Livingstone; 1990.

Roberson MHB. The meaning of compliance: patient perspectives. *Qual Health Res* 1992, **2**(1):7–26.

Roe B, Cullum N. The management of leg ulcers: current nursing practice. In: Cullum N, Roe B, eds. *Leg ulcers: nursing management*. London: Scutari Press; 1995:113–124.

Roe B, Cullum N, Hamer C. Patients' perceptions of chronic leg ulceration. In: Cullum N, Roe B, eds. *Leg ulcers: nursing management*. London: Scutari Press; 1995:125–134.

Roe BH, Luker KA. *Study of the nursing management of patients with leg ulcers in the community: report to Mersey Regional Health Authority*, Liverpool: Department of Nursing, University of Liverpool; 1992. In: Cullum N, Roe B, eds. *Leg ulcers: nursing management.* London: Scutari Press; 1995

Rogers J. *Adult learning, 2nd ed.* Milton Keynes: The Open University Press; 1977.

Skinner EA. *Perceived control and motivation: stress, coping, and competence.* London: Sage; 1995.

Stahlberg D, Frey D. Attitudes I: structure, measurement and functions. In Hewstone M, Stroebe W, Codol JP, Stephenson GM, eds. *Introduction to social psychology.* Oxford: Blackwell; 1994:142–166.

Strauss A, Corbin J, Fagerhaugh S, *et al. Chronic illness and the quality of life, 2nd ed.* St Louis: Mosby; 1984.

Tschudin V. *Counselling skills for nurses, 3rd ed.* London: Bailliere Tindall; 1991.

Weiner B. *Human motivation: metaphors, theories and research.* London: Sage; 1992.

FURTHER READING

Burnard P. *Counselling.* Oxford, 1995, Butterworth–Heinemann.

Dryden G, Voss J. *The learning revolution.* Aylesbury: Accelerated Learning Systems; 1994.

Ewles L, Simnett I. *Promoting health: a practical guide,* 3rd ed. London: Scutari; 1995.

Gibson CH. A concept analysis of empowerment. *J Adv Nurs* 1991, 16:354–361.

Lorig K. *Common-sense patient education: a practical approach,* 2nd ed. Newbury Park CA: Sage; 1996.

Pender NJ. *Health promotion in nursing practice,* 3rd ed. Norwalk, USA: Appleton and Lange; 1996.

Porritt L. *Interaction strategies: an introduction for health professionals,* 2nd ed. Edinburgh: Churchill Livingstone; 1990.

Rankin SH, Stallings KD. *Patient education: issues, principles, practice,* 3rd ed. Philadelphia: Lippincott; 1995.

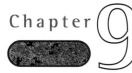
Chapter 9

Pressure Sores

Pressure sores are defined as 'a lesion on any skin surface that occurs as a result of pressure and includes reactive hyperaemia as well as blistered, broken or necrotic skin' (Parish *et al.* 1983). They are complex lesions of the skin and underlying structures and vary considerably in size and severity. Their complexity requires an individualized and interactive approach to decision making and care delivery and this chapter attempts to link the extensive literature on pressure sores to practice by outlining important principles for practice. There is a focus on the interactive decision-making processes involved in assessment, planning and evaluation. Areas of the literature presented include pressure sore pathophysiology, epidemiology and aetiology and are practically applied to the component parts of the nursing process: assessment, planning, care delivery and evaluation.

PRINCIPLES OF PATIENT ASSESSMENT AND CARE DELIVERY

The purpose of baseline nursing assessment is to identify both actual and potential problems which then inform individualized planning and delivery of care. Within the context of pressure sore prevention and management, baseline assessment is commonly associated with the term 'risk assessment'. The focus of risk assessment has been toward the development and use of risk calculators which are in widespread use and provide the basis of pressure sore prevention policies (Waterlow, 1985; Millward, 1990; Watts & Clark, 1993). Such tools, however, are limited in relation to their reliability and validity (Clark & Farrer, 1992; Bridel 1993a; Deeks, 1996) and their use underplays the value of clinical observations as the basis for individual care delivery.

Therefore, within the context of this chapter, risk assessment is used as a general term that includes consideration of many variables including skin assessment, general condition, relevant history and calculation of risk (*see* Box 9.1). There is an abundance of literature to support the assessment process enabling informed decision making regarding initial and ongoing care delivery. The following sections aim to illustrate clearly the application of research and theory to practice.

SKIN ASSESSMENT: FUNDAMENTAL PRINCIPLES

It is important to recognize that skin assessment is a key feature of this assessment process. A risk calculator is meaningless, for example, if a patient has an existing pressure sore. The patient has an actual problem that requires treatment and that treatment will depend on the severity of the sore and the circumstances of the individual.

The skin provides a wide range of signs and symptoms that indicate both potential

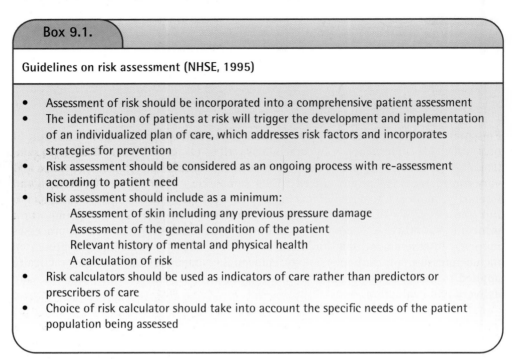

Box 9.1.

Guidelines on risk assessment (NHSE, 1995)

- Assessment of risk should be incorporated into a comprehensive patient assessment
- The identification of patients at risk will trigger the development and implementation of an individualized plan of care, which addresses risk factors and incorporates strategies for prevention
- Risk assessment should be considered as an ongoing process with re-assessment according to patient need
- Risk assessment should include as a minimum:
    Assessment of skin including any previous pressure damage
    Assessment of the general condition of the patient
    Relevant history of mental and physical health
    A calculation of risk
- Risk calculators should be used as indicators of care rather than predictors or prescribers of care
- Choice of risk calculator should take into account the specific needs of the patient population being assessed

and actual problems. It is important to recognize the clinical significance of the indicators of risk requiring a nursing response. Indeed, recent descriptive studies highlight the role of skin observation in the delivery of individualized repositioning schedules (Banks & Bridel, 1995).

Knowledge of the basic anatomical structures and pathological processes involved in the development of pressure sores is essential for interpretation of the clinical signs and symptoms presented. This section highlights characteristics of the skin that both protect and are vulnerable to external forces. It also provides a detailed account of pressure sore pathology and the issues relevant to the interpretation and application of pathophysiological knowledge to practical assessment.

Anatomy and pathology

The tissues involved in pressure sore development are the skin, subcutaneous fat, deep fascia, muscle and bone. These are described in more detail in Chapter 7 and illustrated in Figures 7.1 and 7.2. Key features of the skin and underlying tissue are important in providing protection against external forces:
- Epidermis stratum corneum provides a physical barrier desmosomes and tonofibrils provide strength.
- Dermis dermal papillae provide strength, collagen and elastin matrix buffers external pressure.
- Subcutaneous fat provides mobility and padding (Torrance, 1983).

Despite these characteristics pressure sores do develop mainly as a result of disruption to the vascular network of arteries, arterioles and capillaries. Various parts of the vascular system are vulnerable to occlusion and damage:

- Arteries: arteries are prone to angulation (and therefore occlusion) as they pierce the deep fascia.
- Arterioles: subcutaneous fat has poor tolerance to shearing forces and offers little protection to the arterioles. Subcutaneous fat is poorly vascularized and damage to a small number of arterioles will lead to a large area of fat necrosis.
- Capillaries: capillary walls are fragile and vulnerable to damage and their low intravascular pressure offers little resistance to external load (Bridel, 1993b).

The most comprehensive research, exploring the pathophysiology of pressure sore development is that of Barton and Barton (1981) who examined tissue changes in mice using light and electron microscopy. They determined that pressure sores develop as a result of two processes:

1. Occlusion of blood vessels by external pressure.
2. Endothelial damage of arterioles and the microcirculation caused by the application of disruptive and shearing forces (Barton & Barton, op. cit.).

These two processes, which often occur concurrently, initiate a series of pathophysiological events that may or may not result in tissue damage and the appearance of a pressure sore.

Occlusion

Occlusion of blood vessels results in anoxia and a build up of metabolites. Release of pressure produces a large and sudden increase in blood flow as the anoxia and metabolites act on precapillary sphincters and metarterioles. The increase in blood flow may reach 30 times its resting value (Lamb *et al.*, 1980) and the bright red flush so produced is known as reactive hyperaemia. This is a normal physiological response and is seen commonly in everyday life (after sitting on a chair, for example). This hyperaemic reaction is proportional to the duration of the occlusion and generally lasts 50–75% of the occlusion time (Lewis & Grant, 1925; Goldblatt, 1925).

Krouskop *et al.* (1978) suggested that if the lymphatic vessels of the dependent tissue are intact and excess interstitial fluid, resulting from the acute rise in capillary flow, is removed then permanent tissue changes will not progress. It is hypothesized that tissue changes do progress if external load causes damage to lymphatic vessels or significant squeeze-out of interstitial fluid (Krouskop, 1983) (Figure 9.1).

Subsequent interstitial oedema interferes with metabolite exchange, causes distortion and thickening of tissues compressed between bone and the support surface and further increases the vulnerability of the skin (Torrance, op. cit.). Progressive loss of tissue occurs if the application of pressure is not relieved, the wound extending inward. This is described as a Type 1 pressure sore by Barton and Barton (op. cit.).

Endothelial damage

Endothelial damage of arterioles and the microcirculation occurs as a result of the application of disruptive and shearing forces to the skin and subcutaneous tissues on areas of the body not normally exposed to such forces. Distortion of the blood vessels disrupts endothelial cells and activates intrinsic clotting mechanisms (*see* Figure 1.4). Platelets

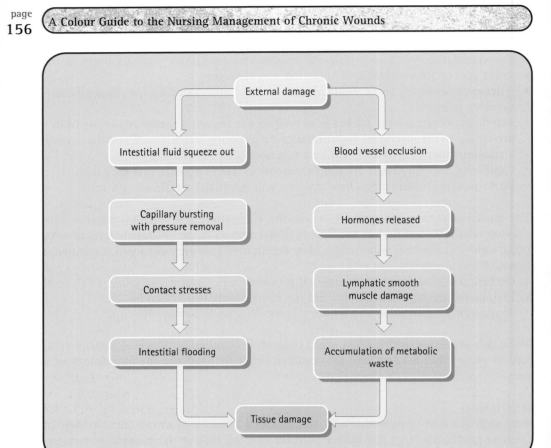

Figure 9.1　Integrated model of tissue damage. (Reproduced from Krouskop, 1983.)

aggregate and occlude the affected vessels causing ischaemic necrosis of dependent tissues. The epidermis may remain intact for a number of days before it sloughs off to reveal the extent of the tissue damage beneath (Barton & Barton, op. cit.). This is described as a Type 2 pressure sore by Barton and Barton (op. cit.) and on presentation such a pressure sore would be classified as a full-thickness sore.

SKIN ASSESSMENT IN PRACTICE

In determining actual and potential problems some definition of the term 'pressure sore' is required. The Clinical Practice Guidelines on the Prevention and Management of Pressure Sores (NHSE, 1995) include a clear recommendation for the recording of pressure sores. They state 'For the purposes of clinical practice the minimum data to be recorded concerning the pressure sore should include the following:

- Classification.
- Site.
- Clinical description (this may include size, colour, depth, exudate, odour and so on.)'

The inclusion of three elements for documentation purposes illustrates the complicated nature of pressure sore description and the variety of factors that inform a clinical decision relating to treatment. From a practical nursing perspective it is necessary to distinguish between actual and potential problems and it may be useful to consider a pressure sore as a physical break in the skin that is related but different to changes in the appearance of the skin (which may or may not be reversible). The former indicates an actual problem, the latter a potential problem. Both require a nursing response.

This reflects debate within the literature regarding the classification of pressure sores and the need to distinguish between intact and broken skin (Lyder, 1991; Reid & Morison, 1994), but there is clear recognition that external force generates a variety of other skin changes that are clinically important (Lyder, op. cit.; Lowthian, 1994; Reid & Morison, op. cit.).

Skin changes

Skin changes may vary from a normal hyperaemic response of short duration (e.g. 5 minutes) to persistent non-blanching discolouration with localized swelling, heat and induration (Lyder, op. cit.; Lowthian, op. cit.). In undertaking clinical assessment of the skin, it is important to relate the pathophysiological events to their visual appearance and consider whether the response observed is normal or abnormal. This enables the clinical significance of signs and symptoms to be determined. Such consideration can only be undertaken within the clinical environment and requires consideration of:

- Circumstances associated with the appearance of the hyperaemic response.
- Duration of the response.
- Presence of blanching under light finger pressure.

For example, the observation of a reddened area on a usually mobile patient who has woken from sleep is unlikely to have any clinical importance. A reddened area observed when repositioning an immobile patient should prompt further observation, including signs of blanching and duration of the reactive hyperaemic response.

Other skin changes described in the literature relate directly to pathology. For example, local oedema, induration, heat, non-blanching hyperaemia, blue, purple or black discolouration (Shea, 1975; Parish *et al.* op.cit.; Lowthian, 1987; Lyder, op. cit.; Reid & Morison, op. cit.). Such signs and symptoms may or may not lead to subsequent loss of the epidermis (Banks & Bridel, op. cit.) but they are clearly linked to the pathology of pressure sore development, indicating lymphatic involvement and capillary disruption (Krouskop, op. cit.). Such changes are clinically important and should prompt relief of pressure (position change and equipment provision).

Although considered clinically important, there is debate regarding the inclusion of these observations within pressure sore classification systems (Lyder, op. cit; Hitch, 1995). Debate seems to focus on the classification of pressure sores for research and audit purposes and difficulties in achieving good inter-rater reliability and validity of definition (Lyder, op. cit.; Healey, 1996).

From a practice perspective, regardless of the classification system used, it is essential that the record of care provides clear descriptions of the skin changes observed and such evidence should direct and support individual patient care.

Classification of pressure sores

A number of authors developed classification systems (Shea, op. cit.; Barton & Barton, op. cit.; Forrest, 1980; David *et al.* 1983; Torrance, op. cit.; IAET, 1987; Lowthian, op. cit.; Lyder, op. cit.; AHCPR, 1992; DoH, 1993; Reid & Morison, op. cit.). In early publications they were developed for research and audit purposes (David *et al.* op. cit.) but are now used within the practice setting as part of prevention policies and associated clinical audit.

The purposes of such tools for practice include:
- Multidisciplinary review (evaluation) of progress.
- Application of clinical trials to practice.
- Development of guidelines for pressure relief.
- Audit of practice.
- Understanding of healing process.

A review of the classification systems reveals that with the exceptions of Barton and Barton (op. cit.) and Forrest (op. cit.), who based their classifications on pressure sore pathology, other authors categorized pressure sores on the basis of clinical appearance and tissue layer affected. The terms 'Grade' and 'Stage' are interchangeable and wound characteristics graded from 2–4 or 5 are similar in category and description with specification of layers of the skin and subcutaneous tissues. Variation is dependent on the grade or stage 1 categorization and whether skin changes are included or excluded.

Categories including the descriptors superficial, partial-thickness and full-thickness wounds are also found within these classifications (IAET, op. cit.; Lowthian, op. cit.; AHCPR, op. cit.; DoH, op. cit.; Reid & Morison, op. cit.). These generally classify breaks in the epidermis or dermis as superficial or partial-thickness wounds and those involving the subcutaneous fat and any tissue beneath as full-thickness wounds. From a practice perspective, classification systems do have limitations because agreement may be poor (Healey, 1995). What is essential is a clear baseline description enabling meaningful care planning and evaluation at periodic intervals; three important categories can be identified for the purposes of assessment, planning and delivery of care:
1. Skin changes that indicate a potential problem and require active preventative care.
2. The presence of a superficial pressure sore involving the epidermis or dermis which heals by regeneration of epithelial cells with a restoration of normal function.
3. The presence of a partial or full-thickness wound extending through the dermis and underlying subcutaneous tissues which heals by granulation.

Key points to consider in relation to skin assessment are summarized in Box 9.2.

Box 9.2.

Skin assessment in practice: key points

- Skin assessment and interpretation of signs and symptoms is the basis of pressure sore prevention and treatment
- External force generates a variety of skin changes that are clinically important, these include:

  Reactive hyperaemia: blanching or non-blanching

  Local oedema

  Heat

  Induration

  Blue, purple or black discolouration
- It is important at clinical level to distinguish between a normal and abnormal skin response
- Documentation of skin changes supports clinical decisions
- In clinical practice a classification system should distinguish between:

  Intact and broken skin

  Superficial and partial or full-thickness wounds

RISK ASSESSMENT: FUNDAMENTAL PRINCIPLES

In conjunction with skin assessment, there are a variety of factors that require particular consideration in the planning of services for patients. Such factors have been determined by a large body of evidence derived from speciality led research exploring both the epidemiology and aetiology of pressure sore development.

Epidemiology

Epidemiology studies are based on the principle that whole populations or representative samples are considered, rather than individuals. Epidemiological research can be broadly divided into prevalence and incidence studies. Prevalence is a measure of the number of people with a disease in a defined population either within a certain time (period prevalence) or at a specific point in time (point prevalence) (Donaldson & Donaldson, 1985). It is a useful indicator of the extent of chronic, long-lived disease and disability.

Incidence is the proportion of individuals who first present with a given problem during a defined period of time in relation to the local population at risk (Minotti, 1978). It is a useful measure of the extent of burden created by short-lived or quickly recoverable diseases or problems.

Prevalence studies have been useful in indicating the extent of the problem within hospital and community settings at local, regional and international levels (Barbenel *et al.* 1977, David *et al.* op. cit., O'Dea, 1993; O'Dea, 1995) and indicate that a large number of hospital and community-based patients have pressure sores.

Early prevalence studies revealed that almost all pressure sores occur below the waist with particularly vulnerable areas being the sacrum, buttocks and heels (Nyquist & Hawthorn, 1987; David *et al.* op. cit.). These areas are not adapted to weight-bearing (Braden & Bergstrom, 1987) and are not normally exposed to unrelieved pressure (Exton-Smith & Sherwin, 1961). These data support observations made in practice and are an example of research that simply reinforces what has been appreciated for years of practice.

Factors that may predispose to pressure sore development, such as age, mobility and incontinence, are identified when pressure sore positive and pressure sore negative groups are compared (Barbenel *et al.* 1977; Barbenel *et al.* 1980; Waterlow, 1988). Investigators also suggest that no one single causative factor exists (Bridel, 1993c).

Incidence studies identify the proportion of individuals who first present with a pressure sore and most commonly involve the study of specific patient groups. Groups sampled include patients in the following categories: acute and long-stay elderly, elective surgical, chronic medical, intensive care, paraplegic, nursing home and fractured neck of femur (Norton *et al.* 1962; Versluysen, 1986; Clark & Watts, 1994; Kemp *et al.* 1990; Stotts, 1988; Clough, 1994; Berlowitz & Wilking, 1989; Bergstrom & Braden, 1992; Ek *et al.* 1991). These studies yield important information both from an epidemiological and aetiological point of view.

The reported incidence of pressure sores ranges from 4.6% to 66%, although most fall within the range of 10–30%. However, from an epidemiological perspective, grade distribution rather than the number of pressure sores is of the most interest. Studies that have sampled a broad range of age groups report that reactive hyperaemia and superficial sores account for more than 95% of all sores (Stotts, op. cit., Kemp op. cit.; Clark & Watts, op. cit.). This perhaps supports further the earlier debate relating to the role of skin assessment and the need to undertake detailed skin assessment with an emphasis on the recognition of skin changes (Lowthian, op. cit.; Banks & Bridel, op. cit.).

Box 9.3.

Factors identified by epidemiological study

- Pressure damage is both reversible and progressive in nature
- For the majority, pressure sores are a short-lived event
- Almost all pressure sores occur below the waist with particularly vulnerable areas being the sacrum, buttocks and heels
- Factors including immobility, age and incontinence are associated with pressure sore development
- Patients with a pressure sore require active prevention
- A high proportion of pressure sores develop within the first 2 weeks after admission
- Increasing length of stay increases the likelihood of sore development

It is worth noting that incidence studies indicate that a high proportion of pressure sores develop in the first 2 weeks after admission to hospital (Stotts, op. cit.; Norton *et al.* op. cit.; Versluysen, op. cit.), but that increasing length of stay increases the likelihood of sore development, although this is related to relative risk (Norton *et al.* op. cit.; Stotts, op. cit.). This is clearly an important consideration in determining the priority given to pressure area care and supports the need for both early and continued assessment.

Broad conclusions drawn from epidemiological study that are directly relevant to practice are summarized in Box 9.3.

Aetiology

Critical determinants of pressure sore development have been classified by Braden and Bergstrom (op. cit.) as being the intensity and duration of pressure and the tolerance of skin to pressure. However, although categorizing factors in this way is useful, it is essential to remember that it is the interaction between the tolerance of the skin and pressure that determines skin response and pressure sore development.

Intensity and duration of pressure

Research in this area is broadly divided into studies concerned with capillary pressure, the application of uniform pressure and the application of localized pressure. The literature highlights the individual nature of the response to external pressure because of variations in the tolerance of the skin as well as providing evidence that the nature of the applied force will have great bearing on outcome. Important considerations in the intensity of pressure and its effect on capillary blood flow include:

- Autoregulatory response. When external pressure is applied to the skin an autoregulation process allows internal capillary pressures to rise correspondingly (Landis, 1993; Bader, 1990).

  It appears that this autoregulation process only breaks down, in individuals with normal circulation, when external pressure exceeds diastolic pressure (Holstein *et al.* 1979). However, in patients with increased susceptibility, occlusion has been reported when pressures of less than 20 mmHg are applied (Bennett & Lee, 1985) and Bader (op. cit.) illustrated an impaired autoregulatory response, shown by limited tissue recovery and decreasing oxygen saturation with each subsequent load application.

- Collagen. It is hypothesized that collagen, which constitutes 99% of dry-weight dermis, buffers external pressure and protects and prevents capillary occlusion. It appears that collagen prevents disruption to the microcirculation by buffering the interstitial fluid from external load, thereby maintaining the balance of hydrostatic and osmotic pressures (Reddy *et al.* 1975; Krouskop, op. cit.).

  It is known that as collagen is removed from tissue, a larger fraction of an externally applied load is transmitted to interstitial fluids which leave the pressurized area (Reddy et al. op. cit.) and, if sufficient, allows cell-to-cell contact and capillary bursting (Figure 9.1). The collagen content of the skin alters with disease and age and therefore the protective capacity of the dermis will vary from individual to individual.

- Pressure application. The situation is further complicated by variations in the application of a given load. Research suggests that an external pressure applied in a uniform or enveloping manner has little if any long-term effect on tissue (Bliss, 1993, Branemark, 1976; Husain 1953). It is the effect of the application of a local or point-pressure on the skin which is of interest in pressure sore aetiology.

- Shear forces. The effect of shear on human skin has been reported by Bennett and Lee (op. cit.). Using a sensor head incorporating four sensors (two pressure, one shear and one blood flow plethysmograph), the authors demonstrated that the primary force generating mechanical occlusion is pressure but that shear plays an important contributory role. Elderly and paraplegic individuals were found to experience greater shear forces and reductions in blood flow than normal people at the same pressure values. This observation provides further evidence of the individual nature of the load–response relationship.

As the number of factors involved in determining capillary occlusion are varied and context-specific, it is not possible to identify a universal pressure threshold above which pressure damage will occur; the literature illustrates the individual nature of the skin response to pressure (Bridel, 1993b). In relation to the duration of pressure applied, time is only important if occlusion has occurred and the literature clearly illustrates that once above a critical pressure and critical time value, the extent of the tissue damage is determined by the time of pressure application and not the intensity (Husain, op cit.; Brooks & Duncan, 1940).

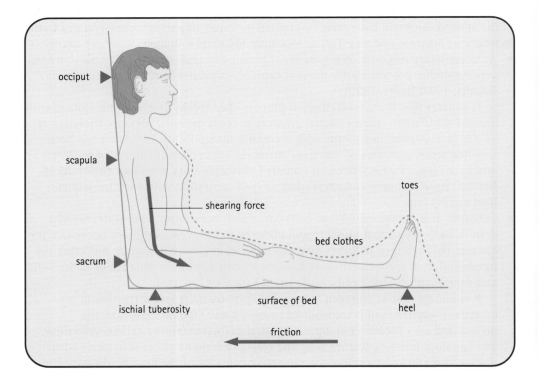

Figure 9.2 Shearing forces, friction and pressure in a semi-recumbent patient (▲ = pressure points). (Reproduced from Morison, 1992.)

Key points highlighted by research relating to the intensity and duration of the pressure required for pressure sore development are summarized in Box 9.4.

Tolerance of the skin

Factors affecting tissue tolerance can be subdivided into extrinsic and intrinsic factors (Braden & Bergstom, op. cit.). Extrinsic factors affect tissue tolerance by impinging on the surface of the skin and include exposure to moisture, irritants and friction. They have received little research interest and their relationship with pressure sore aetiology is not clear. Intrinsic factors affect the ability of the skin and supporting structures to respond to pressure and shear forces by influencing sensation, perception and response mechanisms and altering the structural constituents and perfusion of tissue. The influence of these factors is now discussed.

Extrinsic factors

Moisture. The contribution of moisture is linked to pressure sore development in numerous aetiological accounts with particular reference to incontinence (Braden & Bergstrom, op. cit.). However, Torrance (op. cit.) suggested that other characteristics associated with patients who suffer incontinence, such as old age and reduced mobility, are the link between high-pressure sore occurrence and incontinence. This view is supported by research which does not identify incontinence as a prognostic factor (Ek *et al.* op. cit.).
Skin irritants. The role of starch, altered pH by excessive use of soap and detergent residues in hospital sheets is not clearly determined. A link has been established between the use of these agents and skin irritation since at least the 1960s (Bettly, 1960), and there is general advice within the literature regarding the dangers of using excessive soap (Lowthian, op. cit.; Torrance, op. cit.; Alberman, 1992; Gunnell, 1992), however, the clinical significance in relation to pressure sore development is not understood.

Box 9.4.

Pressure intensity and duration: key points

- There is no universal pressure threshold value above which capillary occlusion occurs
- The threshold pressure value for each person will be dependent on
    the collagen content of the dermis
    the autoregulatory response
    the application of the load and complicating shear force
- If a threshold pressure value is exceeded then duration of pressure application is of greater importance than the intensity of pressure
- The response of the skin to pressure is inextricably linked to factors affecting skin tolerance

Friction. Evidence that friction increases the susceptibility of the skin to pressure ulceration was provided by experimentation on pigs by Dinsdale (1973, 1974). He applied pressure alone and pressure with friction and more ulcers developed in animals exposed to pressure with friction. The effect on the magnitude of pressure was of particular importance with pressure alone requiring 290 mmHg and pressure with friction producing ulcers at 45 mmHg.

Intrinsic factors
Intrinsic factors affecting the ability of the skin and supporting structures to respond to pressure and shear forces are numerous. It is useful to consider the numerous variables within a framework of factors that affect the collagen component of the skin and those affecting tissue perfusion.

That collagen plays a key role in pressure sore aetiology is a relatively recent concept (Krouskop, op. cit.) and requires further research at the cellular level. However, collagen provides a framework which inter-relates other known variables including age, spinal injury, nutritional factors, physiological and psychological stress, steroid administration, poor oxygen saturation, lymphatic drainage and interstitial flow.

For example, the synthesis, maturation and degradation of collagen is determined by age-related changes and steroid administration (Hall *et al.* 1974, 1981), nutrients including protein, carbohydrates, fats, vitamins and trace elements (Bergstrom *et al.* 1986, Brown, 1991; Keighley, 1982) and spinal cord injury (Claus-Walker *et al.* 1973).

Tissue perfusion is affected by a number of intrinsic factors including systemic blood pressure, serum protein, lymphatic drainage, body temperature, smoking and serum haemoglobin as well as factors that potentiate endothelial cell damage and increase platelet thrombosis. Research exploring these variables presents a confusing, sometimes contradictory picture and their clinical application may be limited (e.g. systemic blood pressure [Bridel, 1993b]). From a practical perspective perhaps of most value is knowledge relating to the potential influence of factors affecting the critical closing pressure of blood vessels.

The 'critical closing pressure' is the pressure within a vessel at which it collapses completely and blood flow ceases (Lippold & Winton, 1979). It is determined by an interplay of forces between intravascular pressure (which may be affected by systemic blood pressure and serum protein), muscle contraction and elastic forces of the blood-vessel wall (nutritional factors) and externally applied pressure (collagen, interstitial pressure and lymphatic drainage). In the skin and subcutaneous tissues, the interplay of forces is further complicated by the presence of shear forces (Bennett & Lee, op. cit.). That four variables are involved explains why no individual patient response is the same, although trends are apparent.

Other intrinsic factors affecting tissue perfusion further complicate the picture. Body temperature affects the metabolic rate of tissue and oxygen demand and haemoglobin and smoking affect the oxygenation of tissues (Bergstrom & Braden op. cit.; Holmes *et al.* 1987; Cullum & Clark, 1992; Lamid & El Ghatit, 1983). Also, Barton and Barton (op. cit.) listed a number of factors that potentiate endothelial cell damage and thrombosis including endotoxins, metabolic acidosis, dehydration, burns, thromboplastins (released during surgery), bacteraemia, hypoxia and blood stasis. However, the exact nature of the relationship between these factors and pressure sore development has not been established and again highlights that a complicated interplay of factors are likely to determine eventual outcome.

In more detailed reviews of the literature both Bridel (1993b) and Bliss (op. cit.) concluded that the role of the many extrinsic and intrinsic factors in the aetiology of pressure sore development is largely unclear. From a practice perspective, however, it is important to maintain a general awareness of the many potentiating factors so that 'balanced and informed' decision making can occur at an individual level. A summary of factors thought to be important is provided in Box 9.5.

Box 9.5.

A summary of intrinsic and extrinsic factors related to pressure sore development

- Extrinsic factors:
    Incontinence
    Skin irritants
    Friction
- Intrinsic factors:
    Collagen:
      Age
      Steroid administration
      Spinal injury
      Nutrition
    Perfusion:
      Systemic blood pressure
      Critical-closing pressure
      Serum albumin
      Temperature
      Blood oxygen saturation (haemoglobin and smoking)
      and others

It is clear that extrinsic factors are easily addressed by nursing care, with immediate gain, whereas the intrinsic factors may be difficult to address in the short term and require a multidisciplinary approach.

RISK ASSESSMENT IN PRACTICE

Where baseline skin assessment indicates no existing skin changes or damage then the purpose of further assessment is to identify any potential risk of pressure sore development. The literature relating to the pathology, epidemiology and aetiology of pressure sores provides clear guidance in some aspects of the general assessment of patients' risk, while also indicating that an awareness of the many factors potentially involved in pressure sore development is required to inform clinical judgement and decision making. For example, specific client groups can be identified as generally at risk of pressure sore development and minimum standards can be established at a local level.

Such minimum standards may include the provision of low-risk foam mattresses for an elderly ward or a high-risk mattress supports for an intensive care unit. However, within these environments the probability of pressure sore development will vary and require individual assessment.

Individual assessment should consider the following questions simultaneously:
- Is the patient exposed to prolonged or repetitive pressure (friction and shear)?
- Are there factors present that reduce skin tolerance?

In emphasizing these two elements, the role of clinical judgement (incorporating experience and knowledge of patient circumstance) and risk calculator are clearly distinct, particularly when the risk calculator consists of factors affecting skin tolerance (Waterlow, 1988). However, when considering risk assessment in this way it is essential to remember that it is the interaction between the tolerance of the skin and pressure that determines skin response and pressure sore development.

Exposure to pressure, friction and shear

In considering exposure to pressure, mobility and activity elements of assessment provide baseline data. However, other elements specific to the patient also help risk assessment:
- Knowledge of patient circumstance (e.g. reason for immobility).
- Clinical experience of the medical or surgical condition (e.g. expected post-operative period of immobility).
- Sensory perception (e.g. stimulus to move).
- Motivational and compliance factors (e.g. stimulus to move).
- Position required or favoured by the patient.

These factors are largely ignored by researchers (and risk calculators) yet affect greatly, at an individual level, patient care. For example, a semi-recumbent position generates friction and shearing forces which, as previously discussed, exacerbate the pressure effect (Figure 9.2). Also, sitting generates high pressures over the ischial tuberosities which may be exacerbated if the patient has a tendency to slip forward. Practical problems are also encountered when patients prefer one position and resume their favoured position despite all the efforts or when patients are haemodynamically unstable and are as a consequence too unstable to move.

It is also important to consider immobility and activity factors within the context of the local environment and equipment provision. For example, the type of mattress, chair or other equipment provided within the environment will affect exposure to pressure, friction and shear. Together with other clinical signs and symptoms relating to the skin response, such factors specific to the individual and the environment help in the risk assessment process. The variables involved and the knowledge required of patient factors illustrates that risk assessment is an interactive and dynamic process.

The role of risk calculators

Within the context of the preceding sections the role of risk calculators as central to risk assessment has been challenged. It is suggested that first consideration be given to the skin and its response to pressure to identify actual and potential problems and secondly to consider exposure to pressure, friction and shear. However, the literature highlights the complex nature of pressure sore development and the numerous factors potentially involved. Therefore, within a practice setting, awareness and assessment may be variable.

Risk calculators have been developed in an attempt to provide a structure and consistency to patient assessment and, despite various limitations in respect of their reliability and predictive validity (Bridel, 1994; Edwards, 1995; Smith *et al.* 1995; Effective Health Care, 1995; Deeks, op. cit.), their widespread use (Watts & Clark, op. cit.) would suggest that these tools are valued by clinical nurses and that their limitations are not necessarily important within the clinical environment. Indeed, in a review of 138 pressure sore prevention policies, 90% of policies recommended their use (Watts & Clark op. cit.). Risk calculators provide a number of important practical advantages that can be applied within the context of their limitations when they inform rather that predict or prescribe care (Table 9.1).

Table 9.1.
The benefits and limitations of risk assessment tools

Practical benefits	Practical limitations
1 Raise awareness	1 Do not distinguish between: (a) actual problem (pressure sore) (b) potential problem (skin changes) (c) potential problem (at risk)
2 Provide a minimum standard of risk assessment	
3 Crude indicator of risk	2 Do not distinguish between: (a) pressure factors (b) skin tolerance factors
4 Provide a framework for equipment guidelines	
	3 Are only a snapshot view
	4 Do not consider patient circumstances
	5 Do not predict skin response

In relation to their use, perhaps a number of key principles can be established:
1. Reliability: Recognition that inter-rater agreement (or reliability) of the tools may be poor (Bridel, 1993a; Edwards, op. cit.) or difficult to achieve and will affect patient scores. The implications of user variation should be considered if it greatly affects categorization of no risk or at risk. Also, the grade and experience of staff may be important (Bergstrom *et al.* 1987).
2. Validity. There is increasing data relating to the predictive validity of risk calculators within various settings yet there is no evidence that any one particular score is more accurate than another (Effective Health Care, op. cit). Users should have a general understanding of the margins of error and whether the tool of their choice greatly underpredicts or overpredicts risk.
3. Given points 1 and 2, risk calculators can inform but not prescribe practice.

PRINCIPLES OF CARE DELIVERY FOR THE PREVENTION AND TREATMENT OF PRESSURE SORES IN CLINICAL PRACTICE

Clinical judgement and interpretation of signs and symptoms is essential to pressure sore prevention and treatment. It involves the synthesis of a wide range of factors relating to a patient and should be considered as a continuous process. The principles of prevention and treatment are established by the aetiology literature which clearly indicates priorities for planning of care and apply whether the patient has an existing pressure sore or a potential problem (skin changes or risk factors). Prevention and treatment of pressure sores, therefore, include:
- Relief or reduction of pressure applied.
- Remove extrinsic factors that may exacerbate the pressure effect.
- Alleviate intrinsic factors that reduce tissue tolerance.
- Provide an optimum local environment for healing.
- Ongoing evaluation of the skin response.

Pressure: intensity and duration

The need for relief of pressure has long been established (Norton, 1962; Exton-Smith & Sherwin, op. cit.), and because pressure exacerbated by shear and friction actually cause pressure sores the focus of preventative care and treatment must be towards relief or reduction of these forces. This basic principle of pressure sore prevention and treatment may be achieved in a number of ways using a combination of repositioning or provision of equipment to alter pressure intensity or duration. Care delivered is determined at individual patient level by initial assessment and ongoing evaluation of the skin response.

Consideration is required in relation to the need for pressure relief, intermittent relief or pressure reduction. Patient circumstances will reflect the care delivered.

Positioning

Position is important in a number of ways. The position adopted can achieve complete pressure relief of an area, redistribute pressure, minimize friction and shearing forces and also reduce the pressure applied. Indeed, complete pressure relief can only be achieved by appropriate positioning and requires consideration regardless of the support surface used. For patients with existing pressure sores, it is particularly important to relieve the area from pressure.

Practitioners require an awareness of potential problems associated with the semi-recumbent position and poor seating provision which results in forward slide and the generation of friction and shearing forces. An innovative alternative to the semi-recumbent position is described by Preston (1988) and involves the use of pillows to position the patient at a 30° tilt. This has two important effects: firstly, the position redistributes pressure away from the sacrum and heels and secondly, the pillows maintain the patient in a stable position, thereby minimizing friction and shear. However, there are practical problems associated with this position and physiotherapy input is advised.

In relation to seating, various factors require consideration including chair dimensions and design, that is, height, depth, angle of back support, arm-rest height and height of lumbar support (Lowry 1989). For example, Gilsdorf et al. (1991) reported that arm rests supported between 5% and 9% of the body weight of spinal-cord injured patients. Also, weight distribution is affected by the position of the feet.

Particular difficulties are experienced in maintaining good posture when patients require leg elevation and careful consideration should be given to the value of sitting a patient in a chair as opposed to elevation in bed. Also, when long-term seating is required, in spinal-injured patients, for example, specialist evaluation of the skin response using measures of transcutaneous oxygen tension are indicated (Bader, op. cit.; Coggrave et al. 1994).

Equipment

There is an increasingly diverse and expanding equipment market providing for pressure sore prevention and treatment needs. Very few of the products available have been evaluated using well-designed research methods and there is no 'best buy' (Young, 1992; Effective Health Care, op. cit.). However, within the practice setting there is evidence that the provision of clear guidelines for equipment improves use for preventative purposes and reduces pressure sore incidence (Bale et al. 1996).

As there may be great variability in equipment availability at a local level this review simply identifies the differences in the basic principles of equipment function and provides an outline of design issues for consideration during selection. Specialist equipment can be described as:

- Constant low-pressure system. These reduce the overall pressure applied by moulding to the patient thereby increasing the contact surface area and providing a reduced and more evenly distributed pressure (Effective Health Care, op. cit.).
- Alternating pressure system. These systems consist of inflatable cells that are programmed to inflate and deflate and provide intermittent relief of pressure.

Within these two categories, design and performance are greatly variable and comparing and contrasting equipment is important for clinical practice and decision making. For example, within the alternating-pressure system category, a number of overlays and mattresses are available. However, basic construction is variable in relation to cell design and cycle time, materials used, automated-pressure adjusters and pressures generated. Similarly, constant low-pressure systems include fibre-filled, foam, gel and water overlays and mattresses, as well as complex systems providing air and air with particulate suspension (low air loss and air-fluidized systems) (Effective Health Care, op. cit.). Although the principles of action are the same, the construction and performance of such equipment is highly variable.

Design elements in relation to constant low pressure supports are described by Jay (1995):

- It must conform to bony prominences without resistance.
- It must not have significant memory.
- It must allow patient emersion.
- It must not bottom-out.
- It must relieve the shear forces caused by patient movement.
- It must prevent skin maceration.
- It must address patient comfort.

Many of these may also be applicable to alternating-pressure systems and seating provision. Whatever the support surface and repositioning schedule used, ongoing skin evaluation informs the frequency of turning and repositioning.

Extrinsic and intrinsic factors

The focus of care in relation to extrinsic and intrinsic factors will clearly be determined by the problems of each individual patient, with emphasis given in the first instance to elements of care providing immediate effect (e.g. continence). When patients have a long-term prevention need, and/or existing sores, particularly partial and full thickness wounds, a multidisciplinary approach is required to address factors intrinsic in nature that affect the tolerance of the skin and the healing process. Such factors are discussed in depth in Chapter 2 (nutritional care), Chapter 1 (factors affecting wound healing) and Chapters 5 and 6 (wound management).

Patient education and participation

Emphasis on patient education and participation is receiving increasing support; the basic principles are considered further in Chapter 8. With specific reference to pressure sore prevention and treatment, patient understanding and participation in care may be crucial to the overall outcome of care. For example, the patient's ability to comply with maintaining a position that allows complete pressure relief may allow a superficial ulcer to heal spontaneously or negate the need for 'high tech' equipment. Similarly, when patients are unable to contribute to their own care needs then this should influence both equipment provision and repositioning frequency.

The involvement of patients in the prevention and treatment of pressure sores was clearly recognized during the development of the consensus guidelines (NHSE, op. cit.). As a result, four guidelines relating to education and participation of patients and carers were developed, detailed in Box 9.6.

Box 9.6.

Guidelines on patient and carer involvement and education (NHSE, 1995)

- A multidisciplinary plan of care should be negotiated with individual patients and carers taking into consideration their knowledge and experience
- Patient and carer involvement in assessment of risk should be encouraged
- The strategy for patient and carer education should incorporate the following:
    - Awareness of risk factors and their implications
    - Strategies for prevention
    - Support services available after discharge or transfer from one care setting to another
    - Awareness of equipment usage and operation
    - Written information
- Recognition should be given to patient's and carer's freedom of choice to accept or refuse advice or care

SELF-ASSESSMENT QUESTIONS AND ACTIVITIES

Case Study 1

Mrs Carmichael is 75 years old. She suffers from occasional stress-related urinary incontinence. Her weight is below average for her height and her skin is rather dry. Otherwise, she is in good health and her mobility and activity levels are unimpaired. She is admitted to hospital for a laproscopic cholecystectomy and her expected discharge is post-operative Day 2. The operation lasts 90 minutes and she is then cared for in the recovery room for 1 hour. She returns to the surgical ward, on a trolley, in a supine position. When the nurses transfer her to bed they notice a reddened area over the sacrum, which blanches under light finger pressure. Low risk foam mattresses are the standard provision within this surgical ward.

1(a) During what time period was Mrs Carmichael at particular risk of developing a pressure sore?

(b) Note the risk factors for pressure sore development in this case.

(c) Discuss what measures, if any, you would initiate to prevent pressure induced damage:
   (1) pre-operatively
   (2) peri-operatively
   (3) post-operatively

2. Describe the patient's role in pressure sore prevention in the first 24–48 hours post-operatively.

Case Study 2

Mrs Mills is 80 years old and was recently discharged from hospital to a nursing home. At the time of discharge she had two pressure sores, a partial-thickness wound on the left heel and a superficial wound on the left buttock.

Mrs. Mills had been admitted to hospital 4 months previously because of a right femoral embolus. She had a long-standing medical history of non-insulin dependent diabetes mellitus. Within a 7-day period Mrs Mills underwent surgery on three occasions, culminating in a right leg above-knee amputation. Her post-operative recovery was delayed by wound dehiscence, infection and unstable diabetes but wound healing was achieved by 8 weeks.

In relation to pressure sore development, active prevention was instigated from admission (including assessment, repositioning and provision of a high-risk mattress and gel pad provision intra-operatively). During the first week of hospitalization, a necrotic area developed on the left heel. Later, Mrs Mills' mobility improved, but her posture was affected by elevation of the amputated right leg and a superficial pressure sore developed on her left buttock.

During the initial nursing-home assessment, a granulating and clean partial thickness wound (3 x 3 cm) is noted on the outer aspect of her left heel. The surrounding skin is dry and flaky. A superficial skin break on her left buttock (2 x 3 cm) is also noted. This is moist with a small yellow sloughy area (0.5 x 0.2 cm). Her sacral area is red but blanches with light finger pressure after 1 hour of sitting.

Mobility assessment reveals that she prefers to sit in a chair and is unable to lift herself up to relieve pressure while sitting. Mrs Mills has difficulty in maintaining a sitting posture while her right leg is elevated and she has a tendency to slip forward in the standard chair. While in bed, Mrs. Mills prefers lying in a recumbent position with three pillows. She is able to turn herself on to her left side but complains of not being able to sleep.

Mrs Mills has lost approximately 12 pounds in weight (5.5 kg) since her hospital admission. Her vascular disease is assessed as being secondary to her diabetes mellitus. Her skin is dry, although her general condition and strength are improving. She is still assessed as being at very high risk of developing a pressure sore.

1. List, with reasons, the pressure-relieving measures that you would initiate.

2(a) Note the factors that could contribute to delayed wound healing in this case (see also Chapter 1).

(b) Which of these factors are amenable to change?

(c) What would you do about them?

(d) Should any other healthcare professional(s) be involved in assessing Mrs Mills and what might be the nature of their therapeutic involvement?

See also Advanced Case Studies 1 and 2 on pages 272–275.

REFERENCES

AHCPR. *Pressure ulcers in adults: prediction and prevention.* Clinical Practice Guideline No.3. Rockville: AHCPR Publication No.92-0047; 1992.

Alberman K. Is there any connection between laundering and the development of pressure sores? *J Tissue Viability* 1992, 2(2):55–56.

Bader DL. The recovery characteristics of soft tissue following repeated loading. *J Rehabil Res Dev* 1990, **27**(2):141–150.

Bale S, Finlay I, Harding KG. Pressure sore prevention in a hospice. In: Cherry GW, Gottrup F, Lawrence JC, Moffatt CJ, Turner TD, eds. *Proceedings of the 5th European Conference on Advances in Wound Management.* London: Macmillan; 1996.

Banks S, Bridel J. A descriptive evaluation of pressure-reducing cushions. *Br J Nurs* 1995, 4(13):736–746.

Barbenel JC, Jordan MM, Nicol SM *et al.* Incidence of pressure sores in the Greater Glasgow Health Board Area. *Lancet* 1977, **2**:548–550.

Barbenel JC, Jordan MM, Nicol SM. Major pressure of sores. *Health Soc Serv J* 1980, **90**(2):1344–1345.

Barton A, Barton M. *The management and prevention of pressure sores.* London: Faber; 1981.

Bennett L, Lee BY. Pressure versus shear in pressure sore causation, Chapter 3. In: Lee BY, ed. *Chronic ulcers of the skin.* New York: McGraw Hill; 1985.

Bergstrom N, Braden BJ. A prospective study of pressure sore risk among institutionalised elderly. *J Am Geriatr Soc* 1992, **40**(8):747–758.

Bergstrom N, Braden B, Krall K *et al.* Adequacy of descriptive scales for reporting diet intake in institutionalised elderly. *J Nutr Elderly* 1986, **6**(1):3–16.

Bergstrom N, Braden BJ, Lagussa A, Holman V. The Braden Scale for predicting pressure sore risk. *Nurs Res* 1987, **36**:205–210.

Berlowitz DR, Wilking SVanB. Risk factors for pressure sores: a comparison of cross-sectional and cohort-derived data. *J Am Geriatr Soc* 1989, **37**(11):1043–1050.

Bettly FR. Some effects of soap on the skin. *BMJ* 1960, 1:1675–1679.

Bliss M. Aetiology of pressure sores. *Rev Clin Gerontol* 1993, **3**:379–397.

Braden BJ, Bergstrom N. A conceptual schema for the study of the etiology of pressure sores. *Rehab Nurse* 1987, 12(1):8–16.

Branemark PI. Microvascular function at reduced flow rates. In: Kenedi RM, Cowden JM, Scales JT, eds. *Bedsore biomechanics.* Maryland: University Park Press; 1976:63–68.

Bridel J. Assessing the risk of pressure sores. *Nursing Standard* 1993a, 7(25):32–35.

Bridel J. The pathophysiology of pressure sores. *J Wound Care* 1993b, **2**(4):230–238.

Bridel J. The epidemiology of pressure sores. *Nursing Standard* 1993c, 7(42):25–30.

Bridel J. Risk assessment. *J Tissue Viability* 1994, 4(3):84–85.

Brooks B, Duncan GW. Effects of pressure on tissues. *Arch Surg* 1940, **40**:696–709.

Brown K. The role of nutrition in pressure area care. *J Tissue Viability* 1991, 1(3):63–64.

Clark M, Farrar S. Comparison of pressure sore risk calculators. In: Harding KG, Leaper DL, Turner TD, eds. *Proceedings of the 1st European Conference on Advances in Wound Management.* London: Macmillan; 1992.

Clark M, Watts S. The incidence of pressure sores within a National Health Service Trust Hospital during 1991. *J Adv Nurs* 1994, 20:33–36.

Claus-Walker J, Campos RJ, Carter RE *et al.* Electrolytes in urinary calculi and urine of patients with spinal cord injuries. *Arch Phys Med Rehabil* 1973, **54**:109–114.

Clough NP. The cost of pressure area management in an intensive care unit. *J Wound Care* 1994, 3(1):33–35.

Coggrave M, Rose L, Bogie K. The role of a seating clinic in pressure sore prevention for spinal cord injured subjects. In: Harding KG, Dealey C, Cherry G, Gottrup F, eds. *Proceedings of the 3rd European Conference on Advances in Wound Management.* London: Macmillan; 1994.

Cullum N, Clark M. Intrinsic factors associated with pressure sores in elderly people. *J Adv Nurs* 1992, **17**:427–431.

David JA, Chapman JG, Chapman EJ *et al.* *An investigation of the current methods used in nursing for the care of patients with established pressure sores.* UK: Northwick Park, Nursing Research Unit; 1983.

Deeks JJ. Pressure sore prevention: using and evaluating risk assessment tools. *Br J Nurs* 1996, **5**(5):313–320.

Dinsdale SM. Decubitus ulcers in swine: light and electron microscopic study of pathogenesis. *Arch Phys Med Rehabil* 1973, **54**:51–56.

Dinsdale SM. Decubitus ulcers: role of pressure and friction in causation. *Arch Phys Med Rehabil* 1974, **55**:147–152.

DoH. *Pressure sores – A key quality indicator: a guide for NHS purchasers and providers.* Lancashire: BAPS Health Publications Unit; 1993.

Donaldson R, Donaldson R. *Essential community medicine (including relevant social sciences).* Lancaster: MTP Press; 1985.

Edwards M. The levels of reliability and validity of the Waterlow pressure sore risk calculator. *J Wound Care* 1995, **4**(8):373–378.

Ek A-C, Unosson M, Larsson J *et al.* The development and healing of pressure sores related to the nutritional state. *Clin Nutr* 1991, **10**:245–250.

Effective Health Care. The prevention and treatment of pressure sores. *Effective Health Care* 1995, **2**(1):1–16.

Exton-Smith AN, Sherwin RW. The prevention of pressure sores: significance of spontaneous bodily movements. *Lancet* 1961, **2**:1124–1126.

Forrest RD. The treatment of pressure sores. *J Int Med Res* 1980, **8**:430–435.

Gilsdorf P, Patterson R, Fisher. Thirty minute continuous sitting force measurements with different support surfaces in the spinal cord injured and able bodied. *J Rehab Res Dev* 1991, **28**(4):33–8.

Goldblatt H. Observations upon reactive hyperaemia. *Heart* 1925, **12**:281–294.

Gunnell DJ. Mysterious slapped face rash at holiday centre. *BMJ* 1992, **304**:477–479.

Hall DA, Blackett AD, Zajoc AR *et al.* Changes in skinfold thickness with increasing age. *Age Ageing* 1981, **10**(1):19–23.

Hall DA, Read FB, Nuki G *et al.* The relative effects of age and corticosteroid therapy on the collagen profiles of dermis from subjects with rheumatoid arthritis. *Age Ageing* 1974, **3**(1):15.

Healey F. The reliability and utility of pressure sore grading scales. *J Tissue Viability* 1995, **5**:111–114.

Healey F. Classification of pressure sores. *Br J Nurs* 1996, **5**(9):567–574.

Hitch S. NHS Executive Nursing Directorate – Strategy for major clinical guidelines – Prevention and management of pressure sores: a literature review. *J Tissue Viability* 1995, **5**(1):3–24.

Holmes R, Macchino K, Jhangiani SS *et al.* Combating pressure sores-Nutritionally. *Am J Nurs* 1987, **87**(10):1301–1303.

Holstein P, Neilson PE, Barras JR. Blood flow cessation at external pressure in the skin of normal limbs. *Microvasc Res* 1979, **17**:71–79.

Husain T. An experimental study of some pressure effects on tissues with reference to the bed sores problem. *J Path Bacteriol* 1953, **66**:347–358.

IAET. *Standards of care for dermal wounds: pressure sores.* Irvine: International Association of Enterostomal Therapy; 1987.

Jay E. How different constant low pressure support surfaces address pressure and shear forces. *J Tissue Viability* 1995, **5**(4):118–123.

Keighley JK. Wound healing in malnourished patients. *AORN J* 1982, **35**(6):1094–1099.

Kemp MG, Keighley JK, Smith DW *et al.* Factors which contribute to pressure sores in surgical patients. *Res*

Nurs Health 13:293–301, 1990.

Krouskop TA. A synthesis of the factors which contribute to pressure sore formation. *Med Hypotheses* 1983,
11:255–267.

Krouskop TA, Reddy NP, Spencer WA *et al*. Mechanisms of decubitus ulcer formation — a hypothesis. *Med Hypotheses* 1978, 4:37–39.

Lamb JF, Ingram CG, Johnston IA *et al*. *Essentials of physiology*. Oxford: Blackwell Scientific Publications; 1980.

Lamid S, El Ghatit AZ. Smoking, spasticity and pressure sores in spinal cord injured patients. *Am J Phys Med* 1993, 62(6):300–306.

Landis EM: Micro-injection studies of capillary blood pressure in human skin. *Heart* 1993, 15:209–228.

Lewis T, Grant R. Observations upon reactive hyperaemia. *Heart* 1925, 12:73–120.

Lippold OCJ, Winton FR. *Human physiology, 7th ed*. London: Churchill Livingstone; 1979.

Lowry M. Are you sitting comfortably? Good seating requirements in a patient care setting. *Professional Nurse* 1989, December:162–164.

Lowthian P. Prevention of heel sores. *Lancet* 1982, i:1089.

Lowthian P. Classification and grading of pressure sores. *Care Sci Prac* 1987, 5(1):5–9.

Lowthian P. Pressure sores: a search for a definition. *Nursing Standard* 1994, 9(11):30–32.

Lyder C. Conceptualisation of the stage I pressure ulcer. *J Enterostomal Nurs* 1991, 18(5):162–165.

Millward J. Relieving the pressure. *Nursing Elderly* 1990, 2(4):14–16.

Minotti A. Incidence studies and registers. In: Holland W and Karhausen L, eds. *Health care and epidemiology*. London: Kimpton; 1978.

Morison MJ: *A colour guide to the nursing management of wounds*. London: Mosby; 1992.

NHSE 95. *Clinical practice guidelines: prevention and management of pressure sores*. United Leeds Teaching Hospital Trust, Leeds. Unpublished.

Norton D, McLaren R, Exton-Smith AN. *An investigation of geriatric nursing problems in hospital*. Edinburgh: Churchill Livingstone; 1962.

Nyquist R, Hawthorn PJ. The prevalence of pressure sores within an Area Health Authority. *J Adv Nurs* 1987, 12:183–187.

O'Dea K. Prevalence of pressure damage in hospital patients in the U.K. *J Wound Care* 1993, 2(4):21–225.

O'Dea K. The prevalence of pressure sores in four European countries. *J Wound Care* 1995, 2(4):192–195.

Parish LC, Witkowski JA, Chrissey JT. *The decubitus ulcer*. New York: Masson Publishers; 1983.

Preston KW. Positioning for comfort and pressure relief: the 30 degree alternative. *CARE Science & Practice* 1988, 6(4):116–119.

Reddy NP, Krouskop TA, Newell PH. Biomechanics of a lymphatic vessel. *Blood Vessels* 1975, 12:261–278.

Reid J, Morison M. Towards a consensus: classification of pressure sores. *J Wound Care* 1994, 3(3):157–160.

Shea JD. Pressure sores, classification and management. *Clin Orthopaed* 1975, 112:89–100.

Smith LN, Booth N, Douglas D *et al*. A critique of 'at risk' pressure sore assessment tools. *J Clin Nurs* 1995, 4:153–159.

Stotts NA. Predicting pressure ulcer development in surgical patients. *Heart Lung* 1988, 17(6) Part 1:641–647.

Torrance C. *Pressure sores: aetiology, treatment and prevention*. London: Croom Helm; 1983.

Versluysen M. How elderly patients with femoral fracture develop pressure sores in hospital. *BMJ* 1986, 292:1311–1313.

Waterlow J. A risk assessment card. *Nursing Times* 1985, 81(48):24–27.

Waterlow J. The Waterlow Card for the prevention and management of pressure sores: towards a pocket policy. *Care Sci Prac* 1988, 6(1):8–12.

Watts S, Clark M. *Pressure sore prevention: a review of policy documents*. Nursing Practice Research Unit, University of Surrey, 1993.

Young J. Preventing pressure sores: does the mattress work? *J Tissue Viability* 1992, 2(1):17.

Leg Ulcers

Leg ulceration is a common problem affecting 1–2% of the population in the UK (Laing, 1992). This represents 80 000–100 000 patients with an open ulcer at any one time and a further 400 000 patients with a healed ulcer that is likely to recur (Callam et al. 1985).

The highest prevalence of leg ulceration is in very elderly people (Cornwall et al. 1986). In terms of service provision, this is important in light of the 43% projected increase in very elderly people by the year 2000. This group of patients is also likely to present with ulcers of mixed aetiology which can be particularly challenging to treat (Cornwall et al. op. cit.). Although traditionally leg ulceration has been thought of as a condition of elderly people, it is important to note that 20% of patients develop their ulcer before the age of 40 years (Callam et al. op. cit.), yet very little is known about the impact of leg ulceration on young sufferers and their families.

In recent years, research has shown the considerable suffering associated with leg ulceration and the reduction in quality of life for patients of all ages (Franks et al. 1994; Philips et al. 1994). Risk factors for delayed healing, such as ulcer chronicity and leg ulcer size, highlight the importance of early intervention and appropriate treatment (Franks op. cit.; Philips et al. op. cit.). Other risk factors, such as reduced mobility, are less easy to influence, especially in an elderly population. Social risk factors relating to the patient's environment and lifestyle may also contribute to delayed healing (Franks et al. 1995a,b). This is an area in which further research is required. The long-held belief that socio-economic factors may contribute to leg ulceration has some validity with studies showing that ulceration occurs more frequently in the lower social classes and that healing is delayed in these groups (Fowkes & Callam, 1994). The recurrence rate of ulceration remains depressingly high with 20% of sufferers having more than six episodes of ulceration and many ulcers failing to heal over a period of many years (Callam et al. 1987a).

Major developments in the management of leg ulcers have been made in the past decade. Many new services are emerging that bridge the gap between community and acute care and embrace the multidisciplinary approach (Moffatt et al. 1992). The possibility of improved health outcomes for these patients and the realization of the high cost of care have all contributed to raising the profile of leg ulceration (Bosanquet et al. 1993).

This chapter begins by reviewing the causes of leg ulceration. Understanding the related anatomy and pathophysiology is a prerequisite to understanding the principles of patient assessment and treatment that follow.

CAUSES OF LEG ULCERS

A number of pathological conditions are associated with lower limb ulceration (Table 10.1). Although a minor traumatic incident is usually the immediate cause of the ulcer, the underlying pathology in Western countries such as the UK is usually vascular. In less developed countries ulceration is more often caused by trauma and infection (Landra, 1988). The aetiology of leg ulceration is now discussed.

Venous ulcers

An understanding of the cause of venous ulceration requires an understanding of the anatomy of the venous system of the lower limb and the mechanics of its blood flow.

Anatomy of the venous system and the mechanics of blood flow

The leg consists of three systems of veins: the deep, superficial and perforating veins (Figure 10.1). These contain valves to prevent backflow of blood (Figure 10.2).

Venous return is aided by a combination of mechanisms including calf muscle contraction, variations in intra-abdominal and intra-thoracic pressure. Failure of the valves allows reverse flow of blood causing further damage to other valves, which leads

Table 10.1.
Causes of leg ulcers (Morison & Moffatt, 1994)
1. Principal causes
• Chronic venous hypertension, usually because of incompetent valves in the deep and perforating veins
• Arterial disease, for example, atherosclerotic occlusion of large vessels leading to tissue ischaemia
• Combined chronic venous hypertension and arterial disease
2. More unusual causes (2–5% in total)
• Neuropathy, for example, associated with diabetes mellitus, spina bifida, leprosy
• Vasculitis, for example, associated with rheumatoid arthritis, polyarteritis nodosum
• Malignancy, for example, squamous-cell carcinoma, melanoma, basal-cell carcinoma, Kaposi's sarcoma
• Blood disorders, for example, polycythaemia, sickle-cell disease, thalassaemia
• Infection, for example, tuberculosis, leprosy, syphilis, fungal infections
• Metabolic disorders, for example, pyoderma gangrenosum, pretibial myxoedema
• Lymphoedema
• Trauma, for example, lacerations, burns, irradiation injuries
• Iatrogenic, for example, overtight bandaging, ill-fitting plaster cast
• Self-inflicted

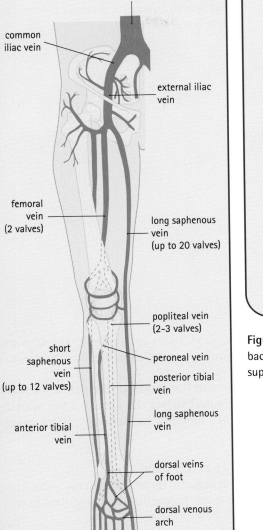

inferior vena cava

common
iliac vein

external iliac
vein

femoral
vein
(2 valves)

long saphenous
vein
(up to 20 valves)

popliteal vein
(2-3 valves)

short
saphenous
vein
(up to 12 valves)

peroneal vein

posterior tibial
vein

long saphenous
vein

anterior tibial
vein

dorsal veins
of foot

dorsal venous
arch

digital vein

Figure 10.1 Veins of the pelvis and lower limb, illustrating the right common iliac vein and its tributaries.

deep vein
(designed to carry venous
blood under pressure)

superficial vein
(designed to
carry venous
blood under low
pressure)

perforating vein
(valve closed as
calf muscle
contracts)

subcutaneous
tissue

skin

semi-rigid fascia enclosing
calf muscle

calf muscle
'pump'

Figure 10.2 Healthy, intact valves prevent backflow of blood from the deep to the superficial veins (Morison & Moffatt, 1994).

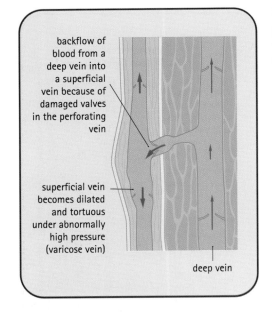

backflow of
blood from a
deep vein into
a superficial
vein because of
damaged valves
in the perforating
vein

superficial vein
becomes dilated
and tortuous
under abnormally
high pressure
(varicose vein)

deep vein

Figure 10.3 An incompetent valve in a perforating vein allows backflow of blood from the deep to the superficial venous system (Morison & Moffatt, 1994).

to the development of varicose veins (Figure 10.3). Damaged valves in the deep and perforating veins are one cause of chronic venous hypertension in the lower limb which leads to venous stasis and oedema.

Venous return is facilitated by ankle movement (extension of the Achilles tendon) and by foot pumps which are activated as the heel strikes the ground when walking (Gardner & Fox, 1986). Limitation in a patient's mobility can seriously affect venous function.

Clinical signs of chronic venous hypertension

Complications arising from chronic venous hypertension, including varicose veins, stasis eczema and lipodermatosclerosis are summarized in Figure 10.4 and described here.

Varicose veins Varicose veins are a common problem, found in 10–20% of the adult population. People in occupations which involve prolonged standing in warm conditions, such as nurses, teachers and warehousemen, are particularly at risk (Table 10.2).

Varicose veins are a sign of chronic venous hypertension in the lower limb, which is usually the result of damage to the valves in the leg veins. The damage may be congenital or acquired (Table 10.3). As a result of such damage, the superficial venous network is exposed to much higher pressures than normal (up to 90 mmHg instead of 30 mmHg). The superficial veins, especially the relatively thin-walled tributaries of the long and short saphenous veins, become dilated, lengthened and tortuous. Approximately 3% of patients with varicose veins go on to develop leg ulcers but not all patients with venous ulcers have varicose veins. It is therefore not clear whether varicose veins and venous ulcers are merely associated conditions with a common

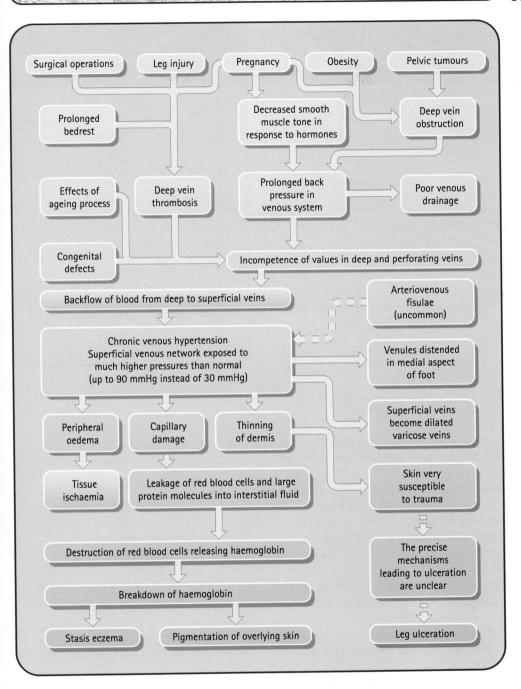

Figure 10.4 Complications arising from chronic venous hypertension. (Reproduced from Morison & Moffatt, 1994.)

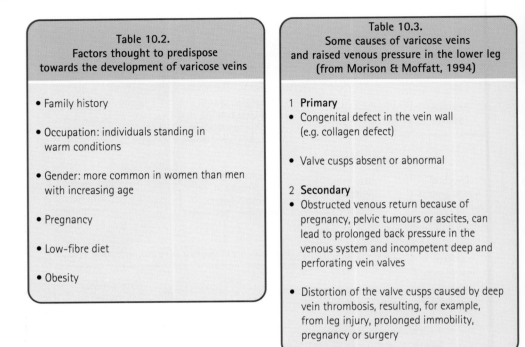

Table 10.2.
Factors thought to predispose towards the development of varicose veins

- Family history

- Occupation: individuals standing in warm conditions

- Gender: more common in women than men with increasing age

- Pregnancy

- Low-fibre diet

- Obesity

Table 10.3.
Some causes of varicose veins and raised venous pressure in the lower leg (from Morison & Moffatt, 1994)

1 **Primary**
- Congenital defect in the vein wall (e.g. collagen defect)

- Valve cusps absent or abnormal

2 **Secondary**
- Obstructed venous return because of pregnancy, pelvic tumours or ascites, can lead to prolonged back pressure in the venous system and incompetent deep and perforating vein valves

- Distortion of the valve cusps caused by deep vein thrombosis, resulting, for example, from leg injury, prolonged immobility, pregnancy or surgery

aetiology or whether varicose veins are a predisposing factor for venous ulcers.

Staining of the skin in the gaiter region
Chronic venous hypertension leads to distension of the blood capillaries and damage to the endothelium, leading to leakage of red blood cells. The breakdown products of haemoglobin cause pigmentation.

Ankle flare
This is distension of the tiny veins on the medial aspect of the foot. It is frequently associated with perforator vein incompetence.

Atrophy of the skin
Thinning of the dermis associated with poor blood supply makes the skin susceptible to trauma.

Eczema
Eczematous changes to the skin are often associated with venous insufficiency and can be aggravated by a number of wound-care products through irritation and allergy, as described in Chapter 7. Secondary infection may occur if the patient scratches persistently.

Table 10.4.
Four theories of the cause of venous ulcers

The fibrin cuff theory
Layers of fibrin laid down as cuffs around the capillary wall causing a diffusion barrier to oxygen and nutrients leading to trophic skin changes (Burnand *et al.* 1982)
Herrick *et al.* (1992) noted that fibrin cuffs were more complex in nature and actively assembled by adjacent connective tissue in response to venous hypertension

White cell trapping theory
Accumulation and activation of white cells in the microcirculation of patients with venous hypertension. Production of toxic metabolites leads to tissue breakdown (Coleridge-Smith *et al.* 1988)

Mechanical theory
Ulceration results from mechanical stress on the patient's limb. High pressure in the capillary bed leads to oedema which in turn raises tissue pressure resulting in stretching of the skin. Ulceration is thought to result from tissue ischaemia (Chant 1990)

The 'trap' growth factor theory
Leakage of fibrinogen and protein-bound growth factors. The growth factors are trapped in the fibrin cuff preventing their use in normal epidermal tissue repair (Higley *et al.* 1995)

Lipodermatosclerosis
This is 'woody' induration of the tissues with fat replaced by fibrosis. The leg often assumes an inverted champagne bottle shape.

Theories of the cause of venous ulcers
A number of theories have emerged that attempt to explain the pathogenesis of venous ulceration. Four of the more popular theories are summarized in Table 10.4. It must be stressed, however, that the precise mechanisms leading to leg ulceration are still the subject of intense debate.

Arterial ulcers

Arterial ulcers are caused by an insufficient arterial blood supply to the limb, resulting in tissue ischaemia and necrosis (Figure 10.5). Occlusion may occur in major or more distal arteries and may be chronic or acute (Table 10.5).

Atherosclerosis is by far the most common cause of arterial ulcers. The process of atherosclerosis involves the deposition and accumulation of fatty material in the walls of arteries to form plaques. The plaques cause narrowing of the lumen of the vessels which results in increased resistance to blood flow. The plaques fissure and haemorrhage leading to thrombosis, embolization and consequent ischaemia (Rose, 1991). Other risk factors that

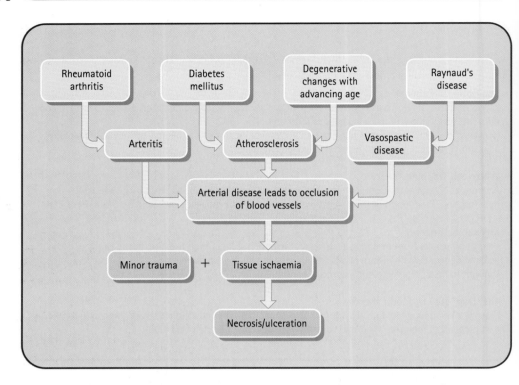

Figure 10.5 Diseases and disorders associated with arterial ulcers: a tentative model. (Reproduced from Morison & Moffatt, 1994.)

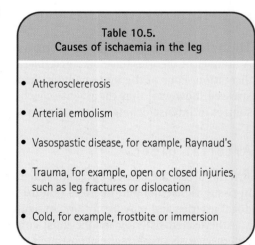

Table 10.5.
Causes of ischaemia in the leg

- Atherosclererosis

- Arterial embolism

- Vasospastic disease, for example, Raynaud's

- Trauma, for example, open or closed injuries, such as leg fractures or dislocation

- Cold, for example, frostbite or immersion

can influence the severity of the atherosclerosis include: male sex, hypertension, hyper-lipidaemia, diabetes mellitus and smoking. Diabetes and smoking are most strongly linked with ischaemia in the legs. Combinations of risk factors, rather than one isolated risk factor, seem to be particularly hazardous.

The most common sites for atherosclerosis in the lower limb are the lower superficial femoral artery (60%) and the aorto-iliac segments (30%), with multiple segment involvement occurring in approximately 7% of patients (Orr & McAvoy, 1987). The degree of ischaemia and the symptoms experienced depend not only on the site of the occlusion but also on the presence or absence of an effective collateral circulation.

Acute ischaemia caused by arterial embolism is potentially the most damaging because the body has not had the time to develop a collateral circulation to compensate. When an occlusion has developed over a prolonged period of time it may cause no noticeable effects for the individual.

At rest, an individual may be able to tolerate up to 70% occlusion of an artery in the lower limb without being aware of any ill effects. On exercise, the increased demands for oxygen in the muscle cannot be met, causing intermittent claudication. In patients with ischaemic pain at rest, the blood vessel is likely to be 90% occluded, indicating a severely compromised arterial circulation.

Critical ischaemia has been defined by the European Working Group on Critical Leg Ischaemia (1992) as

'Persistently recurring rest pain requiring regular analgesia for more than 2 weeks with an ankle systolic pressure ≤ 50 mmHg or toe systolic pressure of ≤ 30 mmHg or ulceration or gangrene of the foot or toes.'

The foot ulcer of a patient presenting with critical ischaemia is illustrated in Figure 10.6.

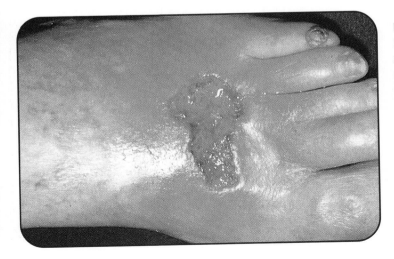

Figure 10.6 Critical ischaemia in an arterial ulcer. (Reproduced from Morison & Moffatt, 1994.)

Clinically, the skin surrounding an arterial ulcer is often shiny and loss of hair, adipose tissue and sweat glands are common. There is no brown staining in the gaiter region unless chronic venous hypertension is also present.

The significance of an arterial component in leg ulcer aetiology is being increasingly recognized. Both Cornwall *et al.* (op. cit.) and Callam *et al.* (1987b) estimated that approximately 21% of patients presenting with a leg ulcer have evidence of arterial insufficiency. This has very important implications for treatment. The accurate differential diagnosis of venous and arterial leg ulcers is essential.

Rheumatoid arthritis and vasculitic ulcers

Leg ulceration is common in patients with rheumatoid arthritis with up to 10% of patients developing an ulcer at some stage (Pun *et al.* 1990). Prolonged use of steroids and susceptibility to trauma often leads to delayed healing in these patients.

In a retrospective study, over an 8-year period of 35 episodes of leg ulceration in 26 patients with rheumatoid arthritis, Pun (op. cit.) found the following causes of ulceration:

- 18.2% vasculitis.
- 45.5% venous insufficiency.
- 45.5% trauma or pressure.
- 36.4% arterial insufficiency.

A deep arterial ulcer in a patient with rheumatoid arthritis is illustrated in Figure 10.7.

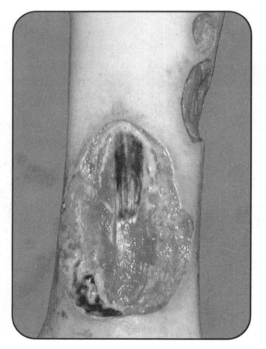

Figure 10.7   A deep arterial ulcer, in a patient with rheumatoid arthritis, with exposed tendon and neurotic tissue visible. (Reproduced from Ruckley, 1988.)

Vasculitic ulcers are also associated with other connective-tissue disorders such as polyarteritis nodosa and systemic lupus erythematosus. The ulcers are usually small, multiple and extremely painful. Healing of these ulcers is likely to be slow and is very much affected by the course of the underlying disease.

Pyoderma gangrenosum is distinctive and characterized by acute necrotizing, rapidly expanding ulceration of the skin as illustrated in Figure 10.8. The ulcer may have an irregular undermined edge and purple margins. There is debate as to whether the underlying cause is primarily vasculitic (Pun *et al.* op. cit.). **If vasculitis is suspected, medical assessment is urgently required.**

Diabetic ulcers

Ulceration of the lower limb, especially the foot, is a common complication for patients with diabetes mellitus (Robertson *et al.* 1986). Delayed wound healing and increased vulnerability to infection are likely (Joseph & Axler, 1990). Gangrene may develop and there is a high risk of the need for lower-limb amputation. However, it has been suggested that 50–75% of amputations are preventable.

The two most common causes of foot ulceration are peripheral neuropathy and peripheral vascular disease (Young & Boulton, 1991). They frequently occur in combination and are complicated by infection. Risk factors for foot ulceration are previous foot ulceration or gangrene, increasing age, peripheral vascular disease, male sex, neuropathy, structural deformity of the foot, nephropathy, retinopathy, living alone and duration of the diabetes.

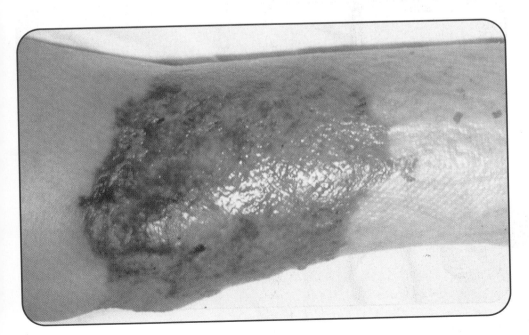

Figure 10.8   Pyoderma gangrenosum. (Reproduced from Morison & Moffatt, 1994.)

Angiopathy in the diabetic patient

In people without diabetes, arterial occlusion or stenosis is commonly found in the iliac and femoral arteries (Figure 10.9), whereas in individuals with diabetes, occlusion usually occurs more distally, affecting the tibial, peroneal and distal arteries (Figure 10.10). Occlusion is likely to be multisegmental, bilateral and to occur more rapidly and at an earlier stage than in someone without diabetes (Levin, 1988). Medial calcinosis occurs in the medial lining of the artery. This can result in difficulties in interpreting non-invasive investigation with Doppler ultrasound. Risk factors for the disease include increasing age, duration of diabetes, smoking, hypertension and hypercholesterolaemia. Microcirculatory damage in people with diabetes occurs frequently, causing damage to the retina, renal glomeruli and digits of the lower limb. Microcirculatory damage occurs more frequently if glycaemic control is poor.

Neuropathy in the diabetic patient

Three main types of peripheral neuropathy occur: sensory, motor, and autonomic.

Sensory neuropathy is characterized by reduced or absent pain sensation in the feet which can result in unnoticed mechanical, thermal or chemical trauma (Figure 10.11).

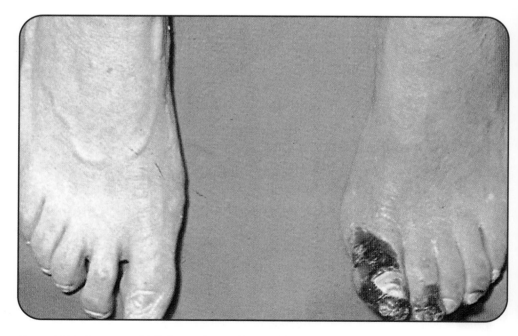

Figure 10.9 Gangrene of left first and second toes with ischaemia of leg caused by occlusion of the deep femoral artery. (Reproduced from Bloom & Ireland, 1992.)

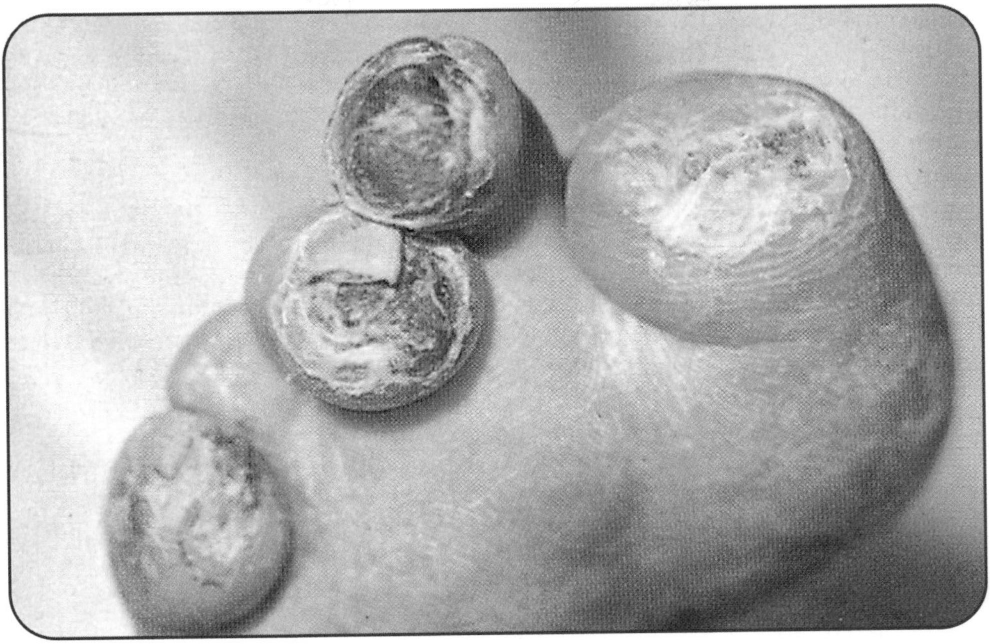

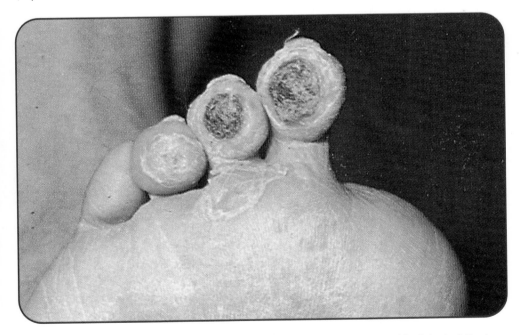

Figure 10.10 Peripheral ischaemia and dry gangrene associated with occlusion of the arcuate vessels of the dorsalis pedis artery; the necrotic areas gradually demarcate and auto-amputate. (Reproduced from Bloom & Ireland, 1992.)

Figure 10.11 Painless destructive damage to neuropathic toes caused when this diabetic fell asleep while warming his feet in front of an electric fire. (Reproduced from Bloom & Ireland, 1992.)

Motor neuropathy results in foot deformity caused by atrophy of the small muscles of the foot causing clawing of the toes and prominent metatarsal heads. A changed gait and repeated prolonged pressure can cause a build up of callus leading to ulceration on the sole of the foot, especially under the first metatarsal head (Figure 10.12), over enlarged bunions and over bony prominences of the toes (Figure 10.13).

Autonomic neuropathy causes alteration in blood flow. The foot is dry, with lack of sweating. The skin cracks and develops fissures allowing entry of fungi and bacteria. Deep perforating ulceration develops below the calluses, leading to infection and abscess formation. The callus may mask the extent of the underlying ulceration. Infection and osteomyelitis are common complications that need prompt and aggressive treatment with debridement and systemic antibiotics.

Other causes of ulceration in the patient with diabetes

Diabetic patients can, of course, develop ulcers because of other pathologies such as chronic venous hypertension. It is crucial to determine the underlying cause of the ulceration for each individual. The role of prevention is particularly important in the diabetic as tissue damage may have devastating consequences.

More unusual causes of leg ulcers

Some of the more unusual causes of leg ulcers are summarized in Table 10.6. Approximately 2–5% of leg ulcers in total are the result of these more uncommon causes.

PATIENT ASSESSMENT

When a patient presents for the first time with a leg ulcer a general patient assessment is required to determine the following:
- The immediate cause of the ulcer.
- Any underlying pathology in the lower limb.
- Any local problems at the wound site that may delay healing.
- Other more general medical conditions that may delay healing.
- The patient's social circumstances and the optimum setting for care.

Assessing the immediate cause of the ulcer and any underlying pathology

It is important to determine the immediate cause of the ulcer to facilitate the development of a plan, with the patient, to prevent recurrence (*see* Chapter 8). It is of paramount importance to go on to determine any underlying pathology.

Assessment of the patient's clinical signs and symptoms, past medical history and simple investigations, normally give sufficient information to determine if an ulcer is the result of any of the following:
- Chronic venous hypertension (approximately 70% of cases).
- Arterial disease (approximately 10% of cases).

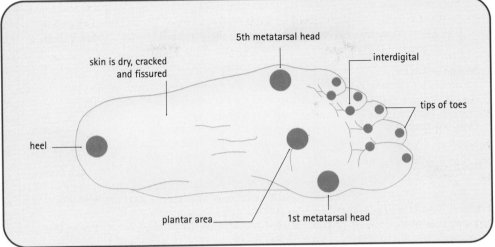

Figure 10.12 Areas of callus formation and neuropathic ulceration beneath calluses. (Reproduced from Morison & Moffatt, 1994.)

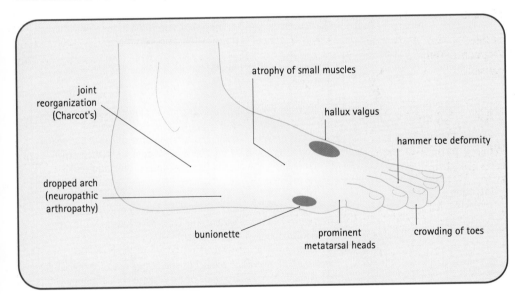

Figure 10.13 The neuropathic foot. (Reproduced from Morison & Moffatt, 1994.)

Table 10.6.
More unusual cases of leg ulcers (from Morison & Moffatt, 1994)

Malignant ulcers	
Squamous cell carcinomas	Can be seen as a primary carcinoma or with an ulcer that undergoes malignant change (Marjolin's ulcer)
Basal cell carcinomas	Usually found on the face but may occur on the leg. Lesion usually presents as a scab which, when knocked, bleeds profusely
Melanomas	Currently on the increase, probably because of exposure to ultra-violet sunlight. These tumours metastasize rapidly. Ulceration of the lesion is indicative of an advanced stage of malignancy
Kaposi's sarcoma, lymhangiosarcoma and bone tumour	Seen often in patients with HIV infection. The lesions can mimic the presentation of a melanoma or of a venous ulcer (Cohen & Prystowski, 1992)
Blood disorders	
Sickle cell disease	Small, perforating ulcers on the lower limb frequently follow a sickle cell crisis. Frequently wrongly described as arterial in origin, they develop because of thrombosis occuring in the veins after sickling. Treatment is therefore compression therapy
Thalassaemia	Small painful ulcers, most commonly in teenagers and young adults
Polycythaemia	Seen in older people usually occurring as atypical ulcers on the foot
Macroglobulinaemias	Rare blood disorders in which ulceration presents as one of many symptoms. Ulceration occurs because of damage in the micro-circulation after the accumulation of large protein molecules
Infection	
Tuberculosis	Currently on the increase. Skin ulceration may present alone but often with chest involvement. The ulcer base is usually grey–pink with irregular, bluish, friable edges
Syphilis	Rare cause of ulceration today but still occurs occasionally. Often presenting in the tertiary stage of the disease with accompaning osteomyelitis. Tends to occur high on the calf or outer aspect of the lower leg (Walzman et al. 1986)
Leprosy	Progressive destruction of digits and ulceration with associated neuropathy, ulcers usually occur on plantar surface
Fungal infection	Occurs in tropical areas associated with malnutrition, poor hygiene and poverty

Table 10.6. (*continued*)

Metabolic disorders Pyoderma gangrenosum	Often accompanies systemic disorders such as ulcerative colitis, Crohn's disease, rheumatoid arthritis or myeloma
Pretibial myxoedema	Rare type of ulceration occurring in patients with myxoedema
Necrobiosis lipodica	Occurs predominantly in patients with diabetes mellitus. Pigmented areas with ulceration in the gaiter region involving secondary infection of the dermis which becomes progressively necrotic
Lymphoedema	i) Primary lymphoedema caused by congenital absence of lymphatic vessels, rarely presenting with ulceration ii) Secondary lymphoedema accompanying venous disease iii) Parasitic elephantiasis caused by filiasis causing lymphatic destruction
Iatrogenic	e.g. Compression-induced ulceration when there is arterial insufficiency or overtight bandaging over a bony prominence when compression is indicated
Self-inflicted ulceration	Deliberate attempts to create or sustain ulceration Possible indicators include: • Ulceration in unusual sites • No other pathology • Immediate improvement when limb is immobilized and protected from damage Evidence of tampering with dressings or bandages is not in itself evidence of self-inflicted injury.

- A combination of chronic venous hypertension and arterial disease. (10–20% of cases).

The differential diagnosis of the more unusual causes of ulceration is more complex and beyond the scope of this chapter.

Specialist assessment is particularly important for patients with diabetes mellitus or suspected arterial disease as the consequences of mismanagement can be catastrophic.

Criteria for referral of leg ulcer patients to the Vascular Surgical Service developed at Charing Cross Hospital in London are given in Table 10.7.

Clinical signs and symptoms

Clinical signs and symptoms of venous and arterial disorders are summarized in Tables 10.8 and 10.9.

Interpretation of the symptoms of vascular disease requires considerable clinical experience. Problems causing pain with walking, such as arthritis, must be differentiated from arterial insufficiency with associated intermittent claudication. It is important to note that, although intermittent claudication most commonly occurs as pain in the calf, high vascular obstruction can cause pain in the buttocks and thighs and may be accompanied by impotence.

Rest-pain usually indicates at least two significant arterial stenoses or occlusions in series. It decreases with dependency of the lower limb and is made worse by heat, elevation and exercise. In the course of peripheral vascular disease, nocturnal, ischaemic pain usually precedes rest-pain. It occurs at night during sleep when peripheral perfusion is reduced.

Table 10.7.
Criteria for referral of leg ulcer patients to the Charing Cross Vascular Surgical Service (from Morison & Moffatt, 1994)

- Patients found to have a resting pressure index (RPI) of 0.5 or below should be referred immediately to the Vascular Surgical Service. Patients should be seen within 1 week of referral (No compression to be applied)

- Patients with an RPI between 0.5 and 0.8 should also be referred for vascular opinion

- Patients with an index of 0.6–0.7 may receive reduced compression (p. 206) (no more than 25 mmHg pressure)

- Young, mobile patients should be referred for a full venous assessment with a view to simple vein surgery

- Patients with recurrent ulceration should be considered for referral for full venous assessment and possible surgery to avoid further recurrence

- All ulcers failing to make satisfactory progress should be referred to the Vascular Surgical Service

- Patients presenting with ulcers when a more unusual cause is suspected should be referred for full investigation

**Table 10.8.
Venous problems: clinical signs and symptoms (from Morison & Moffatt, 1994)**

1 **Prominent superficial leg veins or symptoms of varicose veins, such as:**
- Aching or heaviness in legs, generalized or localized
- Mild ankle swelling
- Itching over varices
- Symptoms caused by thrombophlebitis, localized pain, tenderness and redness (gentle exercise such as walking round the room or repeated heel raising helps to show distension of the veins)

2 **Ankle flare.** Distension of the tiny veins on the medial aspect of the foot below the malleolus

3 **Pathological changes to the skin and tissues surrounding the ulcer, including:**
- Pigmentation. 'Staining' of the skin around the ulcer
- Lipodermatosclerosis. Hardening of dermis and underlying subcutaneous fat, which may feel 'woody'
- Stasis eczema
- Atrophe blanche. Ivory white skin stippled with red 'dots' of dilated capillary loops

4 **Site of ulcer.** Frequently near the medial malleolus, sometimes near the lateral malleolus but can be anywhere on the leg

**Table 10.9.
Arterial problems: clinical signs and symptoms (from Morison & Moffatt, 1994)**

1 **Whole leg/foot**
Symptoms:
- Intermittent claudication: cramp-like pain in the muscles of the leg, brought on by walking a certain distance (depending partly on speed, gradient and patient's weight). The patient gains relief by standing still to rest the ischaemic calf muscles.
- Ischaemic rest pain: intractable constant ache felt in the foot, typically in the toes or heels. Usually relieved by dependency: hanging the leg over the bed or sleeping upright in a chair.

Signs (many are suggestive but not specific to ischaemia):
- Coldness of the foot
- Loss of hair
- Atrophic, shiny skin
- Muscle wasting in calf or thigh
- Trophic changes in nails
- Poor tissue perfusion, for example, colour takes more than 3 seconds to return after blanching of toenail bed by applying direct pressure
- Colour changes: foot/toes dusky pink when dependent, turning pale when raised above the heart
- Gangrene of toes
- Loss of pedal pulses

2 **Site of ulcer**
- Usually on the foot or lateral aspect of the leg but may occur anywhere on the limb, including near the medial malleolus, which is the most common site for venous ulcers

The person gains relief by dangling their feet over the edge of the bed. In diabetic patients severe pain in the legs at night can be the result of diabetic neuropathy, vascular insufficiency or both.

The signs and symptoms of acute arterial occlusion are given in Table 10.10. In the absence of an adequate collateral circulation irreversible damage to skeletal muscle and peripheral nerves occurs within 4–6 hours of severe ischaemia.

Patients known to have severe peripheral vascular disease must be warned to seek immediate medical help should they develop sudden extreme pain in the leg.
For the diabetic patient, peripheral neuropathy is the most significant cause of ulceration. The neuropathy may be sensory, motor or autonomic. The signs and symptoms of diabetic neuropathy are summarized in Table 10.11.

Diabetic neuropathy is frequently bilateral and tends to be symmetrical. Patients are inclined to under-report symptoms of reduced sensation (hypoaesthesia), yet knowledge of such symptoms is crucially important for planning appropriate care and attempting to prevent recurrence of ulceration.

Table 10.10.
Clinical signs and symptoms
of acute arterial occlusion in the lower limb
(from Morison & Moffatt, 1994)

- Pain of sudden onset and severe intensity

- Pallor

- Paraesthesia (numbness)

- Pulselessness (absence of pulses below the occlusion)

- Paralysis (sudden weakness in the limb)

- Polar (a cold extremity)

Table 10.11.
Clinical signs and symptoms
of neuropathy in the diabetic foot and leg
(from Morison & Moffatt, 1994)

1 Foot deformity (e.g. hammer toes), Charcot's foot with collapse of the metatarsal joints giving a 'club foot' appearance

2 Excessive callus formation over bony pressure points, for example, under the metatarsal heads and the plantar surface of the foot

3 Altered sensation (paraesthesia)

- Hyperaesthesia. Excessive sensitivity of the feet which may be so great that the individual cannot bear the slightest touch. The pain may be constant and is often more severe at night, or

- Hypoaesthesia. Diminished sensitivity to pain, vibration, temperature or position. The foot may feel 'dead' or the individual may report unusual sensations when walking, for example, likening it to walking on cushions

4 Reduced or absent sweating, often accompanied by dry skin with cracks and fissures

It is important to note that there are other causes of peripheral neuropathy. These include alcoholism, collagen disorders, pernicious anaemia, malignancy affecting the spinal cord and uraemia.

The importance of specialist vascular assessment for patients thought to have a significant degree of peripheral arterial disease and for patients with diabetes mellitus cannot be overemphasized.

Medical history

Table 10.12 summarizes the factors in a patient's medical history that may throw some light on the underlying aetiology.

Chronic venous hypertension is suggested by a history of varicose veins or thrombotic episodes during surgery or pregnancy.

Callam *et al.* (1987a) found that a history of stroke, transient ischaemic attacks, angina or myocardial infarction increased the probability of arterial impairment in the lower limb and a history of intermittent claudication was almost invariably associated with poor peripheral perfusion.

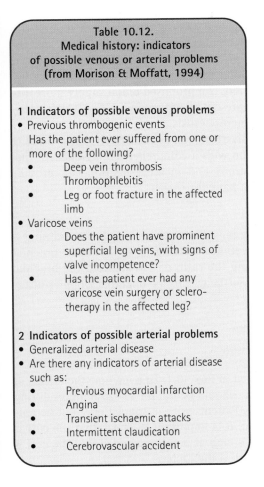

Table 10.12.
Medical history: indicators
of possible venous or arterial problems
(from Morison & Moffatt, 1994)

1 Indicators of possible venous problems
- Previous thrombogenic events
  Has the patient ever suffered from one or more of the following?
  - Deep vein thrombosis
  - Thrombophlebitis
  - Leg or foot fracture in the affected limb
- Varicose veins
  - Does the patient have prominent superficial leg veins, with signs of valve incompetence?
  - Has the patient ever had any varicose vein surgery or sclerotherapy in the affected leg?

2 Indicators of possible arterial problems
- Generalized arterial disease
- Are there any indicators of arterial disease such as:
  - Previous myocardial infarction
  - Angina
  - Transient ischaemic attacks
  - Intermittent claudication
  - Cerebrovascular accident

Palpation of foot pulses

In the past, the presence of palpable foot pulses has been taken as a sign of unimpaired arterial circulation in the lower limb and the absence of pulses as indicative of arterial impairment. This is not an entirely fail-safe test for several reasons.

In a recent study, in which community nurses palpated pulses in 533 ulcerated limbs, no pulses were detectable in 25% of patients for which another simple vascular assessment indicated that it would have been safe to apply compression. Thirty-seven per cent of patients with detectable pulses were demonstrated to have significant peripheral arterial disease. In this study, lack of pedal pulses had a positive predictive value for significant arterial disease in only 35% of patients (Moffatt & O'Hare, 1995a).

This is not just a matter of academic interest. If a patient has a venous ulcer but no palpable foot pulses, withholding compression therapy in the mistaken belief that the patient has significantly impaired peripheral arterial circulation would inevitably delay healing because the underlying problem of chronic venous hypertension would not be corrected.

It is important to note that the dorsalis pedis pulse is congenitally absent in up to 12% of individuals (Barnhorst & Barner, 1968). If the dorsalis pedis pulse is not felt, it is important to palpate the posterior tibial pulse. Oedema is a common problem in patients with ulcers and this can make pulses hard to feel.

There are a number of other clinical situations in which the presence of pedal pulses can give a false impression of a good peripheral arterial circulation. Patients with intermittent claudication may have palpable foot pulses at rest but after a brisk walk the pulses disappear. Further investigations are required to determine the severity of the underlying disease. Patients with diabetes mellitus may have bounding pedal pulses but this does not rule out the possibility of a severely compromised blood supply more distally to the toes. Palpable pulses are usually present in patients with small-vessel disease unless there is co-existing and severe atherosclerosis.

Palpation of pedal pulses remains a subjective test. The use of Doppler ultrasound to record a resting pressure index, in conjunction with a comprehensive assessment that takes account of the patient's signs, symptoms and medical history, can provide objective evidence of the arterial status of the patient.

The resting pressure index (RPI)

A simple vascular assessment technique that can be readily carried out after training is the resting pressure index (RPI). This is sometimes referred to as the ankle-brachial pressure index (ABPI). It involves determining the ratio of the ankle to the brachial systolic pressure with the aid of a simple, hand-held, battery-operated Doppler ultrasound probe in place of a stethoscope.

$$\text{Resting pressure index (RPI)} = \frac{\text{ankle systolic pressure}}{\text{brachial systolic pressure}}$$

The procedure for recording the RPI is described in Box 10.1. To overcome the effects of previous exercise on blood pressure, the patient should lie flat for 15–20 minutes during which time the patient's history can be taken. Patients with dyspnoea may not be able to lie completely flat. This should be recorded. It is important to check that the cuff is an appropriate size and length for the patient's limb. It is recommended that the cuff is 40% of the limb circumference at the mid-point of the limb.

> **Box 10.1.**
>
> Procedure for recording the resting pressure index (RPI)
>
> 1. Ensure that the patient is lying flat for 15–20 minutes and is comfortable and relaxed
> 2. Place the cuff around the arm and apply ultrasound gel over the brachial pulses. Hold the doppler probe until a good signal is obtained. Inflate the cuff until signal disappears and gradually lower pressure until the signal returns. (This is the brachial systolic reading.) Repeat this procedure using the other arm and take the higher of the two readings to calculate the RPI
> 3. Examine the foot and attempt to palpate the posterior tibial and dorsalis pedis pulses
> 4. Secure sphygmomanometer cuff just above the ankle, covering any ulcerated area with clingfilm or a sterile towel. Locate posterior tibial dorsalis pedis and peroneal pulses. Record the ankle systolic pressures. Take the highest of the readings
> 5. To calculate the RPI, divide ankle systolic pressure by brachial systolic pressure

To assess the ankle systolic pressure, the cuff is sited just above the malleolar area. Positioning of the cuff is important. The measurements reflect the pressure required to occlude the artery beneath the cuff and not where the doppler probe is held. Applying the cuff higher up the limb means that an RPI is not being recorded at the ankle. Although it is generally recommended that the Doppler probe be held at a 45–60° angle, it is often necessary to adjust the position if the blood vessel does not lie parallel with the skin. The appropriate ultrasound gel should be used to ensure good transmission of the signal and to prevent corrosion of the probe. A beam of ultrasound waves, emitted by a crystal in the probe, travels to the underlying blood vessels where it is reflected from red blood cells in proportion to the flow velocity of the cells. The returning signal is picked up by a second crystal in the probe.

A normal RPI in a healthy adult is usually greater than 1.0. Patients with a ratio of 0.9–0.95 probably have a mild degree of arterial disease. If the RPI is less than 0.8, there is a significant impairment of blood supply. High compression is contra-indicated in patients with an RPI of less than 0.8 and further vascular assessment is required. Patients with an RPI of 0.5–0.75 frequently suffer from intermittent claudication and below 0.5 ischaemic rest-pain is common.

Patients with a significantly elevated RPI, above 1.5, may have underlying vascular disease such as medial calcinosis. This is found in 10–12% of patients with diabetes. Patients with severe oedema and atherosclerosis (caused by calcification) may have abnormal readings and should be treated with great care. Conditions such as atrial fibrillation may make the procedure difficult and the practitioner may be unsure of the true reading.

If there is any doubt about the significance of the RPI seek medical advice.

Other simple investigations

Some simple investigations that can yield valuable results are summarized in Table 10.13. A wide range of clinical and objective tests for the assessment of the diabetic foot, including tests for pain, vibration and proprioception, are described by Boulton (1988) and Levin (op. cit.).

Further vascular assessment methods

Specialist vascular assessment for both arterial and venous disease may be required but are beyond the scope of this chapter. Morison and Moffatt (1994) and Negus (1991) describe techniques in common use. Increasingly, it is being realized that patients require access to this type of investigation. Services are being developed that bridge the traditional gap between hospital and community, allowing ease of access to patients requiring hospital investigation and treatment (Moffatt *et al.* 1992).

Mixed aetiology ulcers

Between 10 and 20% of leg ulcers do not fall neatly into either the venous or arterial categories. A patient's leg may show all the classic signs of chronic venous hypertension but there may also be underlying arterial problems. The checklist in Table 10.14 can be

---

Table 10.13.
Other simple investigations
(from Morison & Moffatt, 1994)

- BM stix to detect the possibility of undiagnosed diabetes, which is often associated with peripheral arterial problems

- Blood test to test for rheumatoid and antinuclear factors which may indicate potential arteritis or auto-immune disorders; full blood count and estimation of haemoglobin levels

- Patch testing for allergens (e.g. lanolin and parabens) which are present in many commonly used wound-care products

- Tissue biopsy if malignant changes are suspected

- Wound swabs to identify the nature and antibiotic sensitivity of any organisms causing clinical signs of infection

Table 10.14.
Indicators of venous and/or arterial problems in the lower limb (from Morison & Moffatt, 1994)

Indicators of venous problems:

1 Medical history
- Has the patient ever suffered from any of the following: deep vein thrombosis, thrombophlebitis or leg or foot fracture in the affected limb?
- Has the patient ever had any varicose vein surgery or sclerotherapy in the affected limb?

2 Clinical signs and symptoms in the leg
- Prominent superficial leg veins
- Brown pigmentation of the skin around and just above the ankle
- Distension of the tiny veins in the medial aspect of the foot
- Lipodermatosclerosis (hard 'woody' induration of the lower leg)
- Stasis eczema
- Atrophe blanche (skin thin, white and stippled with red dots)

3 Simple vascular assessment/tests
- Pedal pulses present
- RPI > 0.9

Indicators of arterial problems:

1. Medical history
- Are there any indicators of generalized arterial disease, for example, myocardial infarction, angina, transient ischaemic attacks, intermittent claudication, cerebrovascular accident?

2 Clinical signs and symptoms in the leg
- Intermittent claudication
- Ischaemic rest pain
- Pain relief when the leg is lowered below heart level
- Foot dusky pink when dependent, turning pale when elevated above the heart
- Poor tissue perfusion, for example, colour takes more than 3 seconds to return after blanching of toenail bed by applying direct pressure
- Loss of hair, atrophic shiny skin

3 Simple vascular assessment/tests
- Pedal pulses absent or very faint indeed
- RPI < 0.9

useful for summarizing some of the indicators of venous and arterial disease and may alert the practitioner to possible arterial problems when the patient presents with an apparently 'classic' venous ulcer. The severity of the arterial disease will determine which treatment methods can be used safely in these patients.

More unusual ulcers

A small proportion of leg ulcers are not vascular in origin as summarized in Table 10.6. If the wound has an unusual appearance, is in an unusual site or fails to progress, another aetiology should be suspected and the patient should be investigated further

Local wound assessment

After assessing the underlying cause of the ulcer, assessment of the wound itself should be undertaken as described in Chapter 4. This will influence the method of wound cleansing (*see* Chapter 5) and the most appropriate primary wound contact dressing (*see* Chapter 6).

It is helpful to *trace* the ulcer every 2–4 weeks to check progress but the inherent inaccuracies in this simple method should not be forgotten (Johnson, 1993). The surface area may increase as the wound is debrided. Plassmann and Jones (1992) describe a colour-coded, structured-light technique for the three-dimensional measurement of leg ulcers. Such levels of sophistication are, however, rarely available in the clinical setting. Photography is becoming increasingly popular and may be used to encourage patients to follow the progress of the healing process.

The reasons for pain at the wound site should be very carefully assessed as many are easily correctable and correction can significantly improve the quality of the patient's life (*see* Chapter 13).

Assessing other factors that may affect healing

When taking the patient's history and carrying out an assessment of their current general physical condition, it is worth noting any other factors that could contribute to delayed wound healing, such as

- Evidence of, or suspected, malnutrition.
- poor mobility, of whatever cause, which may adversely affect the calf-muscle pump and venous return.
- An occupation or activities that involve prolonged standing, especially in warm conditions.
- Decreased resistance to infection, whatever the cause.
- Poor social circumstances.

The range of local and systemic factors known to affect healing are described in Chapter 1 and are summarized in Figure 1.9. Assessment of the patient's psychosocial problems is also very important (*see* Chapter 4). The patient's occupation and social circumstances should be considered when deciding on the practical arrangements for managing the ulcer and for patient education (*see* Chapter 8).

TREATMENT OPTIONS

Priorities in leg ulcer management

Thorough, systematic and accurate assessment of the patient, the identification of the underlying cause of the ulcer and any local problems at the wound site are prerequisites to planning appropriate care and to preventing avoidable delays in healing. The main management priorities are:

- To correct the underlying cause of the ulcer. This normally means improving the patient's venous and/or arterial circulation in the affected limb.
- To create the optimum local environment at the wound site.
- To improve all the wider factors that may delay healing, especially poor mobility, malnutrition and psychosocial issues.
- To prevent avoidable complications such as wound infection, medicament dermatitis, or tissue damage because of over-tight bandaging.
- To maintain healed tissue.

These principles are described in the context of the aetiology of the ulcer.

Management of venous ulcers

Aims of management

As described, the main cause of venous ulceration is chronic venous hypertension, with very high pressures being exerted on the superficial venous system, usually because of incompetent valves in the deep or perforating veins. The primary aims of venous-ulcer management are therefore:

- To reduce blood pressure in the superficial venous system.
- To aid venous return of blood to the heart by increasing the velocity of flow in the deep veins.
- To reduce oedema by reducing the pressure difference between the capillaries and the tissues.

The use of compression

The best way to achieve these aims is to apply graduated compression from the base of the toes to the knee. The highest pressure (35–40 mmHg) is applied at the ankle, reducing by at least 50% at the knee (Moffatt, 1992).

Methods of achieving graduated compression include the application to the lower limb of:

- Single-layer elastic bandaging.
- Single-layer inelastic bandaging.
- Multilayer bandages.
- Compression stockings.

The advantages and disadvantages of these methods are summarized in Table 10.15.

It is very important to understand the performance characteristics of the different bandages available. Although all are aiming to apply graduated compression, they do so in different ways.

Table 10.15.
Methods of achieving graduated compression (from Morison & Moffatt, 1994)

Method	Advantages	Disadvantages
Single elastic bandages: e.g. Setopress, Surepress, Tensopress (Vin, 1995) (Thomas *et al.* 1986)	1 Pressure is sustained over time (useful for immobile patients) 2 Useful in patients with limited mobility 3 Available on prescription 4 Re-washable	1 Potential risk of excessive high pressures with over extension (many bandages have symbols to help practitioners gauge correct extension) 2 High compression bandage may lack ability to conform to limb contours
Inelastic bandages: e.g. Comprilan, Rosidal K, Elastocrepe (Duby *et al.* 1993) (Charles, 1996)	1 Bandage action enhanced with patient activity 2 Can be applied to patients with mild arterial disease: low resting pressure index 3 Non-allergic 4 Cost-effective 5 Washable	1 Bandage slippage during initial treatment to reduce oedema 2 Not suitable for immobile patients or those with reduced ankle function 3 Restricted availability in the community
Multilayer bandages: e.g. 4-layer bandage systems (Blair *et al.* 1988) (Callam *et al.* 1992)	1 Requires infrequent re-application 2 Adapted for individual limb size and shape, preventing slippage and limb trauma 3 Use of relatively weak bandages in combination avoids excessive rises in sub-bandage pressure	1 Not available on prescription in the community 2 Relatively high unit cost 3 Patient may require a larger size
Elastic compression stockings	1 Pressure profiles of stockings are tested and known 2 A range of compression profiles is available to meet individual needs 3 Much safer than inappropriately applied heavy compression bandages 4 Cosmetically acceptable 5 Useful in preventing recurrence of ulceration	1 Require proper fitting for length, ankle and calf size 2 Initial cost is high but compares well with the cost of elastic compression bandages over 6 months 3 Difficult for patients with restricted movement to apply themselves 4 Compliance rate variable; high compression stockings often poorly tolerated by elderly people but well liked by younger patients who are more mobile

Elastic bandages

These contain an elastomer and are capable of sustaining compression over a long period of time. They are capable of exerting medium to very high compression. There is little variation in pressure with posture or exercise. Although these bandages are generally applied at 50% extension, this can be altered in order to reduce or enhance the pressure required. The manufacturer's recommendations should be read carefully before any bandage is applied for the first time.

Inelastic bandages

These are without elastomer and are generally made of cotton. They are usually applied at 90% extension. Inelastic bandages apply a semi-rigid support to the calf muscle. During exercise, the sub-bandage pressure rises steeply as the muscle contracts against the bandage. At rest, the sub-bandage pressure is relatively low.

Factors affecting the pressure that can be achieved under a bandage are indicated by La Place's Law (Box 10.2).

Table 10.16 shows the practical implications of this equation and how this relates to problems in bandage application. Figures 10.14 and 10.15 illustrate how to apply a bandage in a spiral or in a figure of eight.

It is likely that compression will remain the most important component of treatment for venous and lymphatic disorders. Training in the application of compression bandaging is important and practitioners need to understand the scientific principles that underpin its effective use (Nelson *et al.* 1995b).

Box 10.2.

La Place's Law

Some of the factors affecting the pressure that can be achieved under a bandage are given in the following equation:

$$P \text{ is proportional to } \frac{N \times T}{C \times W}$$

Where
P is the pressure exerted by the bandage
N is the number of layers of bandage
T is the bandage tension
C is the circumference of the limb
W is the bandage width

Criteria for using reduced compression

When the underlying cause of the ulcer appears to be a combination of chronic venous hypertension and poor peripheral arterial circulation, it is the degree of arterial insufficiency that will determine whether compression can be applied. If the RPI is below 0.8, reduced compression (no more than 25 mmHg) can be applied on selected patients, according to the patient's symptoms. Patients with an RPI below 0.5 should not have compression applied.

Frequently, patients will undergo reconstructive surgery or angioplasty to correct arterial impairment. Providing the RPI returns to 0.8, or above, compression can be applied but must be done with care. These patients must be regularly followed up and their RPI checked monthly or more frequently if any change in symptoms occurs. A Duplex scan of the graft or vessel should frequently be undertaken. After correction of the arterial problem, it may be possible to correct any venous abnormality that is amenable to surgery.

Compression hosiery and the prevention of recurrence of a venous ulcer

Compression hosiery is used to control oedema, manage varicose veins, and in the prevention and treatment of venous and lymphatic disorders. They have a number of advantages over bandages, provided that they have been correctly fitted and the patient is able to apply them (Moffatt and O'Hare, 1995b) (Table 10.16).

Compression hosiery is graded into three classes according to the compression exerted at the ankle:

- Class I (14–17 mmHg): Light compression used to treat mild, early varicose veins.
- Class II (18–24 mmHg): Medium compression, for more serious varicosities, for patients who have had acute deep-vein thrombosis and for the treatment and prevention of venous ulceration.
- Class III (25–35 mmHg): Strong compression for severe chronic venous hypertension, severe varicose veins and for ulcer prevention and treatment in patients with very large diameter calves.

Generally, below-knee stockings are sufficient. However, patients with severe post-phlebitic syndrome or lymphoedema may require thigh-length stockings. A study involving provision of Class II stockings to community patients with healed ulcers found that the ulcer recurrence rate at 1 year was 25%. However, in the small percentage of patients who could or would not wear stockings, the recurrence rate was 57% (Moffatt & Dorman, 1995). Another study found that the recurrence rate was lower in patients who wore Class III stockings than those who wore Class II stockings but this group experienced the greatest problems with compliance (Harper *et al.* 1995). The greatest challenge for practitioners is to convince patients that hosiery is the most important factor in preventing their ulcer from recurring.

The recurrence rate for leg ulceration is high (Callam *et al.* op. cit.). Although providing hosiery is the most important aspect, the patient should be seen regularly and requires ongoing support and encouragement to comply with treatment once the ulcer has healed (Moffatt & Dorman, op. cit.). It is essential that the patient understands why he has been given hosiery and this may be reinforced by educational literature.

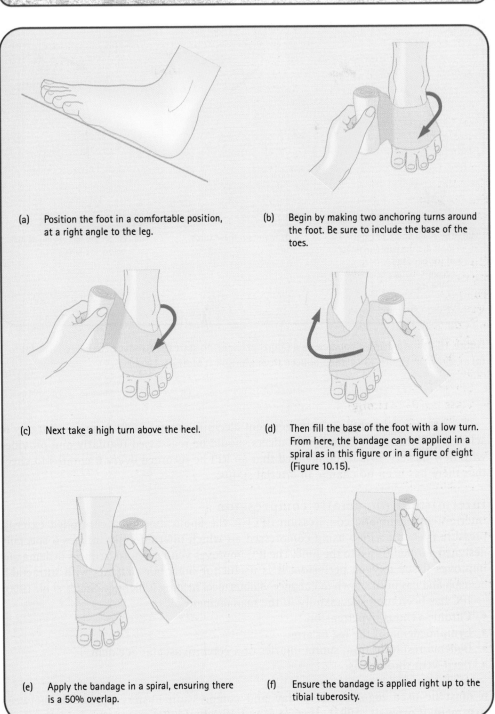

(a) Position the foot in a comfortable position, at a right angle to the leg.

(b) Begin by making two anchoring turns around the foot. Be sure to include the base of the toes.

(c) Next take a high turn above the heel.

(d) Then fill the base of the foot with a low turn. From here, the bandage can be applied in a spiral as in this figure or in a figure of eight (Figure 10.15).

(e) Apply the bandage in a spiral, ensuring there is a 50% overlap.

(f) Ensure the bandage is applied right up to the tibial tuberosity.

Figure 10.14 Applying a bandage in a spiral. (Reproduced from Morison & Moffatt, 1994.)

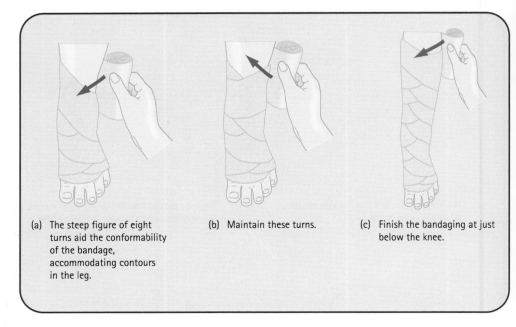

(a) The steep figure of eight turns aid the conformability of the bandage, accommodating contours in the leg.

(b) Maintain these turns.

(c) Finish the bandaging at just below the knee.

Figure 10.15   Applying a bandage in a figure-of-eight. To start the bandage complete steps (a) to (d) as shown in Figure 10.14. (Reproduced from Morison & Moffatt, 1994.)

Younger patients or those with recurrent ulceration may benefit from vein surgery or sclerotherapy. Patients with healed ulcers should be reassessed regularly and provided with new hosiery. It is recommended that an RPI be recorded every 6 months to check that there has been no change in arterial status.

Intermittent pneumatic compression

Intermittent pneumatic compression (IPC) is the application of a controlled external pressure cycle on a limb using compressed air which intermittently inflates a specially designed garment fitted to the limb. The IPC improves venous return, reduces oedema and improves tissue oxygen perfusion. It is useful for immobile patients with intractable oedema and has been shown to enhance venous ulcer healing (Coleridge-Smith *et al.* 1990).

IPC has been used successfully in the management of:

- Chronic venous hypertension.
- Lymphoedema of the leg or arm.
- Oedema resulting from sports injuries or a cerebrovascular accident.
- Deep-vein thrombosis.

It must be used regularly each day and compression hosiery applied in between treatment (Cornwall, 1991). Hazarika and Wright (1981) noted the importance of providing support to elderly patients using IPC to help them to overcome their fear of the equipment. Encouraging compliance with any regime is especially important if treatment is to be effective.

Table 10.16.
The application of La Place's law in practice

Number of layers The more layers applied the higher the sub-bandage pressure	**Problems relating to application** Excessive layers are frequently applied during bandage application, particularly when bandages are joined or excess bandage remains. This may form a tourniquet and prevent venous return.
Bandage tension The greater the extension of the bandage the higher is the resulting sub-bandage pressure Bandage tension is proportional to: • The elasticity of the bandage • How much the bandage is stretched • How many times it has been washed • How long the bandage is in place	Bandages are often overextended as the bandage is being applied to the limb. Common sites for overextension are around the ankle and at mid-calf. Vulnerable points on the limb such as the tibia, malleoli and dorsum of the foot should be protected with padding, particularly when single elastic bandages are used.
Limb circumference The pressure exerted by the bandage is inversely proportional to the circumference of the limb	Thin limbs are at risk of excessive pressure. Bandages are designed to apply the correct pressure to a range of ankle circumferences. The manufacturer's instructions should be carefully read before application. Thin limbs must be protected with padding and the bandage not overextended Large limbs may not receive a therapeutic level of compression and a stronger elastic bandage may need to be applied. Ulcers occurring in the hollow behind the malleoli may receive inadequate compression. Local pressure can be increased by placing a foam or gauze pad over the primary dressing covering the ulcer. **Inverted champagne–bottle shaped legs** Extra padding around the gaiter region may be required to reduce the steep gradient and prevent bandage slippage **Thin limbs** Extra padding around the calf will increase the gradient and reduce the risk of pressure damage
Bandage width The pressure exerted by a bandage is inversely proportional to its width	Higher pressures are obtained with narrower bandages and lower pressures with wider ones. Most bandages are a standard 10 cm in width.

IPC is contra-indicated in patients with:
- A deep-vein thrombosis.
- Severe arteriosclerosis.
- Oedema caused by congestive cardiac failure.
- Severe leg deformity.
- Local gangrene.

Care should be taken if IPC is used in conjunction with elastic bandages, as very high interface pressures may be applied.

Management of arterial ulcers

The prognosis for an elderly patient with an arterial ulcer is much less hopeful than for a patient with a venous ulcer, unless the problem is amenable to surgery or to percutaneous transluminal angioplasty (PCTA).

Of the pharmacological agents, vasodilators are of questionable benefit but oxpentifylline has been shown to be of benefit (Prescott *et al.* 1995). Pain control is often challenging and usually requires the use of opiates.

Effective wound management and the prevention of infection are critical as are a reduction of risk factors such as smoking and hypertension.

Compression bandaging should not be applied as severe damage to the leg can result, as illustrated in Figure 10.16.

Management of ulcers associated with rheumatoid arthritis

The management of a patient with rheumatoid arthritis depends on the underlying aetiology of the ulcer (Pun *et al.* op. cit.). If compression is required it should be applied with great care, avoiding excessive pressure to bony prominences. The long-term use of corticosteroids causes dermal thinning and the limb must be protected from trauma.

Skin grafts are frequently unsuccessful in these patients and often only palliative care can be offered (Pun *et al.* op. cit.). Particular attention should be paid to keeping the skin

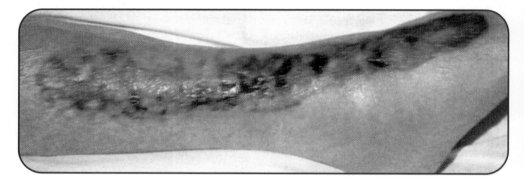

Figure 10.16 A bandage-induced ulcer which led to amputation. (Reproduced from Ruckley, 1988.)

supple with emollients, maintaining mobility and reducing pain. Malnutrition is a frequent problem in these patients as is an increased risk of infection.

Management of the diabetic foot

The long-term management of diabetic patients and the prevention of complications is challenging. It requires a co-ordinated, multidisciplinary team approach and informed patient co-operation.

As described diabetic foot ulcers usually result from the triad of:

- Peripheral neuropathy (the insensate foot).
- Peripheral vascular insufficiency (ischaemia).
- Infection.

According to Levin (op. cit.), management of diabetic foot ulcers requires aggressive treatment. In the short term, this involves:

- Radical local debridement, leaving only healthy tissue.
- Systemic antibiotic therapy to combat any infection after antibiotic sensitivity testing.
- Diabetic control, which, among other effects, optimizes efficiency of the immune system.
- Non-weight bearing for plantar ulcers.

Appropriate wound-dressing selection, discussed in Chapter 6, is important but this is merely an adjunct to the therapies mentioned. If an ulcer is refractory to all treatment, the physician may request a radiograph or bone scan to exclude the possibilities of osteomyelitis or a retained foreign body of which the patient is unaware.

Feet should be kept dry. Soaking the feet causes maceration between the toes and increases the risk of infection. Attention should also be given to rehydrating dry skin around the ulcer and over the lower leg with emollients.

For some patients, it is possible to improve the peripheral circulation through vascular bypass surgery, PCTA, laser treatment and the use of haemorrheologic agents, such as oxpentifylline (Trental), which improves red cell flexibility and blood flow. The combination of endovascular revascularization, growth factor therapy, and comprehensive wound-care protocols can lead to very high limb-salvage rates in specialist centres (Bild et al. 1989; Knighton et al. 1990). However, prevention is infinitely preferable to cure. Some of the risk factors for peripheral vascular disease in diabetic patients are not treatable, such as age and the duration of the diabetes but many risk factors are amenable to change, such as smoking, hypertension, hyperlipidaemia, hyperglycaemia and obesity, and many long-term complications can be significantly reduced when the patient takes responsibility for self-care and has a positive attitude towards health promotion (see Chapter 8).

Patient education is, in fact, the key to preventing foot ulceration. Patients' feet should be inspected at every routine outpatient visit. They should be encouraged to report foot problems as soon as they occur, however minor. The chiropodist should trim the patient's toe nails and treat calluses and other local foot problems.

Patients should be assessed for the need for special footwear to reduce pressure over bony prominences. Extra-depth shoes can be designed to accommodate clawed toes and insoles can be made to reduce plantar pressures (Coleman, 1988). Total-contact casting may be required for the management of diabetic neuropathic ulcers (Sinacore, 1988). Lightweight walking casts are described by Jones (1991).

Diabetic patients can develop ulcers because of chronic venous hypertension in the absence of any history, clinical signs or symptoms of peripheral vascular disease or peripheral neuropathy. Compression should, however, always be applied with caution and under strict medical supervision.

Creating the optimum local environment for healing

There is no doubt that correcting the underlying cause of an ulcer, where possible, is the first priority of leg ulcer management. However, it is also important to select an appropriate dressing to address any local problems at the wound site (*see* Chapter 6). Creating the optimum local environment for healing begins with cleansing the whole leg.

Cleansing the leg

Before applying any kind of dressing to an ulcer, it is important to render the entire leg 'socially' clean. One way to do this is to immerse the leg in a deep plastic bowl lined with a polythene bag and half filled with lukewarm tap water. This helps to remove debris, aids debridement and is comforting to the patient. Alternatively, the ulcer can be cleansed with normal saline.

As discussed in Chapter 5, there is rarely any place for the use of antiseptic solutions except where there is an overwhelming risk of infection and concurrent ischaemia (Thomas, 1991). The use of emollients and the control of varicose eczema are particularly important in the management of patients with venous ulceration as discussed in Chapter 7.

The management of clinical infection

This is dealt with comprehensively in Chapter 3. However, certain leg ulcer conditions require special comment here.

Lymphoedema Patients may require long-term antibiotics because of the progressive destruction of the lymphatics and the build up of waste metabolites and pathogens in the tissues, leading to recurrent bouts of cellulitis. Antibiotic levels within the tissues remain low because of the poor perfusion.

Diabetic foot ulceration Clinical infection is the most serious complication and is frequently caused by synergistic infection by aerobic and anaerobic bacteria. Rampant infection leads quickly to cellulitis and gas gangrene and must be treated aggressively with a cocktail of antibiotics.

Skin grafts frequently fail if infection with haemolytic streptococci or *Pseudomonas* occurs. Antibiotics are often used prophylactically to prevent graft rejection.

There is rarely a place for topical antibiotics in local wound management, even when lower-limb perfusion is poor. The continued overuse of antibiotics is leading to increasing multiresistance and the development of superinfections.

Skin grafting

Pinch or meshed skin grafts can be used to treat large areas of venous ulceration (Poskitt *et al.* 1987). The success of a graft is dependent on the ulcer site being free from pathogens such as haemolytic streptococci, and *Pseudomonas* as well as being free from necrotic tissue. Grafts fail for the following reasons:

- Inadequate blood supply in the recipient area.
- Haematoma that prevents vascular link up and increases the risk of infection.
- Shearing forces that cause the graft to move, severing new vessels.
- Infection.

Frequently, graft failure occurs when a patient is discharged home. This is often because compression was not applied to control venous hypertension and oedema. Returning to a normal life involves a patient in being in an upright position for much of the time and some patients are reluctant to go to bed at night. Patient co-operation and education are vitally important if graft failure is to be avoided.

Correcting more general causes of delayed wound healing

There are many factors that contribute to delayed healing in individual patients, as described in Chapter 1 and summarized in Figure 1.9. All of these factors have the potential to delay wound healing in a patient with a leg ulcer. Four factors, of particular relevance to leg ulcer patients, are restricted mobility, oedema in the limb, malnutrition and psychological problems.

Restricted mobility

Reduced mobility in general and reduced ankle function in particular are significant factors in delaying venous ulcer healing (Franks *et al.* 1995b). Patients should be encouraged to maximize their mobility within the limits of their capability and if they are unable to walk, to carry out ankle extension, flexion and rotation exercises every hour. The physiotherapist may play an important role in increasing patient mobility.

Peripheral oedema

There are many causes of peripheral oedema, including cardiac failure, liver disease, venous and lymphatic disease and malnutrition. Peripheral oedema in a dependent limb can also be encountered in a patient with hemiparesis after a cerebrovascular accident.

Identification of the cause of the oedema is imperative as this will determine treatment. In many cases reducing the oedema by compression is contra-indicated.

Peripheral oedema in the lower limb delays healing by increasing the diffusion distance between blood capillaries and the tissues that they serve. The tissues become starved of oxygen and nutrients and metabolic waste products build up.

Oedema can be improved by exercise and leg elevation. Patients with venous ulceration should be encouraged to sit with their legs elevated above the level of their hips and to raise the end of their beds by 9" (22.5 cm) with blocks. However, care must be taken in patients with severe ischaemia and dependency oedema. High elevation will cause severe pain and further compromise their circulation. Although severe oedema can be reduced by bed-rest and elevation, it is rarely a sensible option, leading to other complications such as stiffened joints, deep vein thrombosis (DVT) and chest infections.

Oedema caused by severe heart failure can occur suddenly. Compression should never be used to reduce this type of oedema as this can exacerbate the condition.

Malnutrition

As with all wounds, malnutrition may lead to delayed wound healing. Malnutrition is a common problem for elderly people for many reasons including poverty, difficulty in getting to the shops or preparing food, loss of interest in diet when living alone, ill-fitting dentures or specific gastro-intestinal disorders. Obese patients can equally be at risk as undernourished patients. Obesity will also contribute to poor ulcer healing through immobility and poor venous return.

The role of nutrition in wound healing is discussed extensively in Chapter 2. Other members of the multidisciplinary team often need to be involved (Taylor & Goodinson–Mclaren, 1992).

Psychosocial issues

Many patients with leg ulcers are elderly, poor and alone. Recent research has shown that social conditions, such as lack of central heating, may play a role in delaying healing (Franks *et al.* op. cit.). Further research is needed in this area to determine the significance of these findings as correlation does not prove causation.

Much has been written about the 'social' ulcer (Wise, 1986). There is no doubt that a minority of patients do have a vested interest in their ulcer not healing but the proportion of patients who actually interfere with the ulcer in an attempt to delay healing is unknown.

If a conscious attempt at self-inflicted injury is suspected the problem must be dealt with sympathetically. The problem may be one of loneliness or fear of losing professional support. Other strategies, such as attending day-care centres or well-ulcer clinics, may help a patient 'let go' of their ulcer. The patient's role in contributing to successful treatment should not be underestimated.

CONCLUSION

Leg ulceration has been described as a 'Cinderella' condition which is unattractive to many health professionals. However, the clinical management of patients with leg ulceration can be a rewarding experience.

The past decade has seen the development of new treatments and initiatives. It is now recognized that significant improvements in healing can be achieved when research-based methods of assessment and treatment are used. There is, however, no room for complacency. Many questions remain unanswered such as the underlying pathology of leg ulcers that fail to heal despite best practice. Interest and excitement in new developments, such as the use of growth factors, has been tempered with caution as the complexity of the situation emerges. Research into the pathogenesis of venous ulceration continues to bring with it the hope that a drug therapy will be developed that breaks the cycle of tissue destruction. Many clinicians also now believe that it is very important to pay close attention to quality of life issues when planning care with patients.

In recognition of the significance of the problem of leg ulceration, the National Health Service Executive have developed clinical guidelines to encourage practitioners and purchasers to adopt the most effective methods of providing care.

SELF-ASSESSMENT QUESTIONS AND ACTIVITIES

Case study 1: A venous ulcer

Mrs Howe is 67 years old. She lives with her husband in a bungalow. She has one daughter who lives locally. She has recently retired from her job as a secretary which she held for 35 years. A year ago Mrs Howe underwent a hysterectomy for carcinoma of the uterus. After this she developed a DVT in her right leg which was treated with Heparin. A few months after this event Mrs Howe noted that her leg had became stained and that her ankles swelled during the day. An ulcer developed spontaneously 4 months ago and has not healed. Clinical examination revealed the presence of other varicosities, on both legs, that had never been treated. Repeated 5-day courses of broad-spectrum antibiotics had been given for reported wound infection. The wound-swab results indicated mixed flora and Pseudomonas aeruginosa.

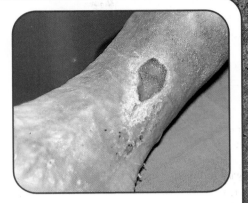

Mrs Howe appears pale and reports an increasing lack of energy. She is fearful about her condition which appears linked to her experience of observing her mother who also suffered from a leg ulcer. The odour associated with the ulcer and her change in mood is having a detrimental effect on her relationship with her husband.

A number of topical agents, including topical antibiotics, have been used to treat her ulcer with little effect. She appears mistrustful of the professionals seeking to help her.

1. *What risk factors are evident in Mrs Howe's case to indicate that she may have a venous ulcer?*
2. *List the investigations that you would routinely perform as part of the assessment of a person with a leg ulcer.*
3. *List six leg ulcer allergens that can cause contact dermatitis in people with venous ulceration (see also Chapter 7).*
4. *What would be your priorities for the management of this patient?*
5(a) *What are the indications for using antibiotics in the treatment of leg ulcers? (see also Chapter 3).*
   (b) *Why would a review of the use of antibiotics seem to be required in this case?*
   (c) *What are the dangers to the patient of inappropriate or prolonged use of antibiotics?*
   (d) *What are the wider implications in the community for the overuse of antibiotics?*
6. *How would you address the quality of life issues raised in the case?*

Case study 2: Ischaemic ulceration

Mr Dawson is 78 years old. He lives in a second floor flat with his wife. He rarely goes out, because of problems of mobility and his difficulty in negotiating stairs. The lifts are frequently broken. His family are supportive if somewhat overbearing and they are extremely anxious about his condition. Mr Dawson retired from his factory job 12 years ago. He has smoked over 20 cigarettes a day for the previous 60 years and he is obese.

Mr Dawson has an ulcer over the dorsum of his foot which is sloughy, deep and punched out. There is surrounding erythema and his foot is cold and oedematous. Foot pulses are absent. He has little calf muscle and shiny, hairless skin on both legs. His toenails are dystrophic.

Mr Dawson began to notice problems when walking 10 years ago. He attributed this to arthritis in both hips although the pain occurred in his thighs and calf. He suffered a stroke 5 years ago after a series of transient ischaemic attacks. He has made a good recovery with only minimal weakness in his left arm. He complains of angina on exercise and his blood pressure is 190/110. His RPI is 0.4 on his right leg and 0.5 on the left. He spends long periods sitting in the chair and often refuses to go to bed as the pain worsens when he lies flat. Some pain relief has been achieved using morphine slow-release tablets and the use of an occlusive dressing.

Urgent admission to a vascular unit is arranged for investigation and treatment. After he has been admitted Mrs Dawson states that she can no longer cope and that he cannot return home.

1. *What are the main risk factors for the development of cardiovascular disease?*
2. *Where are the most common sites for arterial occlusion in the lower limb?*
3(a) *Why does pain develop during exercise in a patient with peripheral arterial disease?*
(b) *What percentage of the blood vessel is normally occluded before a patient experiences rest pain.*
(c) *What methods can be used to improve the arterial circulation in patients with advanced arterial disease?*
4. *What could happen if a compression bandage was applied to Mr Dawson's limb and why?*
5(a) *What risk factors in Mr Dawson's history might be amenable to change?*
(b) *What educational strategies could you use to facilitate Mr Dawson to take more responsibility for his health (see also Chapter 8)?*

6(a) Outline the priorities, from a professional perspective, for Mr Dawson's discharge plan.

(b) How would you involve Mr Dawson and his family in the discharge-planning process?

(c) List the other professionals who may need to become involved if discharge is to be successful and the possible nature of their involvement.

Case study 3: An ulcer associated with diabetic neuropathy

Mr Horn is 53 years old. He has been an insulin-dependent diabetic since the age of 29. He presents to an Accident and Emergency unit with the request that a doctor examine his foot. He is currently receiving laser therapy for diabetic neuropathy and is being investigated for kidney disease. His hospital notes reveal that he is erratic in his attendance at clinics. He has not attended the diabetic clinic or podiatrist for 9 months, despite previous ulceration leading to the amputation of two toes. Discussion with Mr Horn reveals that he has recently experienced a divorce after the collapse of his business. He is now working as a waiter and he is on his feet for up to 14 hours a day. His current foot ulcer developed 3 months ago and he has been applying dry dressings himself. He is now anxious that it is deteriorating. He appears distracted and agitated, reporting that he is due at work shortly and that his boss will not allow him to take time off.

On examination of his feet, pressure marks suggest that his shoes are too tight. Exudate has collected in the inside of his shoes. His feet appear generally unkempt with excessive callous formation over the metatarsal heads and there is a deep, perforating ulcer. The skin on the plantar surface is thick, dry and cracked. His foot feels warm and appears flushed. His pedal pulses are bounding. Mr Horn has no pain in his feet and legs. This has changed in the last few months. Previously, he experienced severe burning pain in his feet and legs which was worse at night.

Routine investigations reveal an RPI of 1.3 on both his right and left leg. His blood-sugar levels are raised. All other investigations are normal.

1. What percentage of patients with diabetes undergo lower-limb amputation and within what time span?

2. What medical, social and psychological factors may have predisposed this patient to recurrent ulceration and may result in the need for further amputation?

3(a) How is sensation assessed in the diabetic foot?

(b) What factors indicate that this patient has an insensate foot?

4(a) What mechanisms within the microcirculation lead to autonomic neuropathy?

(b) What signs and symptoms in this case suggest autonomic involvement?

5(a) How would you establish whether or not this wound is clinically infected? (see also Chapter 3).

(b) Why might a course of systemic antibiotics be indicated in this case?

6(a) What would be the priorities in managing this patient?

(b) List them in order of importance.

7(a) *Patients with diabetes frequently present with gangrenous toes. Why does this occur?*

(b) *What is the role of micro-organisms in causing localized gangrene in the diabetic foot?*

8. *What special considerations need to be taken when assessing the arterial status of a patient with diabetes?*

9(a) *What are the immediate educational needs of Mr Horn?*

(b) *Outline a possible health promotion programme for Mr Horn, indicating the other healthcare professionals who may need to be involved and the likely nature of their involvement (see also Chapter 8).*

For further case studies see Advanced Case Studies 3–6 (pp.276–283).

REFERENCES

Barnhorst DA, Barner HB. Prevalence of congenitally absent pedal pulses. *N Engl J Med* 1968, 278:264–265.

Bild DE, Selby JV, Sinnock P. Lower extremity amputation in people with diabetes: epidemiology and prevention. *Diab Care* 1989, 12:24–31.

Blair SD, Wright DD, Backhouse CM, Riddle E, McCollum CN. Sustained compression and healing of chronic venous ulcers. *BMJ* 1988, 297:1159–1161.

Bloom A, Ireland J: *A colour atlas of diabetes.* London: Mosby; 1992.

Bosanquet N, Franks PJ, Moffatt CJ *et al.* Community leg ulcer clinics: cost effectiveness. *Health Trends* 1993, 25(4):145.

Boulton AJM. The diabetic foot. *Med Clin North Am* 1988, 72(6):1513–1530.

Burnand KG, Whimster I, Naidoo A, Browse NL. Pericapillary fibrin in the ulcer-bearing skin of the leg: the cause of lipodermatosclerosis and venous ulceration. *BMJ* 1982, 285:1071–1072.

Callam MJ, Harper DR, Dale JJ, *et al.* Lothian and Forth Valley leg ulcer healing trial part one, elastic versus non-elastic bandaging in the treatment of chronic leg ulceration. *Phlebology* 1992, 7(4):136.

Callam MJ, Harper DR, Dale JJ, Ruckley CV. Chronic ulcer of the leg: clinical history. *BMJ* 1987a, 294:1389–1391.

Callam MJ, Harper DR, Dale JJ, Ruckley CV. Arterial disease in chronic leg ulceration: an under-estimated hazard? *BMJ* 1987b, 294:929–931.

Callam MJ, Ruckley CV, Harper DR, Dale JJ. Chronic ulceration of the leg: extent of the problem and provision of care. *BMJ* 1985, 290:1855–1856.

Chant ADB. Tissue pressure, posture and venous ulceration. *Lancet* 1990, 336:1050–1051.

Charles H. Developing a leg ulcer management programme. *Professional Nurse* 1996, 11(7):475.

Cohen JI, Prystowski JH. Treatment of ulcerated HIV-associated Kaposi's sarcoma with combination chemotherapy. *Wounds* 1992, 4:208–214.

Coleman WC. Footwear in a management programme of injury prevention. In: Levin ME, O'Neal LW, eds. *The diabetic foot, 4th ed.* St Louis: CV Mosby; 1988:293–309.

Coleridge-Smith P, Sarin S, Hasty J, Scurr JH. Sequential gradient pneumatic compression enhances venous ulcer healing: a randomised trial. *Surgery* 1990, 108:871–875.

Coleridge-Smith P, Thomas P, Scurr JM, Dormandy JA. Causes of venous ulceration: a new hypothesis. *BMJ*

1988, 296:1726–1727.

Cornwall J. Managing venous leg ulcers. *Community Outlook* 1991, May:36–38.

Cornwall J, Dore CJ, Lewis JD. Leg ulcers: epidemiology and aetiology. *Br J Surg* 1986, 73:693–696.

Duby T, Hoffman DS, Cameron J, Doblhoff-Brown D, Cherry G, Ryan T. A randomised trial in the treatment
    of venous leg ulcers comparing short stretch bandages, four layer system and a long stretch paste
    system. *Wounds. A Compendium of Clin Res Practice* 1993, 5(6):276–279.

European Working Group on Critical Leg Ischaemias. Second European Concensus Document on Chronic
    Critical Leg Ischaemia. *Eur J Vasc Surg* 1992, 6:(Supplement A):1.

Fowkes RGR, Callam MJ. Is arterial disease a risk factor for chronic leg ulceration. *Phlebology* 1994, 9:87.

Franks PJ, Bosanquet N, Connolly M *et al.* Venous ulcer healing: effect of socio-economic factors in London. *J
    Epidemiol Community Health* 1995a, 49:385.

Franks PJ, Moffatt CJ, Connolly MI, *et al.* Factors associated with healing leg ulceration with high compression.
    Age Ageing 1995b, 24:407.

Franks PJ, Moffatt CJ, Connolly MJ *et al.* Community leg ulcer clinics: effect on quality of life. *Phlebology* 1994,
    9:83–86.

Gardner AMN, Fox RH. The return of blood to the heart against the force of gravity. In: Negus D, Jantet G, eds.
    Phlebology '85. London: Libbey; 1986:65–67.

Harper DR, Nelson EA, Gibson B, Prescott RJ, Ruckley CV. A prospective randomised trial of Class II and Class III
    elastic compression in the prevention of venous ulceration. *Phlebology* 1995.

Hazarika EZ, Wright DE. Chronic leg ulcers: the effect of pneumatic intermittent compression. *Practitioner*
    1981, 225:189–192.

Herrick SE, Sloan P, McGurk M, Freak L, McCollum CN, Ferguson MWJ. Sequential changes in histological
    pattern and extracellular matrix deposition during the healing of chronic venous ulcers. *Am J Pathol* 1992,
    141(5):1085–1095.

Higley HR, Ksander GA, Gerhardt CO, Falanga V. Extravasation of macromolecules and possible trapping of
    transferring growth factor in ulceration. *Br J Dermatol* 1995, 132:79–85.

Johnson A. Wound assessment. *Wound Management* 1993, 4(1):27–30

Jones GR: Walking casts: effective treatment for foot ulcers? *Practical Diabetes* 1991, 8(4):131–132.

Joseph WS, Axler DA. Microbiology and antimicrobial therapy of diabetic foot infections. *Clin Podiatr Med Surg*
    1990, 7(3):467–481.

Knighton DR, Fylling CP, Fiegel VD *et al.* Amputation prevention in an independently reviewed at risk diabetic
    population using a comprehensive wound care protocol. *Am J Surg* 1990, 160:466–472.

Laing W. *Chronic venous diseases of the leg.* London: Office of Health Economics; 1992.

Landra AD. The tropical ulcer. *Surgery* 1988, 59:1402–1403.

Levin ME. The diabetic foot: pathophysiology, evaluation and treatment. In: Levin ME, O'Neal LW, eds. *The
    diabetic foot, 4th ed.* St Louis: Mosby; 1988:1–50.

Moffatt CJ. Compression bandaging – the state of the art. *J Wound Care* 1992, 1(1):45–50.

Moffatt CJ, Dorman MC. Recurrence of leg ulcers within a community ulcer service. *J Wound Care* 1995,
    4(2):57–61.

Moffatt CJ, Franks PJ, Oldroyd M *et al.* Community clinics for leg ulcers and impact on healing. *BMJ* 1992,
    305:1389–1392.

Moffatt CJ, O'Hare L. Ankle pulses are not sufficient to detect impaired arterial circulation in patients with leg
    ulcers. *J Wound Care* 1995a, 4(3):134–138.

Moffatt CJ, O'Hare L. Graduated compression hosiery for venous ulceration. *J Wound Care* 1995b 4(10):459.

Morison MJ, Moffatt CJ. *A colour guide to the assessment and management of leg ulcers, 2nd ed.* London:
    Mosby; 1994.

Negus D. Diagnosis: methods of investigation. In: Negus D, ed. *Leg ulcers: a practical approach to management.* Oxford: Butterworth–Heinemann; 1991:61–87.

Nelson EA, Harper DR, Ruckley CV *et al.* A randomised trial of single layer and multi-layer bandages in the treatment of chronic venous ulceration. *Phlebology* 1995a, Suppl. 1:915.

Nelson EA, Ruckley CV, Barbenel JC. Improvements in bandaging technique following training. *J Wound Care* 1995b, 4(4):181–184.

Orr MM, McAvoy BR. The ischaemic leg. In: Fry J, Berry HE, eds. *Surgical problems in clinical practice.* London: Edward Arnold; 1987:123–135.

Philips T, Stanton B, Provan A, Law R. Study of the impact on quality of life: financial, social and physiological implications. *J Am Acad Dermatol* 1994, 31(1):49–53.

Plassman P, Jones BF. Measuring leg ulcers by colour-coded structured light. *J Wound Care* 1992, 1(3):35–38.

Poskitt KR, Lloyd-Davies ERV, James A, Walton J, McCollum CN. Pinch grafting or porcine dermis in venous ulcers: a randomised clinical trial. *BMJ* 1987, 294:674–676.

Prescott RJ, Ruckley CV, Harper DR, Gibson B, Nelson EA, Dale JJ. Results of a randomised double blind placebo-controlled trial of oxpentifylline in the treatment of arterial leg ulcers. *Phlebology* 1995, Suppl. 2:171.

Pun YLW, Barraclough DRE, Muirden KD. Leg ulcers in rheumatoid arthritis. *Med J Aust* 1990, 153(10):585–587.

Robertson JC, Daunt SO'N, Nur M. Tissue viability - wound healing and the diabetic. *Practical Diabetes* 1986, 3:14–19.

Rose G. Epidemiology of atherosclerosis. *BMJ* 1991, 303:1537–1539.

Ruckley CV: *A colour atlas of surgical management of venous disease.* London: Wolfe Medical Publications; 1988.

Sinacore DR. Total-contact casting in the treatment of diabetic neuropathic ulcers. In: Levin ME, O'Neal LW, eds. *The diabetic foot, 4th ed.* St Louis: Mosby; 1988:273–292.

Taylor S, Goodinson-McLaren S. *Nutritional support: a team approach.* London: Wolfe; 1992.

Thomas S. Evidence fails to justify the use of hypochlorite. *J Tissue Viability* 1991, 1(1):9–10.

Thomas S. Bandages used in leg ulcer management. In: Cullum N, Roe B, eds. *Leg ulcers, nursing management.* London: Scutari; 1995:63–74.

Thomas S, Wilde LG, Loveless P. Performance profiles of extensible bandages. In: Negus D, Jantet C, eds. *Phlebology.* London: Libbey; 1986:667–670.

Vin F. The physiology of compression: clinical consequences, precautions and contra-indications. In: Negus D, Jantet C, Coleridge-Smith PD, eds. *Phlebology* 1995,(Suppl. 1):1134–1136.

Walzman M, Wade AAH, Drake SM, Thomas AMC. Rest pain and leg ulceration due to syphilitic osteomyelitis of the tibia. *BMJ* 1986, 293:804–805.

Wise G. The social ulcer. *Nursing Times* 1986, May 21:47.

Young MJ, Boulton AJM. Guidelines for identifying the at-risk foot. *Practical Diabetes* 1991, 8(3):103–105.

Other Chronic Wounds

The principles of wound care can be applied to any wound but specific difficulties are apparent with some chronic wounds including malignant wounds, sinuses and fistulae. This chapter details some pathophysiological characteristics of these wounds and considers the literature specific to their care, outlining the multiprofessional nature of decision making.

FUNGATING MALIGNANT WOUNDS

Fungating malignant wounds may arise from primary, secondary or recurrent malignancy (Mosley, 1988). Traditionally, such wounds have been associated with advanced and incurable disease (Mortimer, 1993, Petrek *et al.* 1983) but as specialism within oncology, surgical oncology and radiotherapy develops, increasing success is evident in proactive treatment and invasive palliative procedures for advanced cancer (Grocott, 1995a). Indeed, while considering the management of such lesions, a broad literature is available that illustrates the multidisciplinary nature of medical treatment and decision making and a rapidly improving prognosis for patients with fungating lesions (Kumar & Harding, 1993).

When curative treatment is no longer appropriate or has proved ineffective, there is a change in focus towards palliative care. This is defined by the World Health Organization (WHO):

'The active total care of patients whose disease is not responsive to curative treatment. Control of pain, of other symptoms, and of psychological, social and spiritual problems is paramount. The goal of palliative care is achievement of the best quality of life for patients and their families. Many aspects of palliative care are also applicable earlier in the course of the illness in conjunction with anti-cancer treatment' (WHO, 1990).

From a treatment perspective there is no strict division between curative and palliative care because the same procedure may be used as a curative or palliative measure. The difference relates to the decision-making factors and the balance between treatment side effects and quality of life gain (Mosley, op. cit.).

From a wound-care perspective the focus is clearly palliative and, despite the lack of specific dressings-related research, a number of important principles can be established and are presented within this chapter. First, however, a brief overview of the extent of the problem, pathophysiology and treatment options is given.

Epidemiology, pathology and treatment

Epidemiology

Fungating wounds are most commonly associated with carcinoma of the female breast (Ivetic & Lyne, 1990) but there are a variety of body sites affected by both primary and secondary malignant lesions (Rosen, 1980). With few exceptions, the published material regarding fungating malignant wounds comprises single post-op reports, detailing either treatment or wound-care approaches adopted. Examples are given in Table 11.1.

The prevalence of fungating lesions as a complication of carcinomas is largely unknown. There are few studies that explore the extent of the problem and there is a difficulty in the application of 'old' references (Bloom *et al.* 1962; Haagensen, 1971; Sims & Fitzgerald, 1985) to present day healthcare because of advances in screening and treatment. One recent study indicating the potential size of the problem reported recurrence after treatment of early breast cancer. In a cohort of 525 patients presenting with early breast cancer and treated between 1955 and 1985, with a median 5.3-year follow-up, 55 presented with local recurrence and of these 14 (2.66%) had involvement of breast skin (Stotter *et al.* 1991). However, from an epidemiological perspective this study is limited because late presentation carcinoma patients were not included in the original cohort.

Regardless of the extent of the problem, when patients present with fungating wounds they pose clinical difficulties (Banks & Jones, 1993; Boardman *et al.* 1993; Carville, 1995) and consume considerable nursing time (Sims & Fitzgerald, op. cit.).

Pathology
Fungating malignant wounds result from infiltration of the epithelium by cancerous cells and develop by two processes: ulceration and proliferation (Mortimer, op. cit.). Some wounds show evidence of both processes occurring simultaneously (Grocott, 1995a),

Table 11.1.
Fungating wounds: reported body sites (excluding breast)

Sites affected	Sample Size	Author
Head and neck (squamous cell)	174	Yakubu and Mabogunje, 1995
Nasal	7	Herranz *et al.* 1993
Larynx (spindal cell)	1	Banks and Jones, 1993
Parotid	1	Grocott, 1995a
Axilla (squamous cell)	1	Grocott, 1995b
Shoulder (adenocarcinoma of lung)	1	Boardman *et al.* 1993
Thumb	1	Panebianco and Kaupp, 1968
Abdomen	1	Grocott, 1995a
Sacrum (sacral chordoma)	1	Carville, 1995
Mid-thigh (granular cell)	1	Gokaslan *et al.* 1994

whereas other wounds present as either raised fungating nodules or ulcerating craters (*see* Figure 11.1 and Advanced Case Study 9) (Moody & Grocott 1993; Petrek *et al.* op. cit.). Both types of wound are referred to as fungating malignant wounds but any underlying pathological differences have not been explored or explained (Petrek *et al.* op. cit.).

The development of such wounds is determined by a combination of concurrent and progressive processes that affect blood haemostasis, lymph, interstitial and cellular environments. Local extension of malignant cells distort vascular structures which cause fluctuations in blood flow and generate hypoxic regions within the enlarging tumour. This is complicated by infiltration of lymphatic vessels and poor lymphatic drainage which leads to a rise in interstitial pressure and vascular collapse (Grocott, 1993; Mortimer, op. cit.).

Vascular collapse and variations in tissue perfusion causes infarction, hypoxia and, ultimately, necrosis. This, in turn, enables the development of a further complication, anaerobic infection, which thrives in the necrotic tumour. Such infection is characterized by the symptom of malodour which results from the production of volatile fatty acids as metabolic waste (Mortimer, op. cit.). However, other localized factors also support the colonization of aerobic organisms generating complex bacterial populations (Rotimi & Durosinmi-Etti, 1984).

Poor tissue perfusion and the presence of anaerobic and aerobic infections are of particular importance in the management of these complex wounds.

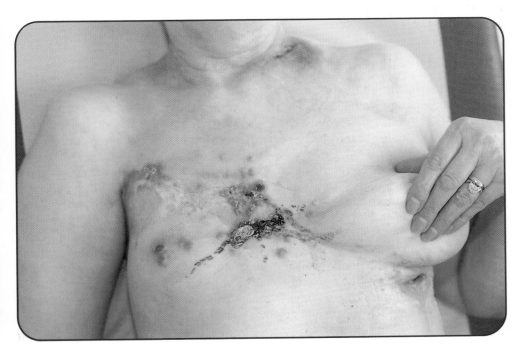

Figure 11.1   A fungating lesion. (Reproduced courtesy of Sue Bale.)

Treatment of the underlying pathology

The treatment of fungating lesions will depend on the underlying tumour pathology (including staging), associated body site, medical knowledge associated with tumour type and combined clinical decision making involving surgeon, oncologist and radiologist. Possible options for treatment include single and combination therapies of radiotherapy, chemotherapy, surgery, hormone therapy, neutron therapy and laser therapy (Grocott, 1995a).

There is evidence of strong multidisciplinary collaboration within the literature, in particular involving breast carcinomas (Piccart *et al.* 1988; Kumar & Harding, op. cit.; Rubens *et al.* 1989) and reviews of the literature illustrate the complexities of decision making with regard to the management of locally advanced disease (Piccart *et al.* 1992; Rubens, 1992).

However, there is a lack of clarity about the true extent of the problem and treatment outcomes for fungating lesions, because of a lack of specificity within study inclusion criteria and staging systems (Piccart *et al.* 1988; Hortobagyi *et al.* 1988; Rubens *et al.* op. cit.; Weshler *et al.* 1990). Indeed, key researchers in the field of breast carcinomas acknowledge the limitations of current research in providing evidence of the real benefits of treatment modalities and the most effective treatment sequence and drug combinations (Piccart *et al.* 1992; Rubens, 1992) and highlight the need for further research and large multicentre clinical trials. Problems encountered in the application of current research are the lack of randomized controlled trials, difficulties in obtaining large samples and the long follow-up time required to determine outcome, during which time new treatment modalities are developed.

The clear message gained from the literature is that much can be done for the treatment and palliation of fungating lesions and referral to specialists in cancer care is essential.

Care of the patient and the wound

There is criticism within the literature about the absence of a research-base to guide the care of fungating wounds (Ivetic & Lyne, op. cit.; Thomas, 1992; Fairbairn, 1994). Indeed, it is suggested that wound-care practice in this field is based on experience rather than any published information and that sharing of experiential learning is rare (Ivetic & Lyne, op. cit.).

However, the recent literature has much to offer in guiding both patient care and wound care. For example: (1) post-op reports illustrate the complexities involved in patient care while illustrating common solutions (Banks & Jones, op. cit.; Boardman *et al.* op. cit.; Carville, op. cit.); (2) reporting of the particular problems patients experience, when living with fungating lesions, gives direction to the focus of care (Collinson, 1993; Sims & Fitzgerald, op. cit.); (3) evidence of the complex bacteriology of these lesions provides direction in relation to reducing odour and exudate (Rotimi & Durosinmi-Etti, op. cit.); (4) knowledge of the properties and performance characteristics of wound-care products enable informed choice (Thomas, op. cit.). It is important to recognize the many elements to research-based care and determine principles as a basis for practice.

Assessment

As previously stated 'the goal of palliative care is achievement of the best quality of life for patients and their families' (WHO, op.cit.). In relation to the care of a patient with a fungating lesion the best possible outcome from care is achievable by focusing on their individual problems (Boardman *et al.* op. cit.; Carville op. cit.).

A review of the literature detailing case studies and experience within clinical practice identifies common themes in relation to patient problems associated with the presence of such wounds (Sims & Fitzgerald, op. cit.; Banks & Jones, op. cit.; Boardman *et al.* op. cit.; Collinson, op. cit.; Grocott, 1993; Carville, op. cit.). Problems affecting quality of life include:

- Excess exudate.
- Malodour.
- Bleeding.
- Fear (as obvious reminder of malignancy).
- Pain at dressing change.
- Bulky dressing materials.
- Inconvenience.

More specifically, excess exudate, resulting in breakthrough soiling and frequent dressing changes, affects independence and social activity; malodour may cause nausea and affect self-esteem and social interaction and bleeding (although rarely severe) may induce anxiety and fear (Collinson op. cit.).

These problems indicate the knowledge-base required for the assessment and planning of care for patients with fungating wounds and illustrate that the goal of achieving 'best quality of life' for many patients will be dependant on an understanding of the underlying pathology and it's application to wound-care practice.

The assessment process should determine the main problems as perceived by the patients. Case study reports illustrate that assessment is a continuous process during the care of patients with fungating wounds because their general and wound conditions fluctuate in response to other palliative treatment and show gradual deterioration (Sims & Fitzgerald, op. cit.; Banks & Jones, op. cit.; Boardman *et al.* op. cit.; Carville, op. cit.).

Assessment frameworks are described by Collinson (op. cit.), Moody and Grocott (op. cit.) and Grocott (1995b), the former two as the basis for clinical practice and the latter for the purposes of research. It is important to distinguish between the information and measurement requirements for research purposes (where wound-characteristic outcomes are required) and the role of assessment for the planning and evaluation of care to achieve patient goals. Collinson's framework has a fungating-wound focus (see Box 11.1), the aim being to 'determine what the patient and their main carers perceived to be the major problems associated with living with a malignant wound' (Collinson op. cit.).

The measurement of fungating wounds receives little attention within the literature, although, in the development of a research tool, Grocott (1995b) describes the difficulties associated with measurement techniques, such as ultrasound imaging and photography and concludes that a patient-led approach may be more suitable. Attempts to measure the depth of a wound, described in Chapter 4, are complicated by the extent of necrotic tissue and there is a risk of haemorrhage with the use of probes. Perhaps the lack of debate regarding wound measurement reflects the main aim of assessment which is to determine the main problems as perceived by the patient.

Box 11.1.

Assessment of malignant wounds (Collinson, 1993)

- Size, site and characteristics of the wound
- Patient's choice of care setting
    home
    hospital
    hospice
- Planned local or systemic treatment
    radiotherapy
    chemotherapy
    hormonal therapy
- Problems associated with current wound management
    pain at dressing change
    frequency of dressing change
    patient satisfaction
- Psychological and social impact of living with a malignant wound

---

An assessment tool relating specifically to odour is described in the literature by Haughton and Young (1995) and provides measurable criteria for a subjective phenomenon (Table 11.2).

Wound care

Common wound-care solutions emerge from the recent literature in relation to symptom control which illustrates that combination dressing regimes are frequently adopted.

Dressings and topical agents are used for the purpose of:

- Debridement.
- Haemostasis.
- Odour control.
- Absorption.

From a long-term management perspective debridement is of primary concern. Necrotic tissue provides an environment in which anaerobic infection thrives with resulting malodour and exudate. Exudate acts as a reservoir for other aerobic organisms that further complicate the malodour. Therefore, removal of necrotic tissue can significantly reduce the problems associated with exudate and malodour (Collinson, op. cit.).

Debridement

Two methods are clearly described within the recent literature. Debridement using a hydrogel (Collinson, op. cit.; Boardman *et al.* op. cit ; Bale & Harding 1990) and a calcium alginate (Collinson, op. cit., Grocott, 1993; Banks & Jones, op. cit.). Collinson (op. cit.) who developed practice protocols, suggests that a hydrogel is effective on

Table 11.2.
Odour assessment scoring tool
(Haughton & Young, 1995)

Score	Assessment
Strong	Odour is evident on entering the room (6–10 feet or 2–3 m from the patient) with the dressing intact
Moderate	Odour is evident on entering the room (6–10 feet from the patient) with the dressing removed
Slight	Odour is evident at close proximity to the patient when the dressing is removed
No odour	No odour is evident, even at the patient's bedside with the dressing removed

eschar, whereas calcium alginate debrides areas of 'soft' necrotic tissue. If the patient is not receiving treatment such as radiotherapy or chemotherapy the debridement 'phase' may continue indefinitely (Collinson op. cit.). More general discussion of methods of debriding open wounds can be found in Chapters 5 and 6.

Haemostasis

Calcium alginates are clearly the dressing of choice for areas prone to bleeding (Collinson, op. cit.; Thomas, op. cit.; Carville, op. cit.) (*see* Chapter 6). However, Grocott (1993) illustrated the need to prevent dressings from drying onto the wound as this can result in bleeding at dressing change.

Malodour

As well as debridement various options are available to reduce malodour. The source of the problem (i.e. infection) may be treated systemically with oral antibiotics (Grocott, 1993) or locally with metronidazole gel (Bower *et al.* 1992; Collinson, op. cit.; Boardman *et al.* op. cit.; Banks & Jones, op. cit.; Thomas & Hay, 1991). Maintaining an intact dressing is an important element in the control of odour (Grocott, 1993; Boardman *et al.* op. cit.) and the use of charcoal dressings is advocated for their odour-absorption properties (Lawrence *et al.* 1993; Haughton & Young, op. cit.).

Absorption of exudate

Various secondary dressings are described within the literature. Factors to consider include:

- Preventing strike-through to reduce the frequency of dressing change and malodour.
- Maintaining a moist environment to minimize pain and bleeding during dressing change.
- Bulk of the dressing affecting movement and body image.

Dressing combinations described include semipermeable films, melolin, pads and Allevyn (Collinson, op. cit.; Grocott, 1993; Banks & Jones, op. cit.; Boardman *et al.* op. cit.). In the case studies describing particularly difficult wound management, the absorbency of Allevyn dressings has been effective in improving patient outcomes (Banks & Jones, op. cit.; Boardman *et al.* op. cit.).

Combination regimes
All reports within the literature describe combination dressing regimes, two are outlined below.

Regime A (Banks & Jones, op. cit.)
Metrotop
Kaltostat
Allevyn cavity
Melolin
Pad
Opsite

Regime B (Boardman et al. op. cit.)
Intrasite or Metrotop
Allevyn cavity
Allevyn hydrocellular sheet
Hyperfix

SUMMARY

An understanding of the pathology of fungating wounds and a knowledge-base, relating to factors expressed by patients as affecting quality of life, together provide a clear direction for wound-care practice.

SINUSES

A sinus is a blind-ended track, lined with epithelium and granulation tissue that extends from the skin to the subcutaneous tissues and may form a sinusoidal cavity (Figure 11.2). Sinuses develop due to the presence of a foreign body and this may be iatrogenic, trauma-related or intrinsic in nature. A sinus may be considered chronic if symptoms are constant or recurrent over a period of several months without indication of spontaneous healing (Søndenaa & Pollard, 1995).

Examples of iatrogenic disease include the development of a post-operative sinus as a result of a non-absorbable suture, retained swab or as a physiological response to a prosthesis. Traumatic injury may leave a residual foreign body, such as glass or metal fragments, which may induce an inflammatory response months or years later. The cause of an intrinsic sinus may result from osteomyelitis and the presence of necrotic bone. Another example commonly reported in the literature is the pilonidal sinus which results from penetration of the skin by keratin plugs and debris, including hair (Søndenaa & Pollard, op. cit.).

Clearly, diagnostic methods and management will depend on the suspected cause of the wound. Healing requires removal of the foreign body and infection, if present, with options for surgical excision and primary closure, surgical excision and healing by secondary intention or curettage and drainage. Such decisions are usually made by members of the surgical team but have broad implications for patient care.

Particular problems can be encountered at an individual level in the management of sinuses, particularly if recurrence occurs. However, little is published in relation to the management of sinuses or the impact of chronic disease on patients, with the exception of pilonidal sinus. This literature contains much debate about management and raises many issues relevant to pre-operative and post-operative preparation and care.

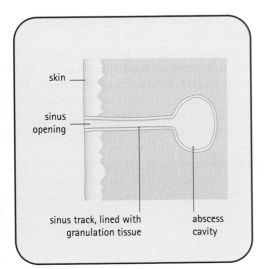

Figure 11.2 A sinus. (Reproduced from Morison, 1992.)

skin

sinus
opening

sinus track, lined with
granulation tissue

abscess
cavity

Pilonidal sinus

Pilonidal sinuses are most commonly a problem associated with the sacrococcygeal area of the body but have also been reported to occur at umbilical (Abdelnour et al. 1994), axilla (Ohtsuka et al. 1994), neck (Miyata et al. 1992) intermammary (Richardson, 1994) and other skin sites (Berry, 1992). The majority of the literature details epidemiology, pathology and treatment for sacrococcygeal pilonidal sinus which is the focus of this review.

Pathology, epidemiology and morbidity

There has been great debate within the literature about the pathology of pilonidal sinuses but they are now considered to be an acquired condition (Berry, op. cit.), whereby keratin plugs penetrate the skin, create a cavity (pit) and facilitate entry of debris, including hair. The debris then stimulates a foreign-body reaction and epithelialization of the cavity which presents as a sinus (Søndenaa & Pollard, op. cit.). It is not known whether recurrence is caused by unrecognized sinuses, overlooked or newly developed pits or post-operative infection (Søndenaa & Pollard, op. cit.).

Pilonidal sinuses are associated with onset of puberty with the majority of patients presenting with the disease at between 20 and 30 years of age (Kooistra, 1942; Clothier & Haywood, 1984; Søndenaa et al. 1995a). As well as age, patient characteristics associated with the condition include obesity, sedentary occupation, local trauma, 'sweaty job' and family history (Clothier & Haywood, op. cit.; Søndenaa et al. 1995a; Berry, op. cit.). Also, more men than women suffer from the disease (Kooistra, op. cit.; Søndenaa et al. 1995a).

Such is the relationship to age and sex that pilonidal sinus is a reported management problem for army populations. During the Second World War, the condition was prevalent amongst US soldiers who referred to it as 'Jeep Seat'; 77 000 patients were admitted to US Army Hospitals (Clothier & Haywood, op. cit.). Also, Karydakis reported that in the Greek army, 4.9% of soldiers had pilonidal sinus in 1960, 25.8% in 1974 and 30–33% 'at present' and suggests the causal link is an associated four-fold rise in weight to height ratio (Karydakis, 1992). It is suggested by Armstrong & Barcia (1994) that pilonidal sinus is a self-limited condition that disappears with age.

Morbidity associated with the disease is variable. Duration of symptoms before presentation were reported to range from 3–516 months (mean 62, median 24) in a patient population of 103 (Søndenaa et al. 1995a). In an early study of 350 patients, the mean duration of symptoms from the onset until the time of admission was 38 months (Kooistra, op. cit.). Of these, 201 (57%) had previous surgery (Kooistra, op. cit.). Indeed, recurrence of disease increases the morbidity for many patients (Clothier & Haywood, op. cit.; Søndenaa et al. 1995a).

Symptoms of pain, discomfort and discharge are those most commonly reported by patients (Søndenaa et al. 1995a; Kooistra, op. cit.), with many (greater than 80%) experiencing pilonidal abscess which may or may not resolve spontaneously with or without antibiotics (Søndenaa et al. 1995a)

Treatment options

A number of retrospective and prospective studies are reported but little consensus exists regarding preventative, first-line and ongoing management. Options for care include the following: conservative treatment (incision and drainage) with active prevention (by shaving and removal of visible hairs from the sinus); incision, curettage and drainage; excision and primary closure (with or without antibiotic administration); and excision and healing by secondary intention (Box 11.2). Within the latter two options, various surgical techniques are described and make comparisons of complication and recurrence rates difficult to interpret.

A further difficulty is the need to distinguish between studies that include patients with pilonidal abscess as well as pilonidal sinus when comparing complication rates between studies. Some studies specifically exclude patients with pilonidal abscess (Khawaja *et al.* 1992; Søndenaa *et al.* 1995b), others include patients with both pilonidal abscess and sinus (Armstrong & Barcia, op. cit.; Lundhus & Gottrup, 1993) and others do not specify exclusion or inclusion criteria and refer continuously to pilonidal sinus throughout the text (Karydakis, op. cit.; Mosquera & Quayle, 1995).

Principles for care are difficult to establish with variation in practice evident in many aspects of patient management, outlined in Box 11.2. Elements of the management

---

Box 11.2.

Practice variation in the management of pilonidal sinus

- **Conservative approach**   shaving, hygiene, patient education

- **Surgical approach**
- (i) **Pre-operative preparation**   bathing/showering, shaving, skin disinfection, anti-biotic: prophylaxis
            no prophylaxis

- (ii) **Surgical options**   incision and drainage: without curettage
            with curettage
            with curettage and phenol
      excision: primary closure
            flap surgery
            specific techniques
            excision and open wound
            (secondary healing)

- (iii) **Post-operative management**   closure method, suture material, dressing, shaving, hygiene, discharge criteria, follow-up time

literature are presented to highlight the difficulty in making an informed, research-based, treatment decision and provide an awareness of factors that require consideration in the pre-operative preparation and post-operative management of this client group.

Conservative treatment and prevention

Conservative treatment and prevention is strongly advocated by Armstrong and Barcia (op. cit) who compared a historical control group of 229 patients (1973–1975), who underwent a variety of surgical procedures, with a group of patients admitted over a 17-year period (1976–1992) during which time a 'conservative therapy' approach was used.

Conservative therapy involved patient education regarding the nature of the condition, the importance of perineal hygiene, hair control (weekly 5 cm strip shave), avoidance of some exercises and simple lateral incision and drainage for acute abscess. The authors reported a gradual reduction in hospital admissions, for pilonidal disease during the 17-year period, from 68 in the first 4 years (1976–1979) to 15 during the last 4-year interval (1988–1991). However, interpretation of these data is limited because of the omission of data detailing admissions as a proportion of those affected and treated on an outpatient basis.

Surgical intervention

Many authors advocate first-line management as excision and primary closure for pilonidal sinus, in preference over excision and secondary (open) wound healing, on the basis of cost (hospital stay) and patient inconvenience (time to heal and time from work) (Khawaja *et al.* op. cit.; Søndenaa *et al.* 1992; Kronborg *et al.* 1985).

The evidence, however, is confused by great variation in complication rates after excision and primary closure from 3 to 61.5% (Kronborg *et al.* op. cit.; Søndenaa *et al.* 1995c) and differences in recurrence rates from 0 to 27% (Søndenaa *et al.* 1995b; Vogel & Lenz, 1992; Lundhus & Gottrup, 1993). There is a paucity of evidence relating to any potential benefits of secondary healing and variation in dressing materials used. The research is confused further by the absence of evidence relating to pre-operative and post-operative variables such as skin preparation, shaving, patient education, suture material and so on. The importance of these variables is unknown, with some studies making specific reference to them and others providing little information.

Tabulated summaries of the studies retrieved are presented at Tables 11.3–11.8 to illustrate the contradiction and conflict within the literature. Where variables are found to be statistically significant (in the randomized controlled trials) the p values are

Table 11.3.
Outcomes: excision and primary closure of pilonidal sinus without antibiotics

Author	Sample	Complication rate n	Complication rate %	Recurrence rate n	Recurrence rate %	Mean hospital stay (days)	Mean healing time (days)	Mean return to work (days)
Karydakis, 1992	6545		8.5	55	0.8	–	–	–
Rossi *et al.* 1993	106		–	3	3.26	5.5	14.6	–

Table 11.4.
Outcomes: excision and primary closure of pilonidal sinus with antibiotics

Author	Sample	Complication rate n	%	Recurrence rate n	%	Mean hospital stay (days)	Mean healing time (days)	Mean return to work (days)
Lundhus & Gottrup, 1993 antibiotic *	56	10	18	15/56	27	2	-	-
Khaira & Brown, 1995 antibiotic **	46	4	9	7/40	17.5	1	-	30/31 within 3–4 weeks

* Pre-operative metronidazole and ampicillin NB. follow-up time 36–64 months
** Intravenous cefuroxime on anaesthetic induction

detailed within the table.

As well as the studies detailed in tabulated form, other surgical techniques are described in the literature. Some detail flap techniques (Khatri *et al.* 1994; Ozgultekin *et al.* 1995) and others combine primary and secondary healing. For example, Muller *et al.* (1992) reported results relating to the Lord–Millar technique (Lord & Millar, 1965) and Mosquera and Quayle (op. cit.) report on Bascom's operation (Bascom, 1980).

One further article (Marks *et al.* 1985) compared the use of metronidazole with no antibiotic therapy in patients with open healing, using the dressing regime described by Wood *et al.* (1977). Interpretation, however, is difficult because of variation in patient characteristics as well as non-random allocation to treatment groups.

Although not a systematic review of the literature, the search used Medline and Cinahl computer databases and also hand searching of the *Journal of Wound Care, Journal of Tissue Viability* and *Proceedings of the European Conferences on Advances in Wound Management* with further retrieval of articles from cited references. The references cited are easily available to clinicians within the field and the 'normal' first option for information retrieval. It must be stressed, however, that this does not purport to be systematic or rigorous as advocated within current Research and Development ideology (Effective Health Care, 1995). The review does, however, highlight the difficulties in the synthesis of research-based clinical decision making and treatment choice and suggests that a systematic review, with rigorous study inclusion and exclusion criteria, is essential to establish 'best practice' and research questions.

Considerations for practice

Considerations for practice can be broadly divided into health promotion advice and symptom control, and surgical preparation and discharge planning. However, the focus of practice will be determined at a local level according to individual general practitioner management, the surgeon's treatment choice or a multidisciplinary approach to patient

Table 11.5.
Outcomes: excision and primary closure
of pilonidal sinus with and without antibiotics

| Author | Sample | Complication rate | | Recurrence rate | | Mean healing |
		n	%	n	%	time (days)
Søndenaa *et al.* 1995b						
antibiotic *	78	34	44	2	2.5	-
control	75	32	43	5	7	-
Søndenaa *et al.* 1995c						
antibiotic **	52	32	61.5	7	13.5	30.8 (11–210)
antibiotic ***	25	15	60	0	-	32.9 (13–88)
no antibiotic	26	16	61.5	0	-	36.4 (13–78)
Vogel & Lenz, 1992						
antibiotic****	40	3	7.5	0	-	-
control	40	21	52.5	0	-	-
		$p < 0.001$				

* Intravenous cefoxitin within 30 minutes of surgery
** Intravenous cloxacillin 30 minutes pre-operatively
*** Intravenous cefoxitin pre-operatively
**** Gentamicin collagen sponge

management based on presenting evidence (literature and patient).

Health promotion options include consideration of diet, exercise, lifestyle factors (such as work and leisure), hygiene and shaving. The latter two must be within the context of local practice and patient management. A majority of patients present with symptoms of pain, discomfort and discharge (Kooistra, op. cit.; Søndenaa *et al.* 1995a), and when an abscess is evident this may or may not resolve by spontaneous perforation, antibiotic administration or both (Søndenaa *et al.* 1995a). Such symptoms require individual assessment and treatment, including information and support about possible treatment and recurrence.

In relation to surgical treatment, given the wide variation in surgical technique, various factors require consideration when making treatment decisions, in particular, the potential impact on lifestyle after surgical intervention (Box 11.3). It is suggested, for example, by Füzün *et al.* (1994) that the surgical technique employed be based on patient preference and employment status. Indeed, patient involvement in decision making and pre-operative discussion of post-operative complications emerges as an

Table 11.6.
Outcomes: primary closure compared with secondary healing of pilonidal sinus

Author	Sample	Complication rate		Recurrence rate		Mean hospital stay (days)	Mean healing time (days)	Mean return to work (days)
		n	%	n	%			
Füzün *et al.* 1994								
primary closure	55	2	4	2/45	4	4.7(3–11)	-	10.7 (9–21)
open wound*	55	1	2	0/46	0	2.4 (3–11) $p < 0.05$	-	17.6 (12–21) $p\,0.05$
Khawaja *et al.* 1992								
primary closure	23	6	26	0/23	0	1	14	19.5
open wound**	23	0	0	0	0	3	41	42
Søndenaa *et al.* 1992								
primary closure	60	16	27	4/56	7	-	22.4	15.4
open wound***	60	23	38	1/59	2	-	85.4 $p < 0.001$	27.3 $p = 0.002$

* Dressings changed daily with 10% povidone iodine
** Gauze soaked in aqueous proflavine changed daily for 1 week and replaced by silicone foam
*** Twice-daily baths and dry dressings

essential component of care.

Post-operative complications reported within the literature include infection, haematoma, pain, wound dehiscence and wound rupture (after primary closure). When primary healing fails, the consensus appears to be that healing should be achieved by secondary intention, with obvious consequences for increased healing time, inconvenience and possible extended time off work. Pre-operative information regarding possible complications and recurrence is an essential element of care, particularly when previous surgery has been employed and the planned surgical technique differs. If excision and healing by secondary intention is planned, then post-operative dressing arrangements, time off work and holiday plans require pre-operative consideration.

From a wound-care perspective, principles of care will clearly be determined by the surgical option of choice. Reference should be made to the physiology of wound healing, the principles of secondary wound healing and principles of surgical wound healing (Chapter 1).

Table 11.7.
Outcomes: primary closure (with and without antibiotics) compared with secondary healing of pilonidal sinus

Author	Sample	Complication rate		Recurrence rate		Median healing time (days)
		n	%	n	%	
Kronborg *et al.* 1985:						
Primary closure	33	3	9	8/32	25	22[1]
Primary closure and antibiotic*	34	1	3	6/31	19	11
Open wound**	32	2	6	4/31	13	66[1]

[1]$p < 0.001$
* Intramuscular clindamycin 1 hour pre-operatively
** Wound packed with petroleum gauze and changed daily

Table 11.8.
Outcomes: secondary healing of pilonidal sinus

Author	Sample	Complication rate		Recurrence rate		Mean healing time (days)	Mean return to work (days)
		n	%	n	%		
Wood *et al.* 1977*	143	not reported		not reported		56 (28–153)	not reported
Matter *et al.* 1995**	50	not reported		18/50	36	30 (10–120)	14 (3–60)

* Dressings: flavine-soaked gauze replaced by foam elastomer dressings 3–4 days post-operatively
** 'The wound packed open' (dressing not specified)

Box 11.3.

Factors affecting the treatment decision for pilonidal sinus

- Patient history
- Presenting symptoms (abscess or sinus)
- Employment status
- Patient choice
- Cost
- Local expertise

FISTULAE

A fistula is an abnormal tract between two epithelial surfaces that connect one viscus to another or a viscus to the skin (Figure 11.3). Fistulas may be either simple, with a single tract or complicated, as shown by multiple tracts (Pringle, 1995). They are associated with a wide range of causes, including disease (commonly malignancy and inflammatory disease), trauma and surgery. They may be spontaneous or planned. Medline classifies in excess of 15 subcategories relating to fistulae but those considered within the context of this chapter are those opening onto the skin and referred to as cutaneous.

The cause of the wound will determine the likelihood of spontaneous closure and general prognosis. For example, fistulae associated with malignancy are unlikely to resolve whereas a post-operative fistula or fistula development during an acute episode of Crohn's disease may well heal. However, with increasingly proactive treatment and palliative care it is not possible to generalize outcome and prognosis. For example, within the speciality of head and neck surgery, good patient outcomes have been achieved even when fistulae are associated with malignancy (Harris & Komray, 1993; Chambers & Worrall, 1994).

Principles of care

Experiential evidence, rather than research, has established the principles of treatment and care relating to fistulae management. The three basic options for treatment and care are simple skin care, creation of conditions to facilitate spontaneous closure and surgical correction (Borwell, 1994). The cause of the wound, its site and the general wellbeing of the patient will determine whether conservative, surgical or combined treatments are adopted (Table 11.9).

Other factors dependent on the type of fistula and associated effluent may require consideration and active treatment. For example, a gastro-intestinal related fistula can result in rapid loss of fluid and electrolytes, which therefore requires careful monitoring and replacement (Pringle, op. cit.). The need for nutritional support (discussed in Chapter 2) requires assessment on an individual basis and may constitute a key component of treatment, particularly for gastro-intestinal related fistulae where dietary

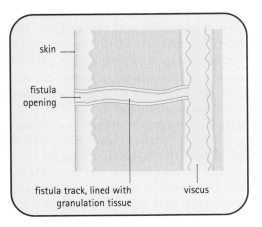

Figure 11.3 A fistula between the skin and a viscus. (Reproduced from Morison, 1992.)

skin

fistula opening

fistula track, lined with granulation tissue

viscus

Table 11.9.
Principles of fistula management

1 Non–active treatment
(a) Protect the skin from fistula effluent
(b) Active palliation of symptoms of importance to the patient
(c) Support the patient and carers

2 Create optimal conditions for spontaneous closure
(a) Protect the skin from fistula effluent
(b) Allow free drainage of the effluent
  • Non-surgical
  • Surgical 'laying open'
(c) Reduce the volume of effluent
  • Surgery (redirect effluent)
  • Diet (gastrointestinal)
  • Drugs (to control primary disease or directly reduce effluent production)
(d) Support the patient and carers

3 Surgical correction of the fistula with primary closure

intake will affect the volume of effluent. Individual needs will be varied, with an emphasis on the mode and characteristics of the nutritional support. For example, total parenteral nutrition may be required for one patient and a high fibre diet advised for another, both with the aim of reducing effluent.

In relation to wound care, particular difficulties are reported in the literature in the management and creation of optimal conditions for spontaneous closure and prevention of sepsis (Devlin & Elcoat, 1983; Pringle, op. cit.; Phillips & Walton, 1992; Harris & Komray, op. cit.; Chambers and Worrall, op. cit.). Indeed, case-study reports highlight the negative impact these wounds have on patient recovery and the huge nursing resource they consume with respect to dressing changes, effluent management and patient support (Pringle, op. cit.; Phillips & Walton, op. cit.).

However, innovations within the field of stoma care have created a large product range that enables skin protection and collection and containment of fistula effluent (Black, 1995; Borwell, op. cit.). Products available can be divided into three categories: skin barriers, filler pastes and appliances; these are described in detail by Black (op. cit.). The literature also reports good patient outcomes after surgery to redirect the effluent and laying open the area to promote healing by secondary intention using Silastic foam (Chambers & Worrall, op. cit.) and amorphous hydrogel (Harris & Komray, op. cit.).

Since fistuale are seen infrequently by many healthcare professionals and pose difficult management problems, a multiprofessional approach is essential to decision-making and individualized care delivery (Elcoat, 1986). An unusual case-study is described (Case study 3) to illustrate the need for a flexible and individualized approach to care.

SELF-ASSESSMENT QUESTIONS AND ACTIVITIES

Case Study 1

Mrs Price is a 59-year-old woman married to a very supportive husband. They have two children and one grandchild. Mrs Price has recently been diagnosed as having breast cancer and elected to have a mastectomy with reconstructive surgery of the breast at the time of operation. For the first postoperative week Mrs Price made an uneventful recovery, both she and her husband were very pleased with the cosmetic result of the plastic surgery. At day 8 the suture-line became dusky-looking and painful and, over the following 48 hours the edge of the graft became completely devitalized and necrotic. This was surgically debrided and the area left to heal by secondary intention, as illustrated. Two days later Mrs Price was discharged to the care of the District Nursing Service.

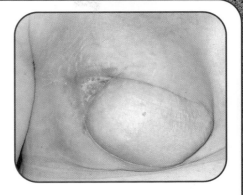

1. *Which dressing products might the district nurse use? Give a carefully reasoned rationale for your choice (see also Chapter 6).*

2. *Could Mrs Price's husband be involved in the wound care?*

3. *Consider the problems this patient might have in relation to body image and how these might be overcome (see also Chapters 8 and 13).*

4. *What is the role of the breast counsellor in caring for this patient?*

5. *Note the likely cause of the wound breakdown in this patient.*

6. *What might have happened if the infection was deep seated and the graft became infected?*

Case Study 2

Mr Brown is 25 years old and has a 6-year history of problems associated with acute episodes of pilonidal abscess and almost continuous discomfort and discharge because of a chronic pilonidal sinus. At the age of 19 he had surgical incision and drainage of the abscess with an uneventful recovery. At the ages of 20 and 22 years his pilonidal sinus was treated by excision and primary closure. In both cases, his recovery was uneventful but he complained that the resultant scar tissue remained sensitive.

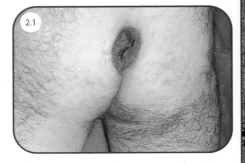

2.1

The sinus recurred 6 months after the last surgical intervention. He discussed

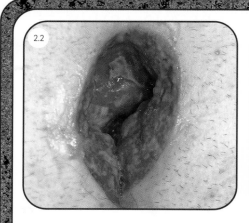

2.2

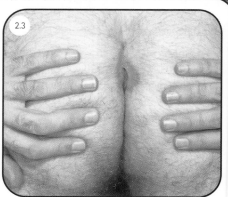

2.3

possible treatment options with the surgeon at an outpatients clinic visit and was re-admitted to hospital for wide-excision and open healing of the wound. Mr Brown fully understood the nature of the postoperative inconvenience that he would suffer and that the healing time would be between 1–3 months. He had discussed with the surgeon the conse-quences of this course of action in rela-tion to time away from work, possible complications and recurrence; no guaran-tee could be offered as to the long-term outcome of the surgery. Mr Brown is active and otherwise in good health.

Pre-operative skin assessment revealed one main sinus with hair visible within it. Two dark cavities to the left of the main sinus were also discovered. The surgery involved wide excision of the main pilonidal sinus and the adjacent tracks (Figs 2.1 and 2.2 above). The wound was packed with povidone iodine-soaked ribbon gauze.

1. Outline, with reasons, the main elements of Mr Brown's pre-operative care.

2.
(a) Why was Mr Brown's sinus packed with povidone iodine-soaked ribbon gauze in theatre?

(b) For how long would it be appropriate to continue with the use of a topical antiseptic, assuming that no complications arise postoperatively? (see also Chapters 5)

(c) Select a dressing regime suitable for Mr Brown once the possible need for the povidone iodine dressing is past (Figure 2.3 above). Consider the properties required of the dressing itself and practical consideration relating to Mr Brown's work and lifestyle and the extent to which he could be self-caring in the longer term (see Chapter 6).

3. What advice should Mr Brown be given in relation to his personal hygiene and skin care prior to his discharge from hospital?

Case study 3

Mr Dawson is a 40-year-old man of no fixed abode. He lived on the streets with a group of three other men in a small North Eastern town and was well known within his regular 'haunts'.

He presented to a GP with approximately 15 small fistulae in the region of his lower back and complained that the smell was resulting in him being increasingly isolated. He was referred to a general surgeon and diagnosed as having ulcerative colitis. Mr Dawson refused admission to hospital and refused the option of surgery and was subsequently referred to the District Nursing Services.

After some delay Mr Dawson attended a district nursing dressings clinic. By this time the number of fistulae had increased to 24 and his skin was excoriated and causing great discomfort. He revealed that his other main problem was smell. The main problem, from a nursing management perspective, was promoting trust and providing care that would simply alleviate the symptoms at minimal inconvenience to Mr. Dawson. He was clear that his lifestyle should not change.

Lifestyle issues were discussed with Mr Dawson who drank heavily and ate little. The district nursing team decided to focus on skin care in the first instance and consulted the community dietician and GP for advice regarding other treatment options. Mr Dawson agreed to visit the GP surgery daily for the first week.

1. Outline the priorities in Mr Dawson's skin care and how these might be achieved in practice.

2. Describe how you would record the findings of the initial wound assessment and subsequent evaluation of the effectiveness of care (see also Chapter 4).

3. Mr Dawson would not discuss his dietary habits with the dietician and refused to change his lifestyle in any other way. Note the ethical issues in this case in relation to patient motivation, compliance and Mr Dawson's right to autonomy (see also Chapter 8).

REFERENCES

Abdelnour A, Aftimos G, Elmasri H. Conservative surgical treatment of 27 cases of ubilical pilonidal sinus. *Lebanese Med J* 1994, **42**(3):123–125.

Armstrong JH, Barcia PJ. Pilonidal sinus disease. *Arch Surg* 1994, **129**:914–919.

Bale S, Harding KG. Using modern dressings to effect debridement. *Professional Nurse* 1990, **5**(5):244–248.

Banks V, Jones V. Palliative care of a patient with terminal nasal carcinoma. *J Wound Care* 1993, **2**(1):14–15.

Bascom J. Pilonidal disease: origin from follicles of hairs and results of follicle removal as treatment. *Surgery* 1980, **87**:567–572.

Berry DP. Pilonidal sinus disease. *J Wound Care* 1992, **1**(3):29–32.

Black PK. Caring for large wounds and fistulas. *J Wound Care* 1995, **4**(1):23–26.

Bloom NJG, Richardson WW, Harries EJ. Natural history of untreated breast cancer (1805–1933). *BMJ* 1962, **2**:213–221.

Boardman M, Mellor K, Neville B. Treating a patient with a heavily exuding malodorous fungating ulcer. *J Wound Care* 1993, **2**(2):74–76.

Borwell B. Nursing management of the patient with a gastro-intestinal fistula. *J Tissue Viability* 1994, **4**(1):23–26.

Bower M, Stein R, Evans TR, Hedley A, Pert P, Coombes RC. A double-blind study of the efficacy of metronidazole gel in the treatment of malodorous fungating tumours. *Eur J Cancer* 1992, **28A**(4/5):888–889.

Carville K. Caring for cancerous wounds in the community: an account of the management of a fungating sacral tumour. *J Wound Care* 1995, **4**(2):66–68.

Chambers PA, Worrall SF. Closure of large orocutaneous fistulas in end-stage malignant disease. *Br J Oral Maxillofac Surg* 1994 **32**(5):314–315.

Clothier PR, Haywood IR. The natural history of the post anal (pilonidal) sinus. *Ann R Coll Surg Engl* 1984, **66**:201–203.

Collinson G. Improving quality of life in patients with malignant fungating wounds. In: Harding KG, Cherry G, Dealey C, Turner TD, eds. *2nd European Conference on Advances in Wound Management*. London: Macmillan; 1993:59–61.

Devlin HB, Elcoat C. Alimentary tract fistula: stomatherapy techniques of management. *World J Surg* 1983, **7**:489–494.

Effective Health Care. The prevention and treatment of pressure sores: how effective are pressure-relieving interventions and risk assessment for the prevention and treatment of pressure sores? *Effective Health Care* 1995, **2**(1):1–16.

Elcoat C. Stoma care nursing, London: Baillière Tindall; 1986.

Fairbairn K: A challenge that requires further research: management of fungating breast lesions. *Professional Nurse* 1994, **9**(4):272–277.

Füzün M, Bakir H, Soylu M *et al.* Which technique for treatment of pilonidal sinus – open or closed? *Dis Colon Rectum* 1994, **37**:1148–1150.

Gokaslan ST, Terzakis JA, Santagada EA. Malignant granular cell tumour. *J Cutan Pathol* 1994, **21**(3):263–270.

Grocott P. Exploratory study into the use of an individually shaped foam dressing for an ulcerating and fungating lesion: patient and professional experiences. In: Harding KG, Cherry G, Dealey C, Turner TD, eds. *2nd European Conference on Advances in Wound Management*. London: Macmillan; 1993:64–69.

Grocott P. The palliative management of fungating malignant wounds. *J Wound Care* 1995a, **4**(5):240–242.

Grocott P. Assessment of fungating malignant wounds. *J Wound Care* 1995b, **4**(7):333–336.

Haagensen CD. *Diseases of the breast, 2nd ed.* Eastbourne: WB Saunders; 1971.

Harris A, Komray RR. Cost-effective management of pharygocutaneous fistulas following laryngectomy. *Ostomy Wound Management* 1993, **39**(8):36–37, 40–42, 44.

Haughton W, Young T: Common problems in wound care: malodorous wounds. *Br J Nurs* 1995, **4**(16):959–963.

Herranz J, Arnal MF, Martinez VJ, Lopez AM. Spindle cell carcinoma of the larynx. *Acta Otorrinolaringol Esp* 1993, **44**(4):305–308.

Hortobagyi GN, Ames FC, Buzdar AU, Kau SW. Management of Stage III primary breast cancer with primary chemotherapy, surgery and radiation therapy. *Cancer* 1988, **62**:2507–2516.

Ivetic O, Lyne PA. Fungating and ulcerating malignant lesions: a review of the literature. *J Adv Nurs* 1990, **15**:83–88.

Karydakis GE. Easy and successful treatment of pilonidal sinus after explanation of its causative process. *Aust NZ J Surg* 1992, **62**:385–389.

Khaira HS, Brown JH. Excision and primary suture of pilonidal sinus. *Ann R Coll Surg Engl* 1995, **77**:242–244.

Khatri VP, Espinosa MH, Amin AK. Management of recurrent pilonidal sinus by simple V-Y fasciocutaneous flap. *Dis Colon Rectum* 1994, **37**(12):1232–1235.

Khawaja HT, Bryan S, Weaver PC. Treatment of natal cleft sinus: a prospective clinical and economic evaluation. *BMJ* 1992, **304**:1282–1283.

Kooistra HP. Pilonidal sinuses: review of the literature and report of three hundred and fifty cases. *Am J Surg* (New Series LV) 1942, 55(1):3–17.

Kronborg O, Christensen K, Zimmermann-Nielson C. Chronic pilonidal disease: a randomized trial with a complete 3 year follow up. *Br J Surg* 1985, **72**:303–304.

Kumar A, Harding KG. Malignant ulcer-rationale of treatment: an experience with fungating breast cancer. In Harding KG, Cherry G, Dealey C, Turner TD, eds. *2nd European Conference on Advances in Wound Management.* London: Macmillan; 1993:61–63.

Lawrence JC, Lilly HA, Kidson A. Malodour and dressings containing active charcoal. In: Harding KG, Cherry G, Dealey C, Turner TD, eds. *2nd European Conference on Advances in Wound Management.* London: Macmillan; 1993:73–74.

Lord PH, Millar DM. Pilonidal sinus: a simple treatment. *Br J Surg* 1965, **52**:298–300.

Lundhus E, Gottrup F. Outcome at three to five years of primary closure of perianal and pilonidal abscess. *Eur J Surg* 1993, **159**:555–558.

Matter I, Kunin J, Schein M *et al.* Total excision versus non-resectional methods in the treatment of acute and chronic pilonidal disease. *Br J Surg* 1995, **82**:752–753.

Marks J, Harding KG, Hughes LE *et al.* Pilonidal sinus excision – healing by open granulation. *Br J Surg* 1985, **72**:637–640.

Moody M, Grocott P. Let us extend our knowledge base: assessment and management of fungating malignant wounds. *Professional Nurse* 1993, **8**(9):586, 588–590.

Mortimer P. Skin problems in palliative care. In: Doyle D, Hanks G, Macdonald N, eds. *Oxford textbook of palliative medicine.* Oxford: Oxford Medical Publications; 1993.

Mosely JG. *Palliation in malignant disease.* Edinburgh: Churchill Livingstone; 1988.

Muller XM, Rothenbuhler JM, Frede KE. Sacro-coccygeal cyst: surgical techniques and results. *Helv Chir Acta* 1992, **58**(6):889–892.

Miyata T, Toh H, Doi F *et al.* Pilonidal sinus on the neck. *Surgery Today* 1992, **22**(4):379–382.

Morison MJ: *A colour guide to the nursing managment of wounds.* London: Mosby; 1992.

Mosquera DA, Quayle JB. Bascom's operation for pilonidal sinus. *J Royal Soc Med* 1995, **88**:45P–46P.

Ohtsuka H, Arashiro K, Watanabe T. Pilonidal sinus of the axilla: report of five patients and review of the literature. *Ann Plast Surg* 1994, **33**(3):322–325.

Ozgultekin R, Ersan Y, Ozcan M *et al.* Therapy of pilonidal sinus with the Limberg Transposition Flap (German). *Chirurg* 1995, **66**(3):192–195.

Panebianco AC, Kaupp HA. Bilateral thumb metastasis from breast carcinoma. *Arch Surg* 1968, **96**:216–218.

Petrek JA, Glenn PD, Cramer AR. Ulcerated breast cancer: patients and outcome. *Am Surg* 1983, **49**(4):187–191.

Phillips J, Walton M. Caring for patients with enterocutaneous fistulae. *Br J Nursing* 1992, **1**(10):495–500.

Piccart MJ, Kerger J, Tomiak E, Perrault DJ. Systemic treatment for locally advanced breast cancer: what we still need to learn after a decade of multimodality clinical trials. *Eur J Cancer* 1992, **28**(2/3):667–672.

Piccart MJ, Valeriola D, Paridaens R, Balikdjian D. Six year results of a multimodality treatment strategy for locally advanced breast cancer. *Cancer* 1988, **62**:2501–2506.

Pringle WK. The management of patients with enterocutaneous fistulas. *J Wound Care* 1995, **4**(5):211–213.

Richardson HC. Intermammary pilonidal sinus. *Br J Clin Pharmacol* 1994, **48**(4):221–222.

Rosen T. Cutaneous metastases. *Med Clin North Am* 1980, **64**(5):885–900.

Rossi P, Russo F, Gentileschi P et al. The pilonidal sinus: its surgical treatment, our experience and a review of the literature (Italian). G Chir 1993, 14(2):120–123.

Rotimi V, Durosinmi-Etti F. The bacteriology of infected malignant ulcers. J Clin Pathol 1984, 37:592–595.

Rubens RD. The management of locally advanced breast cancer. Br J Cancer 1992, 65:145–147.

Rubens RD, Bartelink H, Engelsman E, Hayward JL. Locally advanced breast cancer: the contribution of cytotoxic and endocrine treatment to radiotherapy. Eur J Cancer Clin Oncol 1989, 25(4):667–678.

Sims R, Fitzgerald V. Community nursing management of patients with ulcerating/fungating malignant breast disease. London: RCN Oncology Nursing Society; 1985.

Søndenaa K, Pollard ML. Histology of chronic pilonidal sinus. APMIS 1995, 103(4):267–272.

Søndenaa K, Andersen E, Søreide JA. Morbidity and short term results in a randomised trial of open compared with closed treatment of chronic pilonidal sinus. Eur J Surg 1992, 158:351–355.

Søndenaa K, Andersen E, Nesvik E et al. Patient characteristics and symptoms in chronic pilonidal sinus disease. Int J Colorectal Dis 1995a, 10:39–42.

Søndenaa K, Nesvik E, Gullaksen FP et al. The role of cefoxitin prophylaxis in chronic pilonidal sinus treated with excision and primary suture. J Am Coll Surg 1995b, 180:157–160.

Søndenaa K, Nesvik E, Andersen E et al. Bacteriology and complications of chronic pilonidal sinus treated with excision and primary suture. Int J Colorectal Dis 1995c, 10:161–166.

Stotter A, Kroll S, McNeese M, Holmes F, Oswald MJ, Romsdahl M. Salvage treatment for loco-regional recurrence following breast conservation therapy for early breast cancer. Eur J Surg Oncol 1991, 17:231–236.

Thomas S. Current practices in the management of fungating lesions and radiation damaged skin. Bridgend: The Surgical Materials Testing Laboratory; 1992.

Thomas S, Hay N. The antimicrobial properties of two metronidazole medicated dressings used to treat malodorous wounds. Pharm J 1991, 2:264–266.

Vogel P, Lenz J. Treatment of pilonidal sinus with excision and primary suture using a local, resorbable antibiotic carrier: results of a prospective randomized study (German). Chirurg 1992, 63(9):748–753.

Weshler Z, Brufman G, Sulkes A, Warner-Epraty E, Ben-Baruch N, Biran S, Fuks Z. Radiation therapy for locally advanced breast cancer: prognostic factors and complication rate. Eur J Surg Oncol 1990, 16(5):430–435.

WHO. Cancer pain relief and palliative care. Technical Report Series 804. Geneva: World Health Organization; 1990.

Wood RAB, Williams RHP, Hughes LE. Foam elastomer dressing in the management of open granulating wounds: experience with 250 patients. Br J Surg 1977, 64:554–557.

Yakubu A, Mabogunje O. Skin cancer of the head and neck in Zaria, Nigeria, 1995. Acta Oncol 34(4):469–471.

Quality Assurance

In 1989, the Government published a White Paper called 'Working for Patients' (Department of Health, 1989). This was incorporated by Parliament into the 1990 NHS and Community Care Act. It has led to radical changes in the way that the NHS is organized and financed.

The aim of the changes, first announced in 'Working for Patients', is to raise the quality of healthcare delivered by all GP practices and hospitals to that of the best. The implication, borne out by a number of national clinical and financial audit studies, is that the quality and cost of services offered to patients varies considerably between hospitals and community units and at the individual practitioner level. At the same time patients' expectations of the health service are increasing.

Healthcare professionals are being actively encouraged by the Royal Colleges and by Health Services Management to audit, that is, to systematically and critically review, their practice. Recognition of the benefits of clinical audit is growing within the professions themselves but there is still some confusion about fundamental concepts relating to quality assurance in healthcare and this is not helped by the variety of definitions of some very commonly used terms.

This chapter begins by exploring the concept of quality and the benefits of a high-quality service from the perspective of the patient, the healthcare professional and management. The meaning of terms such as 'quality assurance', 'quality control', 'quality systems', 'standard setting' and 'audit' are explained. A number of debating points have been included within the text to encourage the reader to consider the factors affecting the translation of theory into practice.

WHAT IS QUALITY?

Ovretveit (1992) defined quality in relation to the health services as
'Fully meeting the needs of those who need the service most, at the lowest cost to the organization, within limits and directives set by higher authorities and purchasers'.
This definition of quality incorporates the dimensions of quality described by Shaw (1986): appropriateness, effectiveness, acceptability, accessibility and efficiency (Table 12.1 and Box 12.1) with the legal, ethical and contractual requirements of 'higher authorities' such as the government, professional bodies and the purchasers of services.

Providing a quality service therefore involves the following:
- Meeting or exceeding the expectations of customers.
- Meeting or exceeding professionally agreed standards.
- Improving efficiency and reducing costs.

The 'customer' may be an individual patient, his or her family or the community to be served.

The definition implies that although the customer's view is of central importance, patients are not competent to judge the level of technical excellence of their care, which is the role of healthcare professionals through peer review. The purchaser's role is to assess the health needs of the populations that they serve, to place contracts with providers of services to meet these needs and to get value for money.

Table 12.1.
Dimensions of quality
of healthcare (based on Shaw, 1986)

- Appropriateness. Meeting the actual need of individuals, families and communities

- Effectiveness. Achieving the intended benefit

- Acceptability. Satisfying the patient's reasonable expectations

- Continuity of care and care provider(s)

- Accessibility. Availability not unduly restricted by time, distance or finance

- Efficiency. Maximizing outcomes with the available resources

---

Box 12.1.

Debating point:
Do the dimensions of quality described by Shaw (1986, Table 12.1) apply in practice?

- Some anomalies exist between what is available to patients treated in hospital and people treated at home, for example, certain dressings and compression bandages are not available to community patients through prescription (see Chapters 6 and 10).
- Access to expert care is inevitably dependent on the local availability of resources which includes the availability of healthcare professionals with an expertise in wound care. Particular problems can arise for patients living in remote rural areas and for frail elderly individuals, who may have practical difficulty in attending clinics at some distance from their homes (see Chapter 4 and Table 4.1).
- Development of a wound-care service depends in part on the priority it is given by the purchasing authorities. Who ultimately decides the purchasing authority's priorities?
- Improved efficiency does not necessarily equate with reduced costs overall. Improved efficiency may simply increase demand and a unit's total expenditure.

There will inevitably at times be a conflict of interest between customer-defined quality, professionally defined quality and management's definition of quality (Box 12.2). Any quality system needs to incorporate mechanisms for dealing with this conflict. A quality system encompasses the organizational structure, responsibilities, procedures, processes and resources for implementing quality management (BSI, 1987).

WHY ADOPT A QUALITY APPROACH?

Adopting a quality approach should mean a better service for patients, families, and communities.

The demand for and the cost of healthcare in the Western world is rising at such an alarming rate that it is becoming a very political issue in some countries.

In the USA, healthcare costs rose by $80 billion between 1991 and 1992 to $817 billion or 14% of the gross national product (Berwick, 1992). Costs are rising in the UK too, although less steeply.

The quickest way for any 'firm' to go out of business is to provide a high-quality service without due regard to cost. In a publicly financed health service in which demand is outstripping supply there need to be incentives to increase efficient use of resources (Davies, 1992). Improving the quality of a service can not only reduce needless patient suffering but can also reduce costs, allowing resources to be re-allocated to others in need.

Box 12.2.

Debating point:
How significant a part do patients' views play, in reality, in determining the health care agenda?

- Research suggests that many patients with chronic wounds are passive and may even resist involvement in the decision making process, leaving it to 'the professionals'. How can patients be encouraged to take a more active part in decision making (*see* Chapter 8)?
- Some people argue that if professionals continue to view themselves as the only people able to define and describe technical excellence in healthcare, the passive role of the patient will be perpetuated and the professional will continue to dominate in the professional–patient 'partnership'. Is inequality in the power relationship inevitable (*see* Chapter 8)?
- To what extent do the government reforms give choice to patients in practice? Do the reforms simply increase the power and choice of those able to purchase healthcare on their behalf?

It can do this directly by:

- Increasing the appropriateness of care and reducing unnecessary tests and procedures.
- Reducing avoidable complications and prolonged treatment times.
- Reducing wastage of materials.
- Reducing costs of dealing with complaints.
- Reducing claims for negligence.
- Increasing throughput, where the money follows the patient.

Furthermore, a high-quality service is more likely to retain a motivated, well-trained work force, who are committed to the organization's aims and objectives. Delivering high-quality care is less frustrating and more satisfying for staff and leads to higher morale, better interdisciplinary co-operation and therefore better standards of patient care.

The ethical and professional requirements to act always in the client's best interests are self-evident and the cornerstone of healthcare professionals' codes of professional conduct. Acting in the patient's best interest means allowing individuals to make choices about their health and lifestyle even though their decisions may clash with professionals' views of what is 'best for them'. This raises a number of important issues in relation to compliance and the individual's rights to autonomy, as discussed in Chapter 8.

QUALITY ASSURANCE AND WOUND CARE

The British Standards Institute's definition of quality assurance is 'A management system designed to give the maximum confidence that a given acceptable level of quality of service is being achieved with a minimum of total expenditure' (BSI, op. cit.). Ovretveit defines it as 'All activities undertaken to predict and prevent poor quality'(Ovretveit, op. cit.).
Quality control is a part of quality assurance and is 'The process through which we measure actual quality performance, compare it with a standard and act on the difference' (Juran & Gryna, 1980).

Clinical audit

Clinical audit contributes to quality assurance and involves a cycle of activities (Figure 12.1). The emphasis is on closing the audit loop, that is, rectifying any deficiencies identified and repeating the exercise to see whether in fact anything has changed! Wound care lends itself to audit because

- Large numbers of patients in hospital and the community have a wound at some point in their lives.
- There is a high risk of wounds, such as leg ulcers and pressure sores, becoming intractable with prolonged, inappropriate care (see Chapters 9–11).
- Wounds can cause considerable patient suffering and adversely affect many aspects of quality of life (see Chapter 13).
- Wounds cost the NHS a considerable amount of money.
- Most wounds heal rapidly with appropriate care.

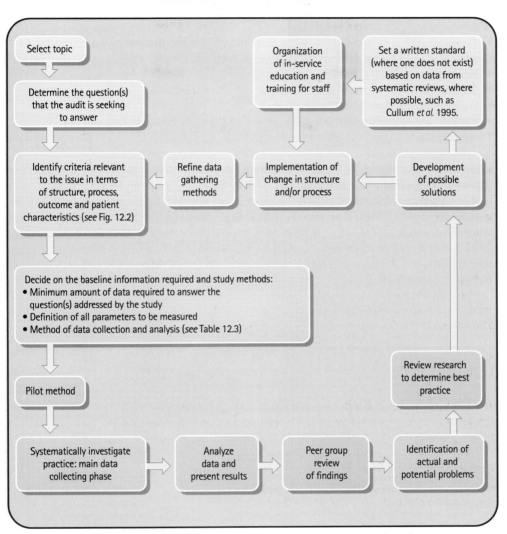

Figure 12.1   The audit process.

The next question to consider is what to audit? Some factors are given in Figure 12.2. The focus should be on measuring outcomes such as:

- Healing rates.
- Quality of life at various points during and after treatment.
- Patient satisfaction with the service.
- Patient understanding of self-help advice to promote healing and prevent recurrence.

Some issues relating to the value of outcome measures, such as patient satisfaction and quality of life, compared with cost and healing rates are noted in Box 12.3.

It is also very important to audit the process of care, as a high-quality process should lead to the optimal outcome for the individual. Morison (1992a) described how the process of wound care was audited in a Community Unit in Scotland. Sixty-nine

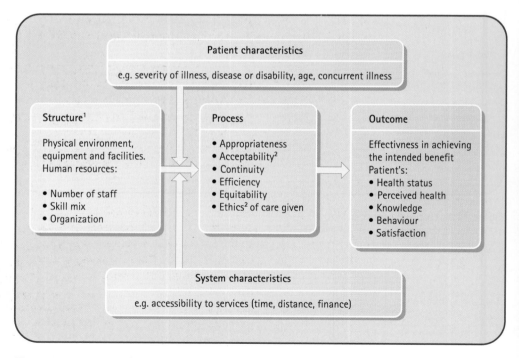

Figure 12.2 What to audit? Examples of factors to consider when developing a programme to measure the quality of care (based on Donabedian, 1969; Shaw, 1986; Hopkins, 1990). (Reproduced from Morison & Moffatt, 1994.)
Notes: ([1]) Simply determine the potential for, or the constraints against, the delivery of high-quality care. ([2]) Ultimately a social construct, influenced by social values.

community nurses (97% of those at work at the time of the study) kept a structured diary for 1 week in which they recorded the nature of each wound, how long the patient had been treated, the number and duration of visits in a week, the wound-care products used and any additional activities undertaken by the nurse at each visit. On a separate questionnaire the staff were asked about the sources of information they used about wound-care products. Most nurses turned to another nursing colleague as the first choice for information and advice. Nurses were also asked about their continuing education experiences and perceived needs in relation to wound care.

Feedback of the results of the audit gave staff considerable insight into their own practice. It highlighted some of the problems of wound-dressing selection (Table 12.2) and the need for a local formulary, which was subsequently developed. The need for a standard on wound assessment in the community was also identified and a standard was developed in one Community Unit.

Box 12.3.

Debating point:

How much value is placed by healthcare professionals and managers on outcome measures relating to patient satisfaction and quality of life when compared with those relating to healing rates or cost?

- Healing rates are considered by some professionals to be the most important outcome to measure. A patient with a healed wound no longer represents a cost to the health service.
- Healing rates are frequently set as targets for achievement with little consideration being given to the factors that can influence them. Risk factors such as wound chronicity, poor mobility and poor general health can all affect how successful treatment can be. There is a danger of generalizing research findings to other populations and of comparing crude outcome data from clinical audit studies without consideration being given to the case mix and the context within which care is being delivered.
- Quality of life and patient satisfaction measures can all too easily be viewed as optional outcome indicators rather than as integral to the evaluation of effective care (see Chapter 13). For patients whose wounds are unlikely to heal, improving quality of life may be the most important yardstick against which to judge effectiveness, as described in Chapter 11 and certain of the advanced case studies.
- Measuring patient satisfaction with treatment is difficult. Patients who are elderly and suffering from chronic illness frequently report high levels of satisfaction with the service. This is often influenced by the relief that someone is taking an interest in them, rather than an appraisal of whether the care is of the very highest quality. Communication and evaluation of satisfaction can be particularly challenging in patients with cognitive or linguistic impairments. Younger patients may have very different expectations and can be more prepared to articulate them.

What is a standard?

A standard is a professionally agreed level of performance that is desirable, achievable, observable and measurable. Measures by which the achievement of a standard can be assessed are

- Structure criteria: resources necessary, for example, manpower, skill mix, equipment, policies and procedures.
- Process criteria: actions taken by staff to achieve the desired outcome.
- Outcome criteria: the desired effect of the care process, for example, patient health status, level of knowledge, skills acquisition, behaviour and satisfaction with care.

The standard-setting cycle (Figure 12.3) is a form of audit in which the minimum standard to be achieved or exceeded is made very explicit for a particular care group (the group of patients to whom the standard applies). More details of the RCN's Dynamic Standard Setting System are given by The Royal College of Nursing (1990).

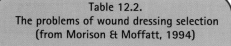

Table 12.2.
The problems of wound dressing selection
(from Morison & Moffatt, 1994)

- There is a bewildering variety of dressings from which to choose

- Many products that look alike have different physical and chemical properties

- Different manufacturers recommend different types of products for the same problem

- Therapeutic traditions may make it difficult to introduce 'new generation' products

- There is a blurring of responsibility between healthcare professionals in relation to prescribing

- Health economics in relation to wound care are complex: products with a higher unit-cost may in fact be very cost-effective

- New products and types of product are appearing on the market every month

- Many wound dressings used in hospital are not available in the community

- There are restrictions in the sizes of many dressings available in the community

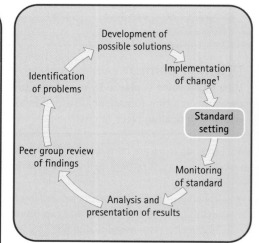

Figure 12.3 The standard setting cycle. (Reproduced from Morison & Moffatt, 1994.) Note: [1]Implementation of change may include modification of the standard.

Success in closing the standard-setting loop (Figure 12.3) and improving patient care depends on ownership of the standard by the staff themselves (Morison, 1992b), on management's commitment to rectifying any deficiencies found and on a reliable and valid method of data collection (Figure 12.4).

Some of the most commonly used methods of measuring quality are listed in Table 12.3. It is very important to obtain professional advice on the method and design of questionnaires and other data-collecting tools. For larger studies, the statistician's advice should be sought on sample size and methods of data analysis before data collection begins! Piloting the method is essential to ensure that it results in the collection of useful and unambiguous data which the people collecting the data understand in terms of definitions used; the method must also be practicable. Issues of confidentiality and data protection must be addressed at the outset.

Creating a climate of enquiry is of paramount importance. Initial resistance to being involved in audit is both natural and understandable (Table 12.4). One definition of

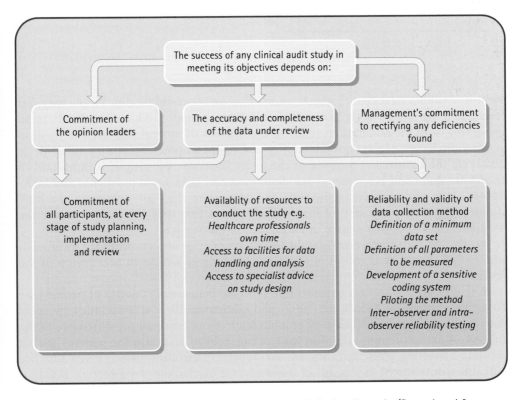

Figure 12.4 Requirements for a successful outcome to a clinical audit study. (Reproduced from Morison & Moffatt, 1994.)

Table 12.3. Examples of commonly used methods of measuring quality (from Morison & Moffatt, 1994)
• Patient satisfaction questionnaires
• Questionnaires to staff
• Audit of documentation
• Direct observation of practice
• Structured diaries recording practice
• Structured interviews with patients
• Structured interviews with staff

Table 12.4. Reasons for resistance to clinical audit (from Morison & Moffatt, 1994)
• Personal threat
• Fear of uses to which data might be put by management
• Time constraints
• Lack of belief in potential benefits
Recognizing resistance:
• Lip service
• Lethargy
• Aggression
• Lack of continuity

audit is 'a calling to account', which has many negative connotations. People may feel threatened by audit, both personally and professionally, which is why it is so important from the outset to develop an atmosphere of mutual support and trust, to address the issues of data confidentiality and to spend time explaining, to all those involved, the nature and purpose of the audit (Morison, op. cit.). It is important to emphasize that audit is not just about identifying problems. Good practice is also high-lighted. It is very satisfying for staff to know when they are achieving the high standards that they are setting for themselves and that they can indeed assure the 'customer' of a specified degree of excellence in the service.

Ideally, the staff themselves should collectively decide the priorities for local audit studies and should be involved in planning the study as well as in peer review of the results.

In reality, there can be a considerable time lag before the majority of people take up a new innovation (Stocking, 1992) and clinical audit is still regarded by some people as new. The commitment of opinion leaders can make all the difference to the success of an audit study. Opinion leaders can help to maintain the impetus during the data-collecting phase but they are also crucial in ensuring that any new practice guidelines, introduced as a result of the study, are carried out (Lomas *et al.* 1991).

THE WAY FORWARD

Clinical audit can be carried out on many levels. It is possible to audit
• A procedure, such as aseptic wound-dressing technique, which is specified in detail in the unit's procedure manual.

- A standard, developed by staff, relating to a particular topic such as wound assessment or pain control.
- An episode of care, such as a planned skin graft.

It is also possible to audit a whole service (Moffatt *et al.* 1992, Stevens *et al.* 1997).

The challenge is to capture accurate and useful data on all patients in an ongoing way or systematically to sample the activity to be audited in a way that ensures that the sample is representative of the population as a whole.

There are very few aspects of healthcare that involve only one professional group and yet uniprofessional audit studies are the most common. There is a move towards multidisciplinary clinical audit which is particularly appropriate in the case of the management of patients with wounds. Experiments in collaborative-care planning (Finnegan, 1991) are evolving to include, in many cases, joint-care planning, a single set of documentation used by all healthcare professionals, with collectively agreed goals and shared audit processes. Patient satisfaction questionnaires may be 'grafted on' to gain an insight into the customer's perspective. It is very rare, however, to find an integrated study that combines the patients', healthcare professionals' and management's perspectives of quality by looking at patient satisfaction, the attainment of professionally agreed standards of clinical practice and value for money.

Once healthcare professionals have become more familiar with standard setting and methods of measuring quality they may decide to introduce a total quality management (TQM) approach which helps to overcome the rather skewed perspective gained from looking at the clinical aspects of care alone.

Total quality management is an approach to creating and maintaining a system of improvement in a complex organization.

TQM goes beyond the processes and practices of quality assurance and quality control. It involves changing the culture of the organization requiring all staff at all levels to be involved in the process of quality improvement. The characteristics and philosophy of TQM are summarized in Table 12.5.

It is impossible to introduce TQM unless there is a quality system in place. The introduction of a quality approach, whether or not this is based on the philosophy of total quality management, requires the development of the following:
- A quality policy. This is a general guide outlining the organization's philosophy and how quality activities will be organized and carried out.
- An overall quality strategy. This is the general, long-term plan for introducing and improving service quality and for changing the orientation of the organization's culture to the pursuit of excellence through a number of quality programmes.
- Quality programmes. These are more short-term plans to achieve certain specific strategy objectives within a given time frame.

Above all, introducing a quality approach requires facilitative leadership (Morison, op. cit.) with the leader acting as the change agent:
- Encouraging staff participation and ownership.
- Explaining the benefits of a quality approach and demonstrating them!
- Removing any perceived threats to staff members' status, responsibility, values, pay and working conditions.
- Improving channels and mechanisms for communication.

Table 12.5.
The characteristics and philosophy of TQM (from Morison & Moffatt, 1994)

- The declared intention to strive for continuous improvement; this means exceeding targets, not just meeting them

- A definition of quality that focuses on meeting the needs of the customer and meeting or exceeding customer expectations

- A total commitment to quality by top management

- Action-orientated measurement systems and translating good ideas originating from staff into action

- An acknowledgement of the interdependency of all staff and the encouragement of collaborative practices

- Investment in staff development

- The recognition that when things go wrong the problem is most likely to be caused by a failure or fault in a process or in systems rather than to be the fault of individuals. The premise is that most people want to do a good job (unless they have been totally demoralized and alienated by management, which indeed indicates faulty processes). The solution lies in identifying the faults in the processes and correcting them rather than blaming individuals

- Systematic elimination of waste, duplication of effort and the use of unnecessary or unproven practices

- Identifying staff-development needs and organizing relevant education and training.
- Identifying and winning over enthusiasts and opinion leaders.

Quality is a philosophy: introducing a quality approach involves changing the hearts and minds of all those involved, directly or indirectly, in patient care so that all are committed to striving for continuous improvement in the service.

SELF-ASSESSMENT QUESTIONS AND ACTIVITIES

(a) *With the help of Table 12.1 and Boxes 12.1–12.3, consider the extent to which Shaw's (op. cit.) dimensions of quality apply in practice in your unit. On what data are you basing your appraisal? What is the quality of these data? What measures have your unit taken to learn more about the patients' views about the service provided and their expectations of it?*

(b) *Imagine that you are a healthcare professional working in the community as part of the primary healthcare team. You begin to be concerned because an increasing number of frail, elderly patients are being discharged back into the community, from the medical and care of the elderly wards of your local hospital, with pressure sores which were not present when these patients were admitted to hospital.*

1. *How do you propose to handle this situation? Who needs to be involved and why?*

2. *What do you anticipate might prove to be the biggest obstacles to bringing about a lasting change for the better in any unit's practice?*

REFERENCES

Berwick DM. Heal thyself or heal thy system: can doctors help to improve medical care? *Quality Health Care* 1992, **1**(supplement):S2–S8.

Bosanquet N, Franks PJ, Moffatt CJ, Connolly MJ, Oldroyd MI, Brown P, Greenhalgh RM, McCollum CN. Community leg ulcer clinics: cost effectiveness. *Health Trends* 1994, **25**(4):145.

BSI. *Quality Systems Part I: specification for design/development, production, installation and servicing (BSI 5750)*. Milton Keynes: BSI; 1987.

Cullum N, Deeks J, Fletcher A et al. The prevention and treatment of pressure sores. Effective Health Care 1995, **2**(1):1–16.

Davies H. Role of the Audit Commission. *Quality Health Care* 1992, **1** (Supplement):S36–S39.

Department of Health. *Working for patients*. London: HMSO; 1989.

Donabedian A. Some issues in evaluating the quality of nursing care. *Am J Pub Health* 1969, **39**(10):1833–1836.

Finnegan E. *Collaborative care planning: a natural catalyst for change*. Birmingham: Resource Management Support Unit, West Midlands Health Region; 1991.

Glasman D. Change management. *Health Service J* 1994, 28th April (1 and 2).

Hopkins A. *Measuring quality of medical care*. London: Royal College of Physicians; 1990.

Juran JM, Gryna FM. *Quality planning and analysis*. New Delhi: McGraw-Hill; 1980.

Lomas J, Enkin M, Anderson GM, Hannah WJ, Vayda E, Singer J. Opinion leaders vs audit and feedback to implement practice guidelines. *JAMA* 1991, **265**(17):2202–2207.

Moffatt CJ, Franks PJ, Oldroyd M *et al*. Community clinics for leg ulcers and impact on healing. *BMJ* 1992,

305:1389.

Morison MJ. Quality assurance and wound care in the community. *Ostomy/Wound Management* 1992a, **38**(8):38–44.

Morison MJ. Promoting the motivation to change: the role of facilitative leadership in quality assurance. *Professional Nurse* 1992b, August:715–718.

Morison MJ, Moffatt, CJ: *A colour guide to the assessment and management of leg ulcers.* London: Mosby; 1994.

Ovretveit J. *Health service quality: an introduction to quality methods for health services.* Oxford: Blackwell Scientific Publications; 1992.

Royal College of Nursing. *Standards of care project. Quality patient care: the dynamic standard setting system.* London: RCN; 1990.

Shaw CD: *Introducing quality assurance, Paper no. 64.* London: Kings Fund; 1986.

Stevens J, Franks PJ, Harrington M. A community/hospital leg ulcer service. *J Wound Care* 1997, **6**(2):62–68.

Stocking B. Promoting change in clinical care. *Quality Health Care* 1992, **1**:56–60.

FURTHER READING

Bardsley M, Coles J. Practical experiences in auditing patient outcomes. *Quality Health Care* 1992, 1:124–130.

Casson S, George C. *Culture change for total quality: action guide for managers in social and health care services.* Brighton: Pitman; 1995.

Courtney D, ed. *Strategic quality management in primary health care: quality improvement at the patient/consumer interface.* Hull: Dept. of Public Health Medicine, University of Hull; 1995.

East L, Robinson J. Change in process: bringing about change in health care through action research. *J Clin Nurs* 1994, 3(1):57–61.

Graham NO. *Quality in health care: theory, application and evolution,* 3rd ed. USA: Aspen; 1995.

Joss R, Kogan M. *Advancing quality: total quality management in the NHS (Health Services Management Series).* Hull: Open University Press; 1995.

Katz J, Green E. *Managing quality: a guide to improving performance in health care,* 2nd ed. London: Mosby; 1996.

Kitson A, Ahmed LB, Harvey G, Seers K, Thompson DR. From research to practice: one organisational model for promoting research-based practice. *J Adv Nurs* 1996, 23:430–440.

Ovretveit J. *Health service quality: an introduction to quality methods for health services.* Oxford: Blackwell Scientific Publications; 1992.

Pearcey PA. Achieving research-based nursing practice. *J Adv Nurs* 1995, 22:33–39.

Redfern SJ, Norman IJ. Measuring the quality of nursing care: a consideration of differing approaches. *J Adv Nurs* 1990, 15:1260–1271.

Sale D. *Quality assurance: for nurses and other members of the health care team.* Essentials of Nursing Management Series, 2nd ed. London: Macmillan; 1996.

Quality of Life as an Outcome Indicator

Over the past 100 years there has been a dramatic decrease in the incidence of infectious diseases in the West, with a corresponding increase in the incidence of chronic diseases. Although in the past treatment was aimed at being curative, it has since been recognized that, in the case of chronic diseases, cure may not be the primary goal; effective management should be the aim. Traditionally, medicine has used survival as its clinical endpoint for success in the management of life-threatening diseases. However, early clinical trials, involving treatment of diseases such as cancer, revealed that patients were being subjected to extreme side effects, often with little benefit in terms of survival. From these observations it was clear that survival was not the only outcome that should be considered but that quality of life could be as important as quantity of life.

Recent changes in the National Health Service have encouraged the process of audit to evaluate the effectiveness of care. The Department of Health's definition (1993) of audit is:

'systematically looking at procedures used for diagnosis, care and treatment ... and investigating the effect care has on outcome and quality of life for the patient'.

Clearly, the measurement of quality of life is important not only for research purposes, but also as a routine part of clinical practice.

This chapter describes some of the terms commonly used in quality of life research and indicates the tools frequently used to measure quality of life. This chapter also describes assessments performed with patients suffering from chronic wounds.

HEALTH AND QUALITY OF LIFE

Before considering in detail the measurement of quality of life, it is helpful to consider some of the terms that are commonly used.

At the heart of medical practice is the concept of 'health'. In 1946 the World Health Organization (WHO, 1958) defined health as

'a state of complete physical, mental and social wellbeing, and not merely the absence of disease and infirmity'.

From this, the state of 'ill health' may be defined as feelings of pain and discomfort or change in usual functioning and feeling. Thus, a person may 'feel' ill without clinical detection of disease. This concept is the key to the assessment of quality of life because it relies on the patient's sense of wellbeing, not a decision made by a doctor weighing up the clinical evidence.

The definition of quality of life is a highly personal one. It is generally acknowledged to be complex and multidimensional and may include such factors as freedom, happiness and financial security (Bulpitt & Fletcher, 1985). As a result of the difficulty of definition in its broadest sense and acknowledging that health affects only part of the individual's lifestyle, health scientists developed tools that look at the areas of life that relate directly to disease and treatment of that disease. In 1988, the term 'health-related quality of life' (HRQoL) was first used to describe the sense of wellbeing that patients experience in their lives which relates directly to their own perceived sense of health (Bullinger, 1993).

The concept of health–related quality of life

Health-related quality of life attempts to assess the impact of a disease and its treatment on disability and daily living. The concept is like that of health because it has a patient-based focus on perceived ability to partake in a fulfilling life. Fulfilment may be challenged by:
- The disease process itself.
- The side effects of treatment.
- Complications associated with both the disease process and its treatment.

In addition, problems may also be associated with the effect other disease processes may have on the patient's wellbeing, particularly changes in psychiatric state. This may be a consequence of the disease or the disease process may be influential in determining the patient's psychiatric state.

With less emphasis on survival as the single goal of treatment, other aspects of HRQoL may be considered as outcomes in their own right:
- The alleviation of symptoms for patients with chronic diseases.
- The restoration of function.
- Ultimately, a return to everyday tasks, employment and increases in activity.

Research into HRQoL has consequently concentrated on understanding how disease processes affect the functional ability as well as the psychiatric state of patients.

Health profiles and health indices

Although it is now generally accepted that it is only the patient who can judge the impact of disease and treatment on his or her health, there is some debate over which areas constitute HRQoL (Price, 1996). Fallowfield (1990) identified four core areas that could describe HRQoL: psychological, social, occupational and physical domains. Others have used similar descriptions but either increased the number of domains or reduced them according to their own judgements (Price, op. cit.).

From these concepts and earlier studies, a variety of HRQoL scales have been developed. Although researchers have accepted that HRQoL is a complex concept, different requirements have led to two distinct types of HRQoL assessment. The most common scales developed have been health profiles. These scales accept that HRQoL is multidimensional and produce outcomes in terms of a number of domains or subscores. Others have attempted to combine different domains to give a global index that attempts to rate patients on a scale from 0 (death) to 1 (best possible health) (Rosser, 1972; Kaplan *et al.* 1976). In most of these scales it is acknowledged that there may be certain states of health worse than death which are assigned negative scores.

The use of indices is very attractive at first glance, in that it gives a single score for each patient and can combine quantity of life with quality of life into an evaluation of treatment outcomes. This method has been used extensively in assessing the relative values of healthcare programmes by assigning cost to quality of life indicators (Quality Adjusted Life Years, QALYs). These can be used across different diseases, to evaluate the cost-effectiveness of different healthcare strategies (Pritchard, 1996). Other health professionals feel that the assessment of HRQoL is too complex to describe in one value and can only be described by a number of scores which represent the selected domains under study into a profile of the patient's lifestyle. In the remainder of this chapter only the use of profiles will be considered because few investigations using health indices have been performed on patients suffering from chronic wounds.

THE DEVELOPMENT OF GENERIC AND DISEASE-SPECIFIC QUALITY OF LIFE TOOLS

Over the past 20 years many tools have been developed to 'measure' quality of life. However, there are relatively few profiles that have received the necessary validation or that have been subjected to repeatability studies to make them scientifically acceptable. In the development of most tools, qualitative data are first collected from patients to determine the key variables and these are then developed into a questionnaire, which is further refined after testing on patients.

There are two types of HRQoL tool, generic tools designed to be used in a variety of disease processes and more specific tools designed for only one disease . Although there is debate over which are the more useful, it is likely that both have their place in wound-care studies.

Generic tools are well-validated methods for use in many clinical and research situations. They have the advantage that comparisons can be made between different patient groups and diseases so that the relative impact of different disease processes on patients can be assessed. They have the possible disadvantage of being insensitive to specific problems experienced by patients which do not fall into the general categories of difficulties associated with disease processes used in generic tools.

Conversely, specific tools have the advantage of being sensitive to factors that are known to be important to patients suffering from the disease under investigation. They have drawbacks in being difficult and laborious to validate and cannot be used for comparison between diseases.

In assessing the benefits of services and treatments to patients it is essential that the tool is sensitive to change. This is particularly important when using generic tools because these frequently combine responses to questions into scores. Real differences may be masked by this aggregation of scores. To assess the value of these scales it is important to test the sensitivity to real changes in the patient's status. An example of this is given in the Riverside Leg Ulcer Project (Franks et al. 1994), in which 12 weeks of treatment led to significant reductions in scores and significantly greater changes in patients whose leg ulcers healed compared with patients whose ulcers failed to heal.

Generic tools to assess health–related quality of life

Table 13.1 describes three frequently used tools to assess quality of life, including the subscores that make up the assessment of HRQoL. These are all generic tools, in that they are designed to be used on a variety of patient groups, irrespective of the disease process under investigation. All may be considered valuable in the assessment of patients' HRQoL.

The Nottingham Health Profile (NHP)

To date, most work on patients with chronic wounds has used this tool (Hunt *et al.* 1986). It is a simple questionnaire that requires patients to answer 'Yes' or 'No' to a battery of 38 questions about their lives. The 'Yes' scores are then weighted according to their relative importance and combined into six subscores that describe the patient's life. The given values are from zero meaning no health problem to 100 being maximum interference. The questionnaire has the advantage of being simple and quick to use, but it does require some skill in weighting the answers and combining them into the final scores.

The Sickness-Impact Profile (SIP)

This was developed as a self-completion questionnaire, in which patients are asked to tick only those statements that they feel are true about themselves (Bergner *et al.* 1981). As with the NHP the scores are weighted and combined to give a total for each subscore. The tool takes approximately 20–30 minutes to complete, making it less useful when a number of patient assessments are required.

Table 13.1.
Three commonly used questionnaires to assess health-related quality of life (HRQoL)

	Nottingham Health Profile (Hunt *et al.* 1986)	Sickness–Impact Profile (Bergner *et al.* 1981)	Short Form 36 (SF-36) (Ware *et al.* 1993)
Questions	38	136	36
Subscores	Emotional reactions Pain Social isolation Sleep Energy level Physical mobility	Sleep/rest Eating Work Home management Recreation/pastimes Ambulation Mobility Body care Social interaction Alertness behaviour Emotional behaviour Communication	Role-functioning Role-physical Bodily pain General health Vitality Social functioning Role-emotional Mental health

The Short Form 36 (SF-36)

This is a relatively new scale comprising 36 simple questions on health and lifestyle (Ware *et al.* 1993). Although the transformed scores have a similar range to the NHP, the scale is reversed, giving zero as maximum interference and 100 as no interference from health problems . It has many protagonists, some of whom consider it to be the 'gold standard' in assessing HRQoL. Although it is undoubtedly a good tool, other scales may be more useful and should be considered in certain situations for particular disorders.

Using generic tools to assess the impact of disease in patients with wounds

Although relatively few studies used generic tools to determine the impact of disease on patients' lifestyle, Lindholm *et al.* (1993) used the NHP to compare 125 patients with leg ulceration matched to age and sex norms from population studies. The median age in this group was 77 years with 59% women. Perceived pain was significantly higher in men than women, with men having five times the score of the age norms and women 2.5 times the age norms. Mobility deficit was also significantly higher in men than women; men had mean scores four times higher than age norms compared with women who had mean scores 1.5 times higher. Emotional wellbeing was also considerably higher in men, being twice the normal value, whereas women had mean scores equivalent to age norms. Both poor sleep and social-isolation scores were double the age norms in men but similar to the norms in women. Clearly, there was an important difference between the sexes in this study, with men appearing to suffer markedly more than women from their ulceration.

Hamer *et al.* (1994) used a case–control design to assess the impact of leg ulceration on patients over the age of 65 years (Hamer *et al.* op. cit.; Roe *et al.* 1995). Eighty-eight patients were recruited from Wirral Health Authority and compared with 70 control patients recruited from health screening of people over 75 years of age. Mean ages were similar between the groups (80 compared with 77 years), and similar sex ratios were evident (66% men compared with 60% women). The mean pain score from the NHP was 45 compared with 15 in control patients ($p < 0.05$), with significantly higher energy-loss scores in the patients compared with the control individuals (58 compared with 24, $p < 0.05$). No significant difference was detected in emotional reactions to health between the two groups. No evidence was given for the impact of leg ulceration on patients' sleep status, mobility or social isolation from the NHP but mobility and social isolation were evaluated using alternative methods.

Using specific tools to assess the impact of disease in patients with wounds

Although generic tools are developed to assess patients irrespective of the disease from which they are suffering, specific tools relate particularly to one disease process. In 1994, Hyland *et al.* (1994) published work on a tool specific to leg ulceration, developed from responses given by patients in Exeter. As with many generic tools, it started through a qualitative process of 22 patients discussing their problems within focus groups. From these discussions, four areas of the patients' lifestyles were identified as being particularly relevant to the problem of leg ulceration:

- Pain.
- Restricted activity.
- Moods and feelings.
- Ulcer preoccupation and treatment.

From the results it was clear that pain intensity varied according to the time and season. Pain also restricted activities such as walking, whereas the need to change the dressing, feelings of embarrassment and coping strategies to avoid further ulceration also prevented patients from performing their usual tasks. Psychological problems expressed themselves as regret about lack of social contact, feelings of depression and reduced will power, helplessness and a sense of uncleanliness. Ulcer pre-occupation was manifested as problems with the uncertainty concerning the outcome and the time scale for treatment.

From these observations a questionnaire involving 54 items was developed; at a later stage the number of items was reduced to 34 after testing with 33 patients. The final questionnaire was then tested on 50 patients with leg ulceration. Of these, 29 (58%) considered themselves to be largely housebound, 16 of the 29 (55%) because of their ulceration. Forty per cent of all patients always had trouble getting on and off buses, whereas 30% always had trouble climbing stairs. Overall, 32% stated that their ulcer always restricted where they travelled.

Avoidance strategies were common in these patients with 38% never standing in crowds, 26% always being afraid of having children on their knees and 34% always avoiding cats. Pain was correlated with sleep-loss and thinking about the ulcer.

Using personal interviews, Phillips *et al.* (1994) attempted to determine the impact of leg ulceration on overall HRQoL in a patient group in the USA. The authors divided their questionnaire into four areas of interest:

- Physical.
- Functional.
- Financial.
- Psychological.

The physical domain included size, depth and duration of ulceration, whereas the functional area examined mobility and ability to perform tasks both inside and outside the house. Financial questions related to the expense of dressings, transport for treatment, and medical fees, whereas the psychological implications of leg ulceration were investigated with questions on such areas as fear, social isolation, anger and depression. The study comprised 62 patients with a mean age of 62 years of which 60% were women. Of the total, 65% reported severe pain; although many had other concurrent diseases, such as heart disease, all thought that their leg ulcer was their most important health problem. Only 20% still worked but it affected their work in all cases. Of the patients who no longer worked, 42% stated that the presence of a leg ulcer had contributed to their decision to give up work. Eighty-one per cent believed that their mobility was adversely affected by their ulcer, whereas 76% believed that their financial situation was similarly affected. The emotional impact of ulceration was great with 68% of patients describing negative emotions such as fear, isolation, depression and negative self-image.

In the Wirral study, patients were asked about the major source of worry with their ulcer (Hamer *et al.* op. cit.; Roe *et al.* op. cit.). For 38%, pain was considered to be the worst thing about having an ulcer, followed by restricted mobility (31%), inconvenience of dressings (10%), exudate (8%) and worry about healing (3%). Most patients were able to walk with or without an aid (76%) or with another person (15%), with most patients seeing family and friends on a daily basis. Although most patients did go out on a regular basis, most felt that they went out less frequently because of their ulcer, chiefly because of pain (56%), reduced mobility (15%), waiting for the nurse to visit (7%) or embarrassment (5%).

The problem of pain

As described, pain is frequently considered by patients with leg ulceration to be their principal concern. Using the shortened McGill pain questionnaire Hamer *et al.* (op. cit.) found that patients most frequently described their pain as 'aching', although the highest intensity of pain was felt by patients feeling a 'sharp' sensation. Using the pain subscore in the NHP, the same study found significantly higher perceived pain in patients than in the control individuals (mean was 45 compared with 15, $p < 0.05$). At the time of the interview, 31% were experiencing pain from their ulcer. In the Exeter study, 26% of patients stated that the ulcer was very painful whereas 30% felt it to be uncomfortable rather than painful or did not notice the pain (Hyland *et al.* op. cit.). In the Riverside Leg Ulcer Project, at their first visit to the clinic 17% of patients described their ulcer pain as continuous, whereas 20% stated that they perceived no pain from their ulcers (Franks *et al.* 1994). After 12 weeks of treatment, only 1% suffered continuous pain compared with 79% experiencing no pain, largely as a result of 52% of the patients having achieved complete healing of all areas of ulceration.

Although there is a paucity of information on HRQoL, in patients suffering from pressure sores, some information has been published on pain associated with dressing changes. In 1992, Butterworth *et al.* (1992) compared two cavity-wound dressings (Allevyn and Silastic foam) in 80 patients. Comfort at dressing change was similar between groups with approximately 90% of assessed changes being pain-free. A similar study by the same group examined a hydrocolloid (Granuflex) with a polyurethane dressing (Spyrosorb) (Banks *et al.* 1994). In all, 40 patients were randomized, of whom approximately 70% described their dressing changes as pain-free. Approximately 70% felt that the dressings were either very comfortable or comfortable when on the leg, with only 15% describing the dressings as uncomfortable. Clearly, there is scope for future research in pain evaluation and pressure sore research, both to assess its impact in patients with sores and as an outcome measure in observational studies and clinical trials.

QUALITY OF LIFE AS AN OUTCOME INDICATOR

There have been relatively few attempts to use HRQoL assessments as outcome measures in studies or trials. However, in 1992, results were published from the Riverside Leg Ulcer Project, which examined psychiatric morbidity and other areas of HRQoL in patients attending community leg ulcer clinics (Franks *et al.* op. cit.). The HRQoL assessments were incorporated into the general plan of the project, which was to implement a research-based system of care into community leg ulcer services through a clinical nurse specialist liaising with a department of acute vascular surgery (Moffatt *et al.* 1992). Over the first 2 years, 475 patients with 550 ulcers were seen. Of these ulcers, 477 were considered venous in origin. The patients assessed for HRQoL had presented at the clinics within the first 6 months of their opening and were suffering from venous ulceration which was then treated by four-layer bandaging (4LB) (Blair *et al.* 1988). In all, 185 patients were recruited, with a mean age of 76 years, 64% of whom were women. The Symptom Rating Test (SRT) was used to assess psychiatric morbidity, this being a well-validated tool (Kellner & Sheffield, 1973). This consists of questions on feelings patients have, the answers to which are combined to give scores for anxiety, depression, hostility, cognitive function and somatic wellbeing. Patients were interviewed at their first visit to their clinic and 12 weeks later, irrespective of whether their ulcers had healed.

After 12 weeks of treatment, 168 patients could be contacted, of whom 52% had ulcers that had healed. In the total patient group, the results showed significant reductions in anxiety, depression and hostility and improvement in cognitive function. It has been suggested that these changes could be associated with the Hawthorne effect (Hamer *et al.* op. cit.; Roe *et al.* op. cit.). However, comparison was also made between patients whose ulcers had healed and patients whose ulcers had failed to heal. In this comparison, there were significantly greater reductions in depression and hostility in patients whose ulcers had healed. These differences could not be explained by the Hawthorne effect because all patients received identical assessment and treatment over the 12 weeks. These results are important, because they suggest that the process of healing the ulcers leads to an improvement in the patients' psychiatric state. It has been suggested that the reverse may be true, that is, change in patients' psychiatric state may have improved the chances of healing. Although this is a possibility, the baseline scores were similar between patients whose ulcers had healed and patients whose ulcers failed to heal. It is therefore more likely to be the healing process affecting the psychiatric state rather than the reverse.

A recent prospective randomized trial of 200 patients suffering from venous ulceration used the NHP to investigate changes over 24 weeks of treatment (Franks *et al.* 1995). The trial was of a factorial design, with all patients randomized to one of two bandage regimens, 4LB compared with a single adhesive compression bandage (ACB) (Granuflex bandage, Convatec), one of two dressings (NA, Johnson & Johnson compared with Granuflex, Convatec), and oxpentifylline treatment (Trental, Hoechst Roussel) compared with a placebo. The results from this trial showed significant improvements in energy, pain, emotion, sleep and mobility in the total group of patients after 24 weeks of treatment. In line with the Riverside experience, there were greater improvements in patients whose ulcers had healed for energy, pain, emotion and sleep domains. When comparing the changes in scores between 4LB and ACB, patients on 4LB experienced significantly greater improvements in energy and mobility than patients on ACB. This result is interesting because it indicates that the improvement in mobility experienced in the 4LB group may not have been directly related to healing of the ulcers.

To date, there has only been one trial in wound care that has considered quality of life factors as a primary endpoint. In a randomized trial of knitted viscose (NA, Johnson & Johnson) compared with hydrocolloid (Granuflex, Convatec) dressings, in patients with arterial ulceration, the trial was stopped after just 22 patients had been entered (Gibson *et al.* 1995). This was because 100% of patients withdrew from the viscose dressing because of ulcer pain, compared with 33% from the hydrocolloid group because of maceration and infection. Clearly, the decision to stop the trial was based purely on the patients' perception of pain, rather than the ability of the two dressings to heal the area of ulceration.

CONCLUSION

This chapter summarizes the current research on health-related quality of life in chronic wound healing. The results of research into chronic ulceration of the lower leg illustrate that the presence of a chronic wound can have a major impact on a patient's life, whether it is through the effects of treatment, social isolation or avoidance strategies. What is also clear is that it is possible to make substantial improvements to the patient's life once the wound has healed. Maintaining an ulcer (that is, preventing further deterioration) is therefore clearly no substitute for healing in these patients.

There is a need for further studies of HRQoL in patients suffering from pressure sores. This is highly problematic because the pressure sore is largely a consequence of some other major morbidity or cluster of factors that have befallen the patient. Despite this, there is a need to establish how much of an impact the sore has on the patient over and above his or her other concurrent problems and the value that the healing of the sore has on changes in the patient's perceived health.

With changes in the NHS and a move towards evidence-based practice and audit, there is a clear need to assess the impact of disease on patients' lives. Although the methods used are relatively simple, there is little evidence that they are being used in everyday clinical practice. Clearly, the patients' perceptions of their health should be evaluated if care is to be truly patient-focused. Methods need to be developed that are scientifically sound, while allowing healthcare professionals to assess the results simply and quickly. This will be a priority in healthcare assessment over the next 10 years.

SELF–ASSESSMENT QUESTIONS AND ACTIVITIES

(a) What is the fundamental difference between specific and generic tools in HRQoL measurement? Can you list the advantages and disadvantages of each type of assessment?

(b) If you were asked to design a study to investigate the effect pressure sores have on HRQoL in patients suffering from a disabling disease, how would you go about it? Consider with whom you would compare the patients with sores. Is it sufficient to compare the population norms, age and sex-matched control individuals or should one consider a group suffering from the same disease but without a sore?

REFERENCES

Banks V, Bale SE, Harding KG. Comparing two dressings for exuding pressure sores in community patients. *J Wound Care* 1994, **3**:175–178.

Bergner M, Bobbitt RA, Carter WB, Gilson BS. The Sickness Impact Profile: development and final revision of a health status measure. *Med Care* 1981, **19**:787–805.

Blair SD, Wright DDI, Backhouse CM, Riddle E, McCollum CN. Sustained compression and healing chronic venous ulcers. *BMJ* 1988, **297**:1159–1161.

Bullinger M. Indices versus profiles: advantages and disadvantages. In: Walker SR, Rosser RM, eds. *Quality of life assessment: key issues in the 1990's.* Dordrecht: Kluwer Academic; 1993.

Bulpitt CJ, Fletcher AE. Quality of life in hypertensive patients on different antihypertensive treatments: rationale for methods employed in multi-centre randomised controlled trial. *J Cardiovasc Pharmacol* 1985, **7**:S137–S145.

Butterworth RJ, Bale S, Harding KG, Hughes LE. Comparing Allevyn cavity wound dressings and Silastic Foam. *J Wound Care* 1992, **1**:10–13.

Department of Health. *Clinical audit: meeting and improving standards in healthcare.* London: HMSO; 1993.

Fallowfield L: *The quality of life: the missing dimension in healthcare.* London: Souvenir;1990.

Franks PJ, Moffatt CJ, Connolly M *et al.* Community leg ulcer clinics: effect on quality of life. *Phlebology* 1994, **9**:83–86.

Franks PJ, Bosanquet N, Brown D, Straub J, Harper DR, Ruckley CV. Perceived health in a randomised trial of single and multi-layer bandaging. *Phlebology* 1995, **1**(Suppl):17–19.

Gibson B, Harper DR, Nelson EA, Prescott RJ, Ruckley CV. A comparison of hydrocolloid and a knitted viscose dressing in the treatment of arterial leg ulcers. *Phlebology* 1995, **1** (Suppl):1071–1072.

Hamer C, Cullum NA, Roe BH. Patients' perceptions of chronic leg ulcers. *J Wound Care* 1994, **3**:99–101.

Hunt SM, McEwan J, McKenna SP. *Measuring health status.* London: Croom Helm; 1986.

Hyland ME, Ley A, Thomson B. Quality of life of leg ulcer patients: questionnaire and preliminary findings. *J Wound Care* 1994, **3**:294–298.

Kaplan RM, Bush JW, Berry CC. Health status: types of validity and the index of well being. *Health Services Res* 1976, **11**:478–507.

Kellner R, Sheffield BF. A self rating scale of distress. *Psychological Med* 1973, **3**:88–100.

Lindholm C, Bjellerup M, Christensen OB, Zedrfeld B. Quality of life in chronic leg ulcers. Acta Derm Venereol (Stockh) 1993, **73**:440–443.

Moffatt CJ, Franks PJ, Oldroyd M et al. Community clinics and impact on healing. *BMJ* 1992, 305:1389–1392.

Phillips T, Stanton B, Provan A, Lew R. A study on the impact of leg ulcers on quality of life: financial, social and psychologic implications. *J Am Acad Dermatol* 1994, **31**:49–53.

Price P. Defining and measuring quality of life. *J Wound Care* 1996, **5**:139–140.

Pritchard C. Using cost effectiveness in allocating resources. *J Wound Care* 1996, **5**:146–149.

Roe B, Cullum N, Hamer C. Patients' perceptions of chronic leg ulceration. In: Cullum N, Roe B, eds. *Leg ulcers: nursing management.* Harrow: Scutari Press; 1995:125–134.

Rosser RM. The measurement of hospital output. *Int J Epidemiol* 1972, **1**:361–368.

Ware JE, Snow KK, Kosinski M, Gandek B. *SF-36 health survey: manual and interpretation guide.* Boston MA: Boston Health Institute, New England Medical Center; 1993.

WHO. *The first ten years.* Geneva: WHO; 1958.

FURTHER READING

European Tissue Repair Society: Consensus on measuring quality of life in chronic wounds. *J Wound Care* 1996, 5(3):139–144.

Wilkin D, Hallam L, Doggett M-A. *Measures of need and outcome for primary healthcare.* Oxford: Oxford University Press; 1993.

Advanced Case Studies

Emphasis has been placed throughout this book on the importance of adopting a holistic, patient-centred approach to wound care, which involves the practitioner using theoretical knowledge in many practical situations. The following case studies have been designed to enable you or those whom you teach to reflect on the complex issues that can be encountered by healthcare professionals, working in diverse care settings including hospitals, nursing homes, hospices and in the community. This chapter includes many commonly encountered but challenging wounds. Some more unusual wounds have also been included here to give you further practice in the application of basic principles in less familiar situations.

HOW TO USE THE ADVANCED CASE STUDIES

You may like to begin by working through selected case studies given here, in order to assess the level of your existing knowledge, before you turn to the appropriate chapters in this book. This approach may appeal particularly to the advanced practitioner. Individuals with less experience may prefer to work through a particular chapter and then to test their knowledge with the help of the simpler case studies, questions and activities at the end of each chapter. The more advanced case studies can then be attempted. These case studies involve the application of knowledge from more than one chapter.

The case studies are grouped into three sections:
- Section 1 – pressure sores (*see* Chapter 9)
- Section 2 – leg ulcers (*see* Chapter 10)
- Section 3 – other chronic wounds (*see* Chapter 11)

The questions relating to each case study are organized into groups. These groups relate to the chapters in this book where particularly relevant information can be found. The chapters to turn to are indicated by the icons on the next page.

Note: **Assessment and treatment methods** You are often asked to state how you set about assessing a patient and the care that you would suggest, based on the information given. Often there is no one correct answer but it is important for you to identify which assessment methods are essential, which are desirable and which are unnecessary and to note methods of treatment that could be hazardous. In all cases, the rationale for suggested assessment and treatment methods should be given, if necessary after consulting the appropriate chapter in this book.

SECTION 1: PRESSURE SORES

Case Study 1:   A pressure sore in a terminally ill patient

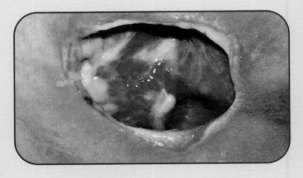

Mrs Adams is 68 years old and has just been admitted to the local hospice for terminal care. She has a diagnosis of cord compression, caused by metastatic cancer of the bone from an unknown primary. On admission she presents with a grade 3 sacral pressure sore, illustrated right, which measures approximately 11cm by 7cm, with a depth of 2.5cm, which she says developed during a recent period of hospitalization. The wound is discharging large amounts of offensive exudate which Mrs Adams says regularly leaks through the outer dressing on to her clothing. Problems with leakage of exudate had kept her confined to the house most of the time. The tissue surrounding the sore is excoriated. This may have been caused by the frequent application and removal of adhesive products, that is, both the dressings and the tapes designed to keep the dressing in place. The wound is causing Mrs Adams considerable discomfort throughout the day. She experiences severe pain at dressing changes, which she has come to dread. Her mobility is limited because of pain from her lower back and chest wall, as well as from the sore itself. Mrs Adams is aware of her diagnosis and the fact that she will not recover but she refuses to discuss the likely course of her disease with staff. She has led a very active life, enjoying cycling, holidays abroad and working with children in a voluntary capacity. Her body image is of great importance to her and she pays special attention to her clothes and hair. On admission she expresses bitterness and anger that the disease has come upon her so suddenly, preventing her from having any quality of life. At times she admits to feelings of both helplessness and hopelessness. Her family express their dissatisfaction with the care that Mrs Adams received while in hospital and believe that her pressure sore was avoidable and the result of poor quality care at that time.

1 a List the factors that may be contributing to delayed wound healing in this patient.
  b Which of these factors are avoidable? How could the effect of any unavoidable factors be minimized?
  c Which of the factors identified are within your sphere of responsibility?
  d Note the other professionals who may need to become involved in Mrs Adams' care and the likely nature of their involvement.

2 a What are the local problems at the wound site?
　b How do you propose to record these?

3 a Note the signs and symptoms that suggest that the wound may be infected.
　b List any investigations that could be carried out to confirm your view that the wound is infected and to identify the nature and antibiotic sensitivity of the causative organism(s). Note how you would collect any samples required.

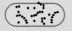

4 a Which method of debridement do you consider would be most appropriate in this case and why?
　b List three alternative methods of debridement that could be used and note the advantages and disadvantages of each.

5 a Which primary dressing do you think would be most suitable? List the properties of the dressing that you are particularly looking for in this case.
　b List three alternative methods that could be used to dress this wound and note the advantages and disadvantages of each, in this particular case.
　c Bearing in mind the condition of the skin surrounding the ulcer, how do you propose to hold the dressing in place?

6 Outline the principles of pressure sore management and describe how you would translate these principles into practice.

7 Mrs Adams' family are clearly unhappy about the care that she received while in hospital, before admission to the hospice. What conditions would need to be met for a patient or her family successfully to establish that professional negligence had occurred?

8 a In relation to the period of care in question, what information would you expect to find incorporated into the nursing records that may justify the appropriateness of the care given to Mrs Adams while in hospital?
　b What might lead you to conclude that the standard of care administered was below a professionally acceptable standard?

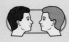

9 How could you involve Mrs Adams and her family in care planning?

10 a What support may Mrs Adams and her family need?
　　b Would you consider involving any other professionals and who do you think should decide who should be involved?

Case Study 2: A pressure sore that developed after a cerebrovascular accident

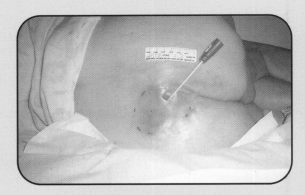

Mrs Graham is 65 years old and is married with three children and seven grandchildren. She had enjoyed a healthy and active life until she suffered a cerebrovascular accident, at home, while gardening. Mrs Graham was admitted to her local hospital where she remained unconscious for the next week.

Over the next 2 weeks she gradually regained consciousness and a dense left-sided hemiplegia began to resolve. While helping Mrs Graham from the bath a nurse noticed a large area of erythema over her sacrum and left buttock. The nurse was surprised that this might be tissue damage as Mrs Graham had been nursed on an alternating airwave mattress since her admission. On closer inspection a small opening was evident near the sacrum. The nurse gently and carefully probed this opening and a large amount of pus and haemoserous fluid drained out, as illustrated above. A sample of this drainage fluid was sent to the microbiology laboratory for culture and sensitivity testing. Meanwhile, the wound was thoroughly irrigated with warm saline and loosely packed with an alginate rope dressing. The large cavity undermining the skin was mapped out on the patient's skin and traced on to an acetate sheet for storage in the notes. The dietician assessed Mrs Graham and discovered that her serum albumin was lower than the normal range. Extra soft food and supplementary feeds were offered to her in an attempt to improve her nutritional status.

1   In the 3 weeks after her cerebrovascular accident Mrs Graham's food intake was clearly limited. Whose responsibility was it to monitor her nutritional status and to correct any deficiencies?

2   List the nutritional factors that may be involved in the aetiology and non-healing of pressure sores.

3   The use of a pressure-relieving mattress was an integral part of this patient's care. However, she still developed a pressure sore. What else might have been done to prevent such tissue damage from occurring?

4   Which method of wound debridement do you consider would be most appropriate in this case and why?

5   How could you protect the area around the pressure sore from the effects of wound exudate?

6   Assuming that this patient recovers sufficiently well to be discharged home, what are the quality of life issues likely to be in relation to her pressure sore?

7   Assuming that the district nurse will be involved with Mrs Graham's care on discharge from hospital, who will bear the burden of the costs of community care? Discuss the implications of people with hospital-acquired problems being charged to the community.

8   Identify issues affecting Mrs Graham's care while in hospital that could be investigated using the audit process.

SECTION 2: LEG ULCERS

Case Study 3:   A venous ulcer with associated dermatological problems

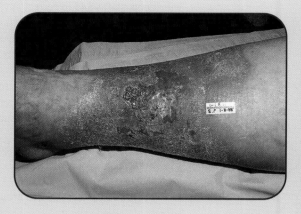

Mrs Scott is an overweight but active 45-year-old woman who works as a shelf-packer in the local supermarket. For the past 5 months Mrs Scott has noticed a brown staining of the skin on her lower leg. After advice from members of the primary healthcare team, Mrs Scott has been wearing an unshaped tubular elastic bandage for support. Since wearing this the skin on her leg has become dry and itchy. Mrs Scott has been applying various emollients, obtained from the local chemist, to her dry skin but the condition has continued to deteriorate. Approximately 4 weeks ago, the area towards the front of Mrs Scott's shin started weeping and then the skin broke down. Initially, Mrs Scott applied an antiseptic cream to this broken area but this did not appear to improve the situation and she felt that she should seek further medical advice. Her GP has just referred her to your outpatient clinic. The clinic has developed an expertise in the management of dermatological aspects of wound care in the lower leg. On examination you find brown pigmentation of the skin around the gaiter area and an ulcerated area approximately 10 cm above the medial malleolus. The ulcerated area is surrounded by a well-demarcated area of acute eczema. After a Doppler-ultrasound examination it is established that Mrs Scott has an adequate arterial blood supply.

1   List five circumstances that might have caused the loss of skin integrity on Mrs Scott's leg and the interventions that might have prevented them.

2   Consider the problems that you will need to address in the management of Mrs Scott's leg ulcer and list the interventions that you will employ to achieve your objectives.

3   Which other disciplines might need to be involved in Mrs Scott's care and management. Give reasons for your choices.

4   Summarize the interventions that you will need to employ, after healing to maintain skin integrity.

5 a   Do you think that the eczema on Mrs Scott's leg is an endogenous or exogenous eczema? Give reasons for your choice.
  b   How do you propose to manage the eczema?

6 a   Describe the nutritional factors that may affect healing in chronic venous-leg ulceration.
  b   What are the implications for this patient's assessment and intervention?

7   Patient education is an integral part of wound and skin-care management. What advice would you give to Mrs Scott that could improve the chances of the ulcer healing and prevent recurrence, and how would you set about giving this advice? (see also Chapters 8 and 10).

8   This is not the first time that a patient has been referred to you from this particular GP's practice, where the underlying cause of the ulcer has clearly not been diagnosed and where the care suggested has been inappropriate or ineffective. You are the most senior nurse and you are in charge of the day-to-day running of the outpatient clinic.
  a   How do you propose to handle this situation? Who needs to be involved and why?
  b   What do you anticipate might prove to be the biggest obstacles to bringing about a lasting change in practice for the better?

Case Study 4: A venous ulcer where there are problems with lymphatic drainage

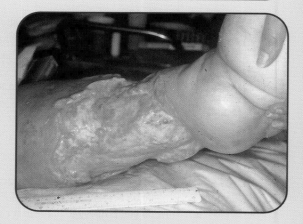

Mrs Cooper is 64 years old and lives in a small, immaculate, cottage with her husband. She has spent the past 3 years in bed because of leg ulceration. Her history of leg ulceration extends back 40 years to the birth of her daughter. With each episode of ulceration she notes that the swelling increases and that bouts of severe infection are more frequent. On examination, Mrs Cooper has deep circumferential leg ulcers on both legs and there is evidence of lymphatic damage with excessive oedema and pronounced skin folds. Her ankle circumference is 43 cm. The non-pitting oedema extends into her thighs. The ulcers produce copious exudate and require dressing twice daily by the district nurse. It is estimated that approximately 1 litre of exudate is lost from these ulcers each day. As a result of the ulceration it is impossible to palpate pedal pulses or to record a resting pressure index. Routine blood tests reveal a haemoglobin level of 8 g/dl and a normal erythrocyte sedimentation rate (ESR). Mrs Cooper finds her ulceration very painful, particularly at the time of dressing changes. Mr Cooper now sleeps in an adjoining bedroom. Mrs Cooper says that this is because she does not sleep well and she disturbs him. Mr Cooper, however, says that he finds the odour from her ulcers intolerable and he is afraid that he will damage her legs further should he knock them. Mrs Cooper is extremely dependent on the community nurse and is unhappy when the nurse who normally visits her is unable to attend and another nurse comes in her place.

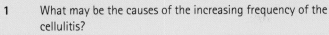

1   What may be the causes of the increasing frequency of the
     cellulitis?

2   Assuming that Mrs Cooper's arterial status is found to be normal:
  a Would elastic or inelastic compression bandages be more
     appropriate for her? Give your reasons.
  b What special precautions must be taken before applying
     compression to Mrs Cooper's limbs?
  c Mrs Cooper's ankle measures 43 cm. What does this tell you about
     the compression that can be achieved using a bandage designed to
     apply pressure when the ankle size is 18–25 cm?
  d How would you overcome this problem and ensure a therapeutic
     level of compression is applied?
  e What other techniques may be useful to reduce excessive oedema in
     this case?

3 a How will you assess Mrs Cooper's nutritional status?
  b What are the likely consequences of Mrs Cooper's anaemia and how
     could this be treated?

4   How could you protect the area around Mrs Cooper's leg ulcer from
     the effects of excess wound exudate?

5   Devise a dressing regime for Mrs Cooper's leg ulcers, giving reasons
     for your choices.

6   What strategies could you use to break the cycle of dependence
     that has developed between Mrs Cooper and the district nurse who
     normally visits her?

Case Study 5:   A Marjolin's ulcer (squamous-cell carcinoma)

Mrs Quinn is 74 years old and has for the past 3 years lived in a residential home. She was admitted to the home with Alzheimer's disease and an increasing inability to cope alone in the community. She has no family and receives few visitors. The staff report that her confusion is worsening and her short-term memory is very poor.

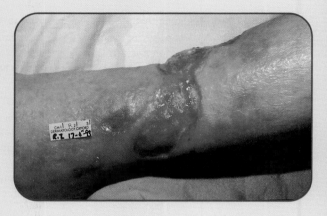

She becomes agitated and aggressive in unfamiliar surroundings and when there is a change to her routine. Her appetite is poor and she has lost 8.5 kg (21 lbs) in weight in the previous 6 months. Mrs Quinn's general health is poor. She suffers from chronic bronchitis, particularly in the winter. She has a leg ulcer which has been present for 6 years. Her medical records show that she has had at least four episodes of leg ulceration with each episode taking longer to heal. On examination Mrs Quinn has evident pigmentation in the skin surrounding the ulcer which is in the gaiter region. The base of the ulcer is necrotic and the wound margins are elevated. There is no evidence of healing and the wound exudate is foul smelling. The new GP covering the home examines her and decides to refer her for further investigation. A biopsy is taken and confirms a squamous-cell carcinoma. Staff report that Mrs Quinn appears to be having increasing pain in her back and hip.

1   What percentage of leg ulcers undergo a malignant change?

2   List the factors that might lead you to suspect that malignant changes had occurred in an ulcer where vascular problems may or may not be present concurrently.

3   What evidence is there in this case that there could be metastatic spread to other organs?

4   What ethical dilemmas may need to be overcome in deciding on a treatment plan for this lady?

5   What treatment options exist for a patient with a squamous-cell carcinoma originating in a leg ulcer?

6 a   Which method of debridement do you consider would be most appropriate in this case and why?
    b   List three alternative methods of debridement and note the advantages and disadvantages of each.

7   How would you dress this wound? Give the reasons for your choice.

8 a   Identify the signs and symptoms of possible protein–energy malnutrition (PEM).
    b   What risk factors may have precipitated malnutrition in this case?
    c   Identify the priorities in Mrs Quinn's management from a nutritional perspective.
    d   Identify key stages in the delivery and evaluation of her nutritional support. With reference to your own practice, reflect on the scope of your professional responsibilities for undertaking activities related to these stages.

Case Study 6:   A tropical ulcer associated with tuberculosis

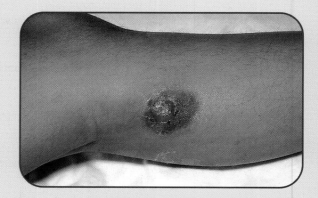

Miss Stanmore is 26 years old and has recently returned from a 6-month visit to Africa. During her stay she developed appendicitis and peritonitis. She required major surgery and a blood transfusion but otherwise made an uneventful recovery. On return to the UK she became unwell. She complained of feeling excessively tired, of losing weight and of having no appetite. Her temperature had risen to 38.2°C and she reported night sweats. On examination she has a small lesion just below her knee which has ulcerated and is surrounded by pigmented skin. Miss Stanmore assumes that the lesion originated from a mosquito bite, however, it does not irritate her. She had been taking antimalarial treatment during her stay in Africa. After examination of her ulcer at the local dermatology outpatient clinic, Miss Stanmore is admitted to hospital for further investigations and treatment. Protein–energy malnutrition (PEM) is suspected. Miss Stanmore is complaining of a number of mouth ulcers and she is suffering from glossitis.

1 a List the factors that could contribute to delayed wound healing for this patient.
  b Which of the factors identified are within your sphere of responsibility?
  c Note the other professionals who may need to become involved in Miss Stanmore's care and the likely nature of their involvement.

2 a What percentage of ulcers have a non-vascular origin?
  b List eight causes of non-vascular ulceration.

3 a Miss Stanmore's ulcer is thought to be caused by tuberculosis. What other diseases can lead to an ulcer of similar presentation?

b What investigations will be required to confirm the underlying aetiology of the ulcer?

4 a What treatment is Miss Stanmore likely to receive in relation to her tuberculosis and for how long is treatment likely to be required?

b How would you treat the ulcer?

c List the infection control measures that would have been required when Miss Stanmore was admitted to the ward.

5 How would you set about learning more about the care of patients with ulcers that are the result of a cause which is only rarely encountered in the UK?

6 a List the baseline indicators of nutritional status that should be measured in this case and give your reasons.

b Summarize the effects of PEM on body systems in general and explain how wound healing may have been impaired as a consequence of PEM in this case.

c List the indicators of possible micronutrient deficiency.

d Outline the nature of the nutritional support that Miss Stanmore is likely to require.

7 Miss Stanmore has been advised to have an HIV test. What counselling should be made available to her before this occurs? Who might become involved?

8 a List the factors evident on admission that suggest that Miss Stanmore could be at high risk of developing a pressure sore, although she is young and relatively mobile.

b What measures would you take to prevent pressure sores from occurring?

SECTION 3: OTHER CHRONIC WOUNDS

Case Study 7:   A facial defect with a fungating lesion of the nose

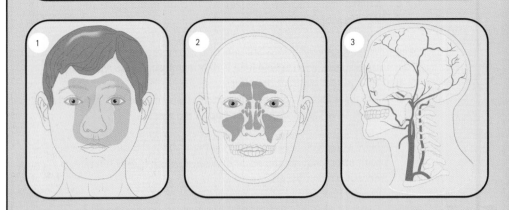

Mr Dickson (aged 59 years) was admitted to the hospice with a large facial defect. He had a 4-year history of nasal problems and the consultant ear nose and throat (ENT) surgeon had made a provisional diagnosis of a Wegner's lymphoma but multiple biopsies had failed to confirm the diagnosis. In spite of numerous investigations and a course of radiotherapy the disease progressed, affecting the connective tissue and necessitating extensive surgical removal of his nose and some surrounding tissue. Before his admission to the hospice, histology had shown that the nature of the lesion had changed and Mr Dickson had a squamous-cell carcinoma. The tumour had extended posteriorly, eroding the nasal and left maxillary sinus. He had proptosis of his left eye and decreasing vision. On admission Mr Dickson's main problems were pain in his face, poor vision in his left eye and apprehension about his right eye, difficulty with drinking liquids, which tended to rise above his prosthesis into the tumour space and reduced mobility and independence. From the beginning, Mr Dickson wanted to carry out his own wound care. Once the staff had gained his trust, he was happy to accept assistance and advice. He was on a regime of antibiotics as a precaution against wound infection. The wound was redressed daily before insertion of his prosthesis. When in situ the prosthesis allowed him to eat and drink. As his disease destroyed more of his face, the prosthesis had to be altered to fit more accurately, however, for the last few months of his life the prosthesis had to be left out, causing more distress and difficulty for Mr Dickson when eating or communicating. Mr Dickson's left eye became totally eroded by the disease and staff became worried about infiltration of his right eye. The radiologist came to assess the situation and Mr Dickson was transferred to hospital, briefly, for radiotherapy to try to halt further progression of the tumour. Mr Dickson enjoyed playing chess and was able to continue doing so for many months after his admission.

1 Figure 1 illustrates the extent of Mr Dickson's facial defect on admission (blue), and 15 months later (red). With the help of Figures 2 and 3, which show the positions of the principal facial sinuses and the main blood supply to the face, consider the potential problems that staff would need to be prepared for as the tissues eroded.

2 What support and information would you need to plan for:
a The patient.
b His family.
c The staff.
d Other visitors and volunteers?

3 How might you involve Mr Dickson and his family in the planning and carrying out of his care?

4 Identify the priorities in Mr Dickson's management from a nutritional perspective.

5 Briefly, note how Mr Dickson's energy, nitrogen and micronutrient requirements may be determined.

6 Identify the other healthcare professionals with whom you may need to liaise to ensure that effective nutritional support is provided.

7 Once Mr Dickson's defect was so extensive that the prosthesis could no longer be used, what dressing regime do you consider would be most appropriate and why (what are the problems at the wound site and what is it that you are trying to achieve)?

8 How could you protect the surrounding skin from further damage?

9 A colleague presents you with an article that she has just found in a specialist wound-care journal, which reports on the efficacy of a new primary wound care dressing that could be of value in this case. By what criteria would you judge this report? What would you do next?

Case Study 8:   A dehisced surgical wound

Mr Banks is a 45-year-old businessman living alone after a recent divorce. For many years he has been moderately obese and he has lived a busy, stressful lifestyle. A diagnosis of cholecystitis was recently made and Mr Banks was admitted for laparotomy and cholecystectomy. Keyhole surgery was not an option in this case. The immediate post- 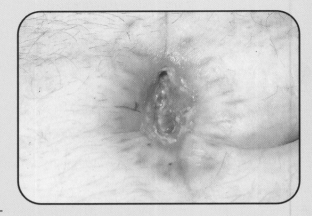 *operative recovery period was uneventful and Mr Banks was discharged, 4 days after his surgery, to his mother's home. Ten days after his operation Mr Banks noticed a reddened area on the suture line. As the district nurse was about to visit, to remove the sutures, Mr Banks was not unduly concerned and he took no action. On removing the sutures a pocket of pus discharged and, on cleaning the wound, the suture line was seen to have dehisced in part. A bacteriological swab was sent for culture and sensitivity testing and Mr Banks was started on a course of broad spectrum antibiotics. Three days later the wound was clean and beginning to show signs of granulation tissue formation, as illustrated above. There was some controversy among members of the primary healthcare team about the most appropriate dressing to use once the wound was clean.*

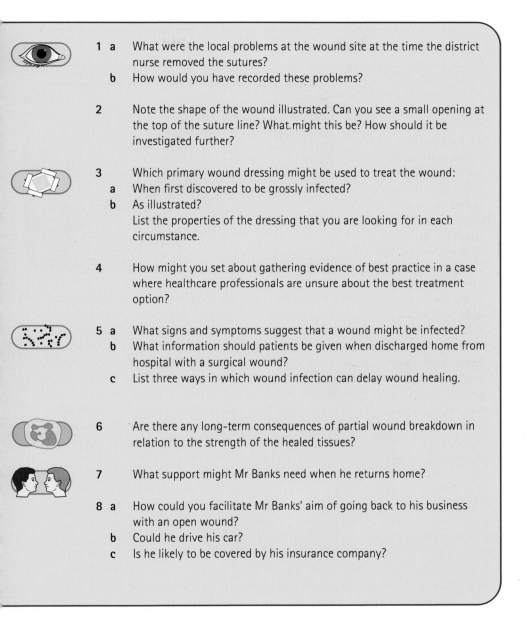

1 a What were the local problems at the wound site at the time the district nurse removed the sutures?

b How would you have recorded these problems?

2 Note the shape of the wound illustrated. Can you see a small opening at the top of the suture line? What might this be? How should it be investigated further?

3 Which primary wound dressing might be used to treat the wound:

a When first discovered to be grossly infected?

b As illustrated?

List the properties of the dressing that you are looking for in each circumstance.

4 How might you set about gathering evidence of best practice in a case where healthcare professionals are unsure about the best treatment option?

5 a What signs and symptoms suggest that a wound might be infected?

b What information should patients be given when discharged home from hospital with a surgical wound?

c List three ways in which wound infection can delay wound healing.

6 Are there any long-term consequences of partial wound breakdown in relation to the strength of the healed tissues?

7 What support might Mr Banks need when he returns home?

8 a How could you facilitate Mr Banks' aim of going back to his business with an open wound?

b Could he drive his car?

c Is he likely to be covered by his insurance company?

Case Study 9:   A fungating breast carcinoma

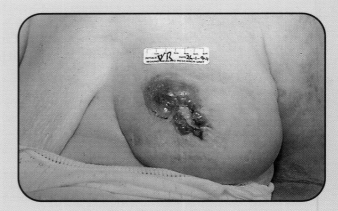

Miss Kilpatrick is a 60-year-old spinster living with her sister. Recently retired from an active career as an accountant, she had taken on the responsibility of school governor to a local primary school. She enjoyed playing golf, walking the dog and playing bridge with her friends. Her menopause began at the age of 49 and around this time Miss Kilpatrick noticed small changes to her left breast, namely a discharge from her nipple, tenderness and a hardness within the breast itself. She had known her male GP for many years and she was too embarrassed to approach him. Miss Kilpatrick ignored the mass in her breast which, over the next 5 years, increased in size and began to ulcerate. Initially, she was able to cope with the discharge by using tissues and lint on the area, however, the discharge became more profuse and offensive as the ulceration increased in size. Her sister, noticing the odour, confronted her and Miss Kilpatrick broke down in tears and showed her sister, who was horrified at the extent of the ulcer and called the GP. The GP arranged for the district nurse to visit, to assess and manage the wound and he also arranged an urgent appointment at the local oncology centre. The district nurse spent time, during her initial assessment visit, in reassuring both sisters and she was not judgmental about the condition and the extent of the ulcerated area. Using rectranicole gel to eliminate the anaerobic bacteria causing the offensive odour, the ulcer became odour-free within 48 hours. An amorphous hydrogel was used in conjunction with this to debride the sloughy surface of the wound. Within 14 days the area was clean and odourless. An alginate dressing was offered and accepted as a dressing material which Miss Kilpatrick could change for herself and the day-to-day management of the ulcer was shared between the district nurse and herself. Local radiotherapy was offered by the oncology centre and Miss Kilpatrick chose to undergo a 3-week course of treatment in the outpatient department. Although offered as a palliative treatment, the benefit locally was a shrinking of the ulcer and a reduction in the exudate level, for which Miss Kilpatrick was very grateful. Full palliative support was given by the palliative care team, who monitored her progress together with the district nurse.

1 Outline the principles of managing fungating wounds. Note how healthcare professionals translated these principles into practice in this case.

2 What special advice might Miss Kilpatrick have required? What information would you give, when and how?

3 Why do you think that an intelligent and active person such as Miss Kilpatrick did not wish to seek treatment?

4 What was the attitude of the GP, the district nurse, oncologist and the palliative care team to the situation in which the patient had found herself?

5 The district nurse was the constant carer throughout this patient's care. Discuss how she could interact with the other healthcare professionals involved, while acting as the patient's advocate.

6 a What effects had Miss Kilpatrick's fungating wound had on the quality of her life?
  b Note the ways in which Miss Kilpatrick's quality of life began to improve during treatment.

7 If you were asked to design a study to investigate the most commonly experienced effects of fungating wounds on patients' quality of life, how would you set about this?

Case Study 10:   Perineal hidradenitis suppurativa

Miss Shaw is a 24-year-old graduate who lives alone in a flat in an inner city. At the time of puberty she began to develop large boils in her perineal area over a 2-year period. Her GP had managed these boils with a combination of broad-spectrum antibiotics and by occasionally lancing the larger boils in the surgery. During her teenage years Miss Shaw had found it difficult to make and maintain relationships with boys, feeling extremely embarrassed about having multiple abscesses in her perineum. She felt different and dirty, opting not to participate in sports and many of the other activities enjoyed by teenagers. This

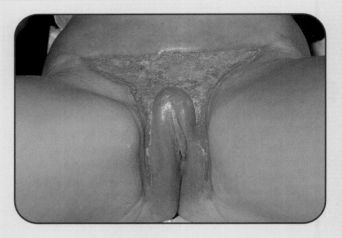

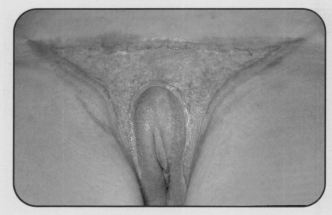

disease was affecting both her emotional development and her quality of life. Multiple courses of antibiotics and the use of analgesics increased her feelings of being different from other teenagers. On several occasions she was referred to the local hospital for excision and drainage of the abscesses under a general anaesthetic. A range of investigations had excluded diabetes. A pattern emerged over the following 18 months where the abscesses were found to be worse premenstrually. At this stage she was referred to the professor of surgery at the university hospital. A diagnosis of hidradenitis suppurativa was made based on a physical examination, history and review of the previous investigations. The nature of this disease was explained to Miss Shaw and her mother who had accompanied her to the outpatients clinic. Extensive local wide excision was discussed and Miss Shaw was given an outpatient appointment for the next month to give her time to consider whether she wished to accept the offer of radical surgery. After deciding to accept surgery, Miss Shaw underwent local wide excision of the affected area and subcutaneous tissues of the perineal area, as illustrated.

The named nurse allocated to Miss Shaw had spent time pre-operatively talking to her about her post-operative management and what she might expect. Photographs of other patients taken throughout their healing phase were shown to Miss Shaw and a patient who had undergone this surgical procedure came into the ward to talk to her about it. A haemostatic alginate dressing was used in the immediate post-operative period and Miss Shaw was catheterized until she was able to begin mobilization 3 days after the operation. At this time a silicone-foam dressing was poured into the wound and Miss Shaw was taught how to cleanse and disinfect both the wound and the dressing. On day 7 she was discharged to her mother's home. Initially, the district nurse visited to help with the dressing changes and to support the family. However, within 2 weeks Miss Shaw returned to her own flat and felt able to manage the day-to-day dressing changes for herself. Over the next 3 months her wound gradually healed; the district nurse visiting weekly to make a new dressing and to assess the progress of the wound. When healing was complete Miss Shaw had maintained full mobility and range of movement of the excised areas with an acceptable cosmetic effect. Within 6 months of surgery she had the confidence to apply for, and be successful in gaining employment. Subsequently, she made many friends at work and began developing relationships with other people of her own age.

1. What effects had Miss Shaw's hidradenitis suppurativa had on the quality of her life?

2. Patient education was an important issue throughout this patient's care. Note down the many teaching techniques that were employed from the time of diagnosis through to discharge. In each case note the principal healthcare professional involved and the nature of their involvement.

3. Which of the methods do you employ in your practice? List the advantages, disadvantages and practical difficulties of each.

4. Patient compliance was high in this case. Why do you think that this was? (think about the disease process and her quality of life pre-operatively, her involvement in dressing changes and wound management and the choices that she was offered from the time of diagnosis onwards).

5   Identify key stages in the delivery and evaluation of the nutritional support required by this patient when in hospital and on discharge.

6   Your unit is now regarded as having developed a particular expertise in the management of challenging wounds such as this. You decide to audit the service provided. In the first instance you have decided to limit your study to patients presenting with hidradenitis suppurativa.

a   Identify issues affecting patient care that could be addressed using the audit process.

b   Who needs to be involved and why?

c   What data do you propose to collect?

d   Who is going to collect the data and how?

e   Who is going to analyse the data?

f   Outline the key features of the change management process should the data suggest that some improvements in the quality of care are required.

Index

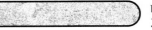